Critical Issues
in Global Health

Critical Issues in Global Health

C. Everett Koop

Clarence E. Pearson

M. Roy Schwarz

Foreword by Jimmy Carter

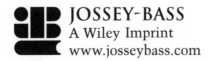

JOSSEY-BASS
A Wiley Imprint
www.josseybass.com

Published by Jossey-Bass
A Wiley Imprint
989 Market Street, San Francisco, CA 94103-1741   www.josseybass.com

Jossey-Bass books and products are available through most bookstores. To contact Jossey-Bass directly call our Customer Care Department within the U.S. at 800-956-7739, outside the U.S. at 317-572-3986 or fax 317-572-4002.

Jossey-Bass also publishes its books in a variety of electronic formats. Some content that appears in print may not be available in electronic books.

Library of Congress Cataloging-in-Publication Data

Critical issues in global health / C. Everett Koop, Clarence E. Pearson, M. Roy Schwarz [editors]; foreword by Jimmy Carter.—1st ed.
    p. cm.—(The Jossey-Bass health care series)
    Includes bibliographical references and index.
    ISBN 0-7879-4824-1 (hardcover)
    ISBN 0-7879-6377-1 (paperback)
    1. World health. 2. World health—Case studies. 3.Medical geography.   I. Koop, C. Everett (Charles Everett), 1916–   II. Pearson, Clarence E.   III. Schwarz, M. Roy   IV. Series.
RA441 .C75 2000
362.1—dc21   00-055498

FIRST EDITION
PB Printing   10 9 8 7 6 5 4

Contents

Tables, Figures, and Exhibits

Tables

Figures

Exhibits

About the C. Everett Koop Institute

Throughout his long and distinguished career as a surgeon, educator, and international health advocate, Dr. C. Everett Koop has tirelessly dedicated his life to improving the health of the global community. In 1992, Dr. Koop returned to his alma mater as a faculty member of the Dartmouth Medical School and founded the C. Everett Koop Institute. The institute is committed to promoting the health and well-being of all people. Working under the influence of Dr. Koop's presence and vision, the staff and students at the institute have implemented several local and national health initiatives.

Over the years, the Koop Institute has established several distinct groups, including the Center for Education Through Innovation, the Center for Healing and the Arts, and the Center for Educational Outcomes. These programs are devoted to a wide array of projects, ranging from local arts-based caring at the Dartmouth-Hitchcock Medical Center to informational Web page production. The institute also sponsors local lectures and events, publishes academic papers, and provides evaluative feedback and recommendations to educational institutions. The Koop Institute is currently designing programs that challenge the traditional conceptions of health education.

Through education, service, and communication, the Koop Institute provides innovative solutions to the problems we face in human health today. It is the institute's belief that the power of education is founded on the strength of human relationships and the ability to communicate effectively. In its brief history, the Koop Institute has expanded considerably and fine-tuned its efforts to reach an increasing number of people.

If you would like more information about the Koop Institute's programs or would like to further its founder's legacy with a contribution, please contact the institute directly:

The C. Everett Koop Institute at Dartmouth
7025 Strasenburg Hall
Hanover, NH 03755
Telephone: (603) 650–1450
Fax: (603) 650–1450
E-mail: koop.institute@dartmouth.edu
Web site: http://koop.dartmouth.edu

About the National Center for Health Education

The National Center for Health Education was created in 1975 in response to an urgent need for a private nonprofit organization that could coordinate education for health efforts nationwide. Its current mission is to lead the nation in the implementation of lifelong comprehensive health education for our children and youth.

Established at the recommendation of a special presidential commission, it was developed with the objective of "raising the level of health citizenship." The center was conceived as a flexible, problem-solving mechanism in health education that would encompass five major functions: advocacy, convening, technical assistance, research and evaluation, and information exchange. For the twenty-five years, the National Center for Health Education has performed these roles, helping people—especially children—gain control of their own health through education and action.

The National Center for Health Education is committed to improving the health of all Americans through education, and it has focused its major efforts on school health education through its Growing Healthy curriculum. The most widely used K–6 health curriculum in U.S. schools, Growing Healthy is the most widely tested and the most effective of all curricula now being used. In recent years, the center has expanded its international activities as more and more countries around the world are requesting assistance in the development and implementation of programs affecting the health and well-being of their citizens through education.

If you would like additional information about the National Center for Health Education programs or consulting services, or if you would like to make a contribution to the organization, please contact:

National Center for Health Education
72 Spring Street
New York, NY 10012
Telephone: (212) 334–9470
Fax: (212) 334–9845
E-mail: nche@nche.org
Web site: http://www.nche.org

Foreword

A study of history can help us shape the future. It is not just a matter of avoiding the repetition of past mistakes but also one of laying a foundation for future successes. As we face the challenges of global health, I am both encouraged and concerned by what I have observed in the twentieth century.

We can be encouraged by scientific developments, which have produced a crescendo of powerful health tools. We now have vaccines and therapeutic agents of great potency and improved safety, and better and even safer products will be forthcoming with each passing year. Practitioners of tropical medicine, who bemoaned the adverse effects inherent in treating various helminthic and parasitic diseases thirty years ago, never expected a drug such as Mectizan, which is extremely effective and so safe that it has been given to tens of millions of people for the treatment of onchocerciasis, or river blindness. They also never dreamed that a major pharmaceutical firm, Merck and Company, would contribute the medicine free "to every endemic village, for as long as it is needed."

We can be encouraged by the development of global organizations. We started the twentieth century without a United Nations, a World Health Organization, a World Bank, or UNICEF. Those who are inclined to criticize these organizations have no idea of the peace, the good health, and the improvements in development that have resulted because we now have the ability to shape global perspectives and develop unified actions.

We can be encouraged by the involvement of individuals and organizations of all kinds with the common objective of improving health. We began the twentieth century with a tradition of a few religious organizations sending missionaries to provide health services to developing areas of the world. We begin the twenty-first with many other powerful groups involved in this task. Service organizations such as

Lions, Rotary, and Kiwanis bring resources and people to focus on specific problems. Literally thousands of nongovernmental organizations (NGOs) concentrate on a broad spectrum of health and development issues. Bilateral assistance from government to government is now so common that we forget how rare it was a century ago. And that, of course, is how taxpayers, even those who have little interest in remote areas, become global citizens. Many corporations now are involved, like Merck, in making helpful gifts of their products. To this we can add the contributions of numerous private foundations and generous individuals, such as Ted Turner and the Gates family.

We can be encouraged by developments in rapid transportation and communications. Because of media networks like CNN, the plight of the hungry and suffering is more likely to be recognized, and the world is more likely to respond. The digital revolution is changing our ability to deliver advice and assistance to almost any place and at any time.

Finally, we can be encouraged by the proven results of these efforts. Life expectancy has continued to increase throughout much of the world. Global infant mortality rates have been cut in half in the past forty years. Other specific problems have been dramatically solved. Measles mortality has been greatly reduced; smallpox has disappeared; guinea worm and polio are on the verge of joining the ranks of eradicated diseases.

But the news is not all positive. HIV/AIDS is taking an enormous toll in Africa and parts of Asia, and the cost of treatment is beyond the capability of most affected people. Tobacco is now the single most lethal agent in the world, and political and economic pressures are blocking efforts to arrest this spreading plague. Environmental degradation is a progressive problem, especially among those least able to counter its effects. Malnutrition is still a fact of life for millions of children everywhere, and many other afflictions are being targeted only spasmodically, if at all.

There is a great need for more cooperation and concerted action by well-meaning organizations. We must face the embarrassing fact that there is no systematic approach to improving global health care.

These realities must cause us to increase our efforts to bring more science, more global and bilateral assistance, and more generous help from international agencies, governments, corporations, NGOs, and service agencies to bear on health problems, especially in the developing nations.

The miracles of science could and should be shared equally in the world. There is a growing chasm between those of us who are rich, powerful, and healthy and those who are poor, weak, and suffering from preventable diseases. If we are to improve health, we must concentrate on existing disparities in opportunities, resources, education, and access to health programs. Only to the extent that we can eliminate these inequities will our dreams for global health in the twenty-first century be realized.

Plains, Georgia   JIMMY CARTER
April 2000

~

Introduction

Health has always been important to individuals and to nations, but as the third millennium of the Common Era dawns, the expectation of what improved health might bring to both individuals and nations is greater than it has ever been before. It also carries a higher price tag. As nations grapple with the limits on resources necessary to meet their health goals, paradoxically, some of the most innovative things can probably now be done in developing countries.

Those of us who have been interested over the long term in the prospects of adequate health care for developing nations have been thwarted by the fact that the situation seemed extraordinarily difficult due to the lack of an infrastructure. Today, however, thanks to the computer, the Internet, and the cellular telephone, the need for the complex infrastructure we had come to rely on in decades past has all but disappeared. The future looks brighter than at any time in memory as the World Health Organization, charitable groups, and even individuals are making plans to use the Internet to bring health to the developing world with an enthusiasm that is, well, contagious. We have recognized the shrinking of the planet in other walks of life, but the shrinking of the world for the benefit of health is something different and something eagerly anticipated.

Industrialized nations still face the dilemma of reaching populations with the message of preventive medicine when they seem more attentive to the glamorous world of therapeutics; indeed, the more esoteric, creative, and innovative a new therapy is, the more likely it is to become popular. My own experience as a physician who practiced for almost forty years and then served in the Public Health Service for eight additional years as the Surgeon General of the United States has led me to believe that we need to make the message of preventive medicine more glamorous if we are to reap the benefits of prevention, which is generally cheap and effective.

Although infectious diseases plague the developing countries, immunization is catching on, and acute infectious diseases are being successfully treated with newer antibiotics. Smallpox has been conquered, and polio and measles have all but disappeared from the United States and are theoretically eradicable worldwide. Unfortunately, we can never make comparisons between the industrialized nations and the rest of the world without recognizing the extraordinary roles that poverty and lack of education play in holding back progress in less developed nations. Although the gap between the haves and the have-nots may increase in some facets of life, it is my firm belief that newer technologies, including the computer and the Internet, will bring healer and patient closer together and nations closer together as they seek in concert to overcome the old diseases that plague us all as well as to be ready on the front line for new diseases not yet widely encountered.

The need for closer networking among all nations points up the need for expanded funding and authority of the World Health Organization. In the more than half a century that WHO has been in operation, what it has accomplished is impressive, but what could be achieved with more money, more resources, and more innovation is also extraordinarily apparent. If we lost WHO, we would have to reinvent it tomorrow. The health needs of the world would demand it—as the chapters in this book clearly show.

ORGANIZATION OF THE BOOK

This book has been organized into three major parts. Part One, "Countries, Continents, and the World," opens with a global view of the world's health by our distinguished Secretary General of the World Health Organization, Dr. Gro Harlem Brundtland. Chapters focusing on the major regions of the world written by experts with experience on the ground provide a truly worldwide view. Part One also includes portraits of four countries—China, India, Russia, and the United States—representing the largest and most populated areas of the world. Mexico and Canada are included as neighbors of the United States, a key player in global health and economics.

Part Two, "The Organizational Landscape in Global Health," highlights the pressing health issues—including communicable and infectious diseases, tobacco control, and environmental health—that currently affect the world and their anticipated outcomes. It also discusses the processes and applications—such as research, health promotion and disease prevention, and financing—related to health issues. These chapters are written by leading scholarly professionals who are specialists in these areas.

Part Three, "Organizations, Management, Leadership, and Partnerships," gives a *raison d'être* to assist the reader in searching for the best and most cost-effective ways of solving the many global health issues and problems we will face during the coming century.

The final chapter in Part Three suggests some specific follow-up actions for consideration by the opinion leaders of government, business, and the nonprofit sector as they strive to answer the question "What's next?"

ORIGINS OF THE BOOK

One of the most remarkable aspects of putting this book on global health in the twenty-first century together was the fact that of the seventy-five internationally renowned medical and public health experts we asked to participate, seventy-five enthusiastically accepted. No author contributing to this volume is a second choice because our first choice was not available. I don't know of any other compendium that can say that. The contents of this book will find different niches among different readers, to be sure, but all readers will benefit from the global perspective they will be able to synthesize from this remarkable and diverse group of experts. My thanks go to each of them, not only for taking the time to prepare the manuscripts, but also for sharing their valuable expertise in this major communicational undertaking. The promptness with which manuscripts were submitted has been exemplary and unprecedented in my experience.

ACKNOWLEDGMENTS

The difficulty in thanking the many people who made this volume possible is that if I try to remember them all, I will inadvertently leave out somebody who was extraordinarily important. Nevertheless, taking that risk, I want first to thank my two coeditors, who really did most of the work. Special thanks go to Laurie Norris, who had general oversight of the project and worked indefatigably to bring it to a satisfactory conclusion. Andy Pasternack, Health Editor for

Jossey-Bass Publishers, contributed a different sort of expertise to help us put this volume together. Finally, the collective thanks of the editors go to the staff at the Koop Institute, at the National Center for Health Education (Clarence Pearson's associates), and at the China Medical Board (Roy Schwarz's associates), whose attention to detail and ability to network with each other made this book possible.

Hanover, New Hampshire   C. EVERETT KOOP, MD, ScD
April 2000

Critical Issues
in Global Health

PART ONE

Countries, Continents, and the World

CHAPTER ONE

The Future of the World's Health

Gro Harlem Brundtland

Gro Harlem Brundtland, MD, *took office as Director-General of the World Health Organization on July 21, 1998. Born in Oslo, Norway, she served for ten years in the Norwegian public health system as a medical doctor and master of public health before turning to a political career. She was appointed Prime Minister of Norway in 1981 and has held that office three times, most recently between 1990 and 1996.*

As we look back at the twentieth century, we can see that the great and numerous health achievements it contained constitute one of the biggest social transformations of our times—truly a health revolution. Living conditions have improved dramatically for the large majority of the human race. The past few decades have witnessed extraordinary gains in life expectancy. Today, a substantial majority of the world's population faces a relatively low risk from infectious diseases of any sort. Health care has grown from an undifferentiated domestic activity into a vast industry absorbing 9 percent of world wealth—more than $2 trillion annually.

However, as we look forward into the new century, we must not lose sight of a darker legacy that the century just ended has left us.

More than a billion of our fellow human beings have not benefited from the health revolution. The single most important challenge now, at the beginning of the twenty-first century, must be to help lift these billion people out of poverty. I believe that with vision, commitment, and successful leadership that we could, in the first decade of this century, see many of the world's poor people no longer suffering the burden of premature death and excessive disability, and that alone would significantly reduce poverty.

Dramatically reducing the high rate of mortality and morbidity suffered by the poor will mean focusing more on interventions that we know can achieve the greatest possible health gain—such as giving renewed attention to diseases such as tuberculosis, malaria, and HIV/AIDS. There is also a great need to invest more in reducing maternal mortality. Whereas only one woman in more than four thousand in Europe or the United States risks dying in childbirth, that ratio can be as high as one in sixteen for women in the poorest countries of the world.

One of the lessons learned in the twentieth century is that successes achieved in public health often lead to new challenges. So if we do succeed in curbing poverty and giving all people a real chance to climb the ladder of social and economic development, new health threats will follow nevertheless. These threats will be due in part to the fact that people live longer, that their lifestyles are changing, and that they become exposed to such hazards as tobacco.

If the tobacco epidemic were to remain unchecked, the number of smokers could be expected to rise from 1 billion today to about 1.6 billion some twenty years from now. That would increase the number of tobacco-related deaths from 3.5 million today to close to 10 million in 2020, with almost all of those extra deaths occurring in the developing world. Half of those who die from tobacco die in middle age. And in addition to the lives cut short, tobacco accounts for a vast amount of disease and disability and places a huge burden on health systems.

In any event, a major transition in the way that health systems are structured and financed will have to take place in a very short space of time and often under very severe financial restraints. We need to develop ways in which the financial burdens of medical needs are more fairly shared, leaving no household without access to care or exposed to economic ruin as a result of health expenditure. Health systems will need to respond with greater compassion, quality, and efficiency to the increasingly diverse demands they face.

The progress made in the twentieth century points to the real opportunity for reaching these goals, but opportunity entails responsibility. Working together, we can transform lives now debilitated by disease and fear of economic ruin into lives filled with realistic hopes. Doing so requires that we place health at the core of the global development agenda, where it belongs.

Improvements in health have helped spur human and economic development in the past, and they will continue to do so in the future. I have always believed that we cannot make real changes in society unless the economic dimension of the issue is fully understood. I believe that combating poverty through better health is sound economics. For example, a five-year difference in life expectancy between two otherwise similar countries can increase the rate of economic growth in the healthier country by half a percent per year. The cumulative effect of such a difference is significant in development terms.

The World Health Organization is now collecting, analyzing, and circulating the evidence that investing in health is one major avenue toward poverty alleviation. Creating such an evidence base is vitally important. The expanding knowledge base is what made the twentieth-century health revolution possible. Knowledge improves health through two mechanisms. The more obvious one is the invention of specific technologies, such as the production and administration of drugs and vaccines, but knowledge is also the basis for health-promoting behaviors. People wash their hands because of their knowledge of microbes; they quit smoking because they grasp the evidence that tobacco kills.

Scientific knowledge is therefore relevant to all people, and our challenge is to spread that knowledge and make it more integral to the way people lead their lives. Within this knowledge base, continuously renewed and expanded, we must find the answers to bring in the excluded billions and to make the right decisions on how to help them out of poverty.

Although the generation and application of new knowledge about diseases and their control have yielded substantial successes, many problems and challenges of course remain. Some problems emerge from the reduction in mortality from infectious disease and accompanying declines in fertility: the very successes of the past few decades will inexorably lead to a "demographic transition" from traditional societies where almost everyone is young to societies with rapidly increasing numbers of middle-aged and elderly. With this transition, a new set of diseases rises to prominence—cancers, heart disease, stroke, and mental illness figure prominently among them. Available interventions against these diseases, including preventive ones, yield less decisive results than we have achieved for most infectious diseases. And their costs can be very high.

Many countries are consequently facing a double burden: they must deal with the disease problems of the poor while simultaneously responding to rapid growth in noncommunicable diseases. Large numbers of other individuals, both poor and nonpoor, fail to realize their full potential for better health because health systems allocate resources to interventions of low quality or of low efficacy related to cost. Increasing numbers of people forgo or defer essential care or suffer huge financial burdens resulting from an unexpected need for expensive services. The continuing challenges to health ministries and to countries thus remain enormous.

New problems constantly arise, as we have witnessed in the emergence of the HIV epidemic, the threat of resurgent malaria, and the unexpected magnitude and consequences of the tobacco epidemic. Achieving better health for all is an ever-changing task. Success will make a major difference in the quality of life worldwide.

Global leadership and advocacy for health remain critical missing ingredients in the formula for making a difference and conveying evidence to the highest level of government. We need to remind prime ministers and finance ministers that they are health ministers themselves and that investments in the health of the poor can enhance economic growth and reduce poverty. Leadership must motivate and guide the technical community to bring today's powerful tools to bear on the challenges before us.

FOUR CHALLENGES

In my view, four main challenges need to be addressed to improve the world's health in the twenty-first century.

First and foremost, there is a need to reduce greatly the burden of excess mortality and morbidity suffered by the poor. The Organization for Economic Cooperation and Development's Development Assistance Committee has established the target of halving the number of people living in absolute poverty by the year 2015. This goal is attainable, but it will require major shifts in the way that governments all over the world use their resources. It will mean focusing more on interventions that we know can achieve the greatest health gain possible within prevailing resource limits. It will mean giving renewed attention to diseases like tuberculosis, which disproportionately affect poor people, as well as malaria and HIV/AIDS, which we now recognize as major constraints on economic growth.

Women and children suffer poverty more than men; there is therefore a need for greater investment in reducing maternal mortality and finding ways of improving maternal and childhood nutrition. Reducing the burden of excess mortality and morbidity also means revitalizing and extending the coverage of immunization programs—still one of the most powerful and cost-effective technologies at our disposal. The elimination of poliomyelitis in the Americas in the past decade and great progress in control elsewhere hold out the promise that polio will join smallpox as a disease known only to history.

The new focus on reducing the burden of disease suffered by poor people is not just a call to governments alone. To make real inroads into absolute poverty will mean harnessing the energies and resources of the private sector and civil society as well. We need to be clear about what the world should be aiming to achieve and the resources needed to meet global goals. I believe that there is a good case for negotiating realistic national and international targets as a means of mobilizing resources, concentrating international attention on the most important problems, and ensuring proper monitoring of progress and achievement.

Second, there is a need to counter potential threats to health resulting from economic crises, unhealthy environments, and risky behavior. Tobacco addiction is one of the single most important threats. It is not just an issue for the North: over 80 percent of all smokers today live in developing countries. A global commitment to tobacco control can potentially avert scores of millions of premature deaths in the next half century, and its success can point the way for effective control of other threats.

Preparing effective responses to emerging infections and countering the spread of resistance to antimicrobial drugs will help insure against the prospect of a significantly increased infectious disease threat. Beyond countering specific threats, promotion of healthy lifestyles underpins a proactive strategy for risk reduction: cleaner air and water, adequate sanitation, healthy diets, and safer transportation—all are important. And all are facilitated by stable economic growth and by ensuring that females as well as males have opportunities to increase their educational attainment.

Third, there is a need to develop more effective health systems. In many parts of the world, health systems are ill equipped to cope with present demands, let alone those they will face in the future. The institutional problems that limit health sector performance are often common to all public services in a country. But despite the importance of these concerns, they have been relatively neglected by governments and development agencies alike.

We now recognize that dealing with issues such as pay and incentives in the public sector, priority setting and rationing, and unregulated growth in the private sector constitute some of the most challenging items on the international health agenda.

Changes in health systems development points are taking place in all parts of the world—changes that respond to different problems in different ways. The pressure for change provides the opportunity for reform. But reform requires a sense of direction. In my view, the broad goal of better health for all should guide reform. Beyond this, however, there is a need to be clear about the desirable characteristics of health systems. The goal must be to create health systems that can do all of the following things:

- Improve health status

- Reduce health inequalities

- Enhance responsiveness to legitimate expectations

- Increase efficiency

- Protect individuals, families, and communities from financial loss

- Enhance fairness in the financing and delivery of health care

There are limits on what governments can finance and on their capacity to deliver services and to regulate the private sector—hence the need for public policies that recognize these limits. Governments should retain responsibility for setting broad policy directions, for creating an appropriate regulatory environment, and for providing financing. At the same time, they should seek both to diversify the sources of service provision and to select interventions for the resources each country chooses to commit that will provide the maximum gains in health levels and their most equitable distribution. At an international level, we need collectively to improve our capacity for humanitarian assistance and for responding to complex emergencies when national health systems cannot cope.

Finally, there is a need to invest in expanding the knowledge base that made the twentieth-century health revolution possible, thereby providing the tools for continued gains in the new century. Governments of high-income countries and large, research-oriented pharmaceutical companies currently invest—and will continue to invest—massive resources in research and development catering to the needs of the more affluent.

Much of this investment benefits all humanity, but at least two critical gaps remain. One involves research and development associated with the infectious diseases that overwhelmingly affect the poor. The other concerns the systematic generation of an information base that countries can use in shaping the future of their own health systems.

The challenges outlined here constitute an agenda for the world community as a whole: for governments and development agencies alike. Even as the lead agency in health, WHO recognizes that the agenda is too broad for this organization alone. We therefore have to be realistic and start to define how WHO can contribute most effectively to this agenda in coming years.

We intend that four interconnected strategic themes should guide the work of the whole organization. The first two concern *where* we focus our efforts. The second two concern *how* we work.

1. We need to be more focused in improving health outcomes.

2. We need to be more effective in supporting health systems development.

3. We need to be more impact-oriented in our work with countries.

4. We need to be more innovative in creating influential partnerships.

SETTING PRIORITIES

The theme of improving health outcomes runs through everything we do. Our first priority must be to reduce—and then eliminate—the debilitating excess burden of disease among the poor. I am particularly concerned that we focus on health interventions that will help lead populations out of poverty.

- We are committed to reducing the burden of sickness and suffering resulting from communicable diseases. WHO's Roll Back Malaria project is central to this approach. But we will also contribute as effectively as possible to combating the global epidemics of HIV/AIDS and tuberculosis and to completing the eradication of poliomyelitis.
- We need to step up our ability to deal with the rising toll of noncommunicable diseases. Special attention will be given to cancer and cardiovascular diseases. WHO's Tobacco Free Initiative is supporting and leading this approach.
- We will pay more attention to the delivery of high-quality health care for children, adolescents, and women.
- The WHO is committed to making progress on the issues of population and reproductive health, with a special focus on maternal mortality and adolescent sexual and reproductive health.
- We will put the spotlight back on immunization as one of the most cost-effective health interventions.
- We need to intensify our efforts to reduce the enormous burden of malnutrition, especially in children.
- We will continue to support countries in their quest for access to affordable and high-quality essential drugs.
- We will work to see that mental health—and particularly the neglected scourge of depression—is given the attention it deserves.
- We need to be better at responding to increasingly diverse kinds of emergencies and humanitarian crises.
- We will develop our capacity within WHO—and in collaboration with others—to give advice on crucial health care financing issues.
- We need to be able to deal more effectively with intersectoral issues—particularly the threats to health that result from environmental causes.

The purpose of our work is to improve people's lives, reduce the burdens of disease and poverty, and provide access to responsive health care for all. We must never lose this vision. The twentieth century has left us with a great deal of unfinished business. But it also showed what could be done. In terms of achievements in health, the challenge before us is to build on the recent past to provide a better, healthier future.

CHAPTER TWO

Africa

Adetokunbo O. Lucas

Adetokunbo O. Lucas, MD, *was formerly a professor of international health at the Harvard School of Public Health and is now a visiting professor at the London School of Hygiene and Tropical Medicine. He is currently the Chair of the Global Forum for Health Research, an organization whose main aim is to stimulate health research on problems affecting the poor.*

Health and disease have had a profound effect on the history and development of Africa south of the Sahara. In no other part of the world have the occurrence and distribution of human and animal diseases played such a prominent role in shaping critical historical events. The distribution of tropical diseases influenced the relationships of the local populations to the external world and largely determined patterns of European settlement. The high mortality from malaria, yellow fever, and other tropical diseases among explorers and other European visitors to West Africa earned the region the title of "White Man's Grave." This prevented Europeans from settling in West Africa, though they were able to establish significant settlements in southern Africa and in the highlands of East Africa. Not only did tropical diseases affect foreigners, but they also influenced internal conflicts and relationships in Africa. These maladies also had a devastating effect on the indigenous people, ravaging the populations with disease and disability and in extreme cases threatening the survival of some communities. Diseases of farm animals, such as trypanosomiasis, limited the availability of animal proteins, an important contributing cause to malnutrition (Lucas, 1989; Gilles and Lucas, 1998).

Health in Africa: Status and Determinants

In the past century, the African region has achieved significant health gains; mortality rates in infants and children have declined, other health indicators have improved, and some endemic diseases have been brought under control (UNICEF, 1998; see Table 2.1). In spite of these gains, sub-Saharan Africa still lags behind other parts of the world (Feacham and Jamison, 1991). Furthermore, recrudescence of some diseases that had been controlled, the emergence of new infections such as the HIV/AIDS, and the steady increase in chronic, noninfectious diseases are threatening and eroding earlier gains (Akinkugbe, 1992; Adult Mortality and Morbidity Project, 1997).

Several factors account for the relative poor health status of Africans:

- *Local geographical and ecological factors* in parts of Africa favor parasitic and other infectious agents and their vectors.
- *Poverty* limits the ability of governments to provide expensive technologies and the ability of populations to acquire them.
- *Poor infrastructure* accounts for a lack of essential services for maintaining good health, such as housing, an adequate supply of safe water, and food security.
- *High fertility* strains national resources and is associated with high-risk pregnancies and abortions.
- *Low literacy rates,* especially among women, limit access to knowledge and information that people need to promote, protect, and restore their health.
- *Civil wars and unrest* disrupt orderly development, displace populations, and damage infrastructure.
- *Inefficient, corrupt, and unstable governments* fail to organize effective health services and are not committed to the goal of equity and social justice.

Region/Group	Child Mortality Rate (deaths of children under age five per 1,000 live births)	Maternal Mortality Rate (deaths per 100,000 live births)	Childhood Malnutrition (percent)	Total Fertility Rate	Primary Education (percent)
Sub-Saharan Africa	183	980	31	6.5	48
Middle East and North Africa	86	100	24	5	81
South Asia	13	560	60	4.4	50
East Asia and Pacific	57	190	26	2.6	81
Central America and Caribbean	48	140	17	3.5	66
South America	54	210	8	3.0	48
Industrialized Countries	11	13	n.a.	1.8	96

Table 2.1. Comparative Statistics: Mortality, Malnutrition, Fertility, and Education.
Source: UNICEF, 1998.

THE CHALLENGE OF THE TWENTY-FIRST CENTURY

In the twenty-first century, the challenge will be to consolidate the gains that were made during the twentieth, to eliminate traditional health problems (infectious diseases aggravated by malnutrition); to deal with the persistent threat of new infections and the recrudescence of ancient scourges like tuberculosis; and to tackle emergent problems. To achieve these goals, the region must adopt a broad range of measures:

- Radical reform of health systems to improve efficiency, cost effectiveness, and equity
- Capacity strengthening to help policymakers and health workers manage diversity and change
- Promotion of health research to guide decisions on local issues and to participate with the global scientific community in efforts to develop new and improved technologies
- Rationalization of international technical cooperation that is designed to promote self-reliance

REFORM OF THE HEALTH SECTOR

The health sector in most African countries is in urgent need of reform aimed at achieving sustained purposeful change to improve efficiency, equity, and effectiveness of the health sector. The World Bank and other agencies have drawn attention to common failures of health systems in developing countries and specifically in the African region (The World Bank, 1993, 1994). African ministries of health have adopted various modular programs that were designed by the World Health Organization (WHO) and UNICEF, including GOBI-FFF (growth monitoring, oral dehydration, breast feeding, immunization, family planning, female education, and supplementary feeding of pregnant women), the child survival package, the control of diarrheal diseases and acute respiratory infections, expanded programs for immunization, and the essential drug program. The World Bank (1993) prescribed a list of cost-effective public health and clinical interventions. It is difficult to synthesize this plethora of vertical programs into realistic national health systems.

Simple characterizations of the health situation in Africa have prompted some experts to propose equally simplistic solutions, but closer analysis shows considerable variation and complexity in the nature and determinants of the health profiles of African people and in the level of available resources—financial, institutional, and human. There is also a tendency to present a static picture of the African situation despite clear evidence that significant changes are occurring in all parts of the continent. The reformed health sector must take note of the complexity and diversity of the health picture in Africa as well as the dynamic changes that are occurring in the region. Rather than blindly applying prepackaged, stereotyped formulas, the reformed health sector must base its strategies on critical analyses of needs and opportunities, and it must carefully adapt its programs to the local situation.

Attempts at reforming the health sector in African countries have encountered many obstacles, especially tensions resulting from the conflicting claims of various interested parties. For example, communities have reacted negatively, even violently, when governments have introduced charges for services that were previously offered for free (Shaw and Griffin, 1995). Doctors and other professional groups often demand the acquisition of expensive high technologies in situations where basic needs have not been met. Public opinion also often favors investment in hospitals and other curative services but makes little demand for preventive services that are usually more cost-effective. The success of health reform in Africa will depend on the extent to which health planners can forge a clear consensus about goals and strategies. The ideal climate for reform of the health sector is one in which there is a strategic alliance among key stakeholders: the civil society, the government, the private sector, health professionals, and other partners including traditional healers.

CAPACITY DEVELOPMENT

Africa has made much progress in training doctors, nurses, and other health professionals, but the shortage of trained personnel still limits the development of the health sector there. Much of the training has been along traditional lines aimed at equipping staff with clinical and other technical skills. For the health sector in Africa to tackle the challenging problems of the twenty-first century most effectively, analytical and management capacity must be enhanced at all levels of the health services. The new breed of health officials in Africa must be equipped to deal with complexity, diversity, and change.

One common source of tension is the conflict between clinical specialists, who often demand relatively large resources for their narrow specialties, and health planners, who take a broader picture of community needs. Training programs for clinical specialists in Africa should extend the curricula beyond technical biomedical skills to broader issues of health policy and management. A good example is an innovative postgraduate training program for obstetricians in Ghana. To assure awareness of broader issues in maternal health, trainees are assigned to a district hospital and become involved in community maternal health services (Martey and others, 1995; Martey and Hudson, 1999).

HEALTH RESEARCH

Research is increasingly recognized as a tool for guiding the development of health policies aimed at achieving efficiency, cost effectiveness, and equity. Findings from epidemiological, social, and behavioral research help define the pattern, distribution, and determinants of health and disease, thereby providing the basis for setting priorities and designing interventions. Health policy and health systems research will help optimize the strategies as well as the monitoring of performance and impact.

It is also necessary to intensify biomedical research aimed at developing new and improved tools for tackling health problems for which cost-effective technologies are not currently available. African institutions have limited resources for applying the powerful tools of biomedical research in the search for new drugs, diagnostic tools, vaccines, and vector control measures. A variety of international programs have been established to bridge this gap by mobilizing resources from the international network of scientific institutions, including the pharmaceutical industry. Key international initiatives in health research include the United Nations Development Programme (UNDP)/World Bank/WHO Special Programme for Research and Training in Tropical Diseases (TDR), the Council for Health Research and Development (COHRED), the European Commission program for Health Research with Developing Countries, and the Global Forum for Health Research (GFHR) (Godal, Goodman, and Lucas, 1998). African governments should make appropriate responses to these international initiatives and participate effectively. Specifically, they should orient their research establishment to take fullest advantage of the global effort and to assimilate research advances into their health services (Commission on Health Research for Development, 1990; Osuntokun and Hashmi, 1992; World

Health Organization, 1996; European Commission, 1997; Global Forum for Health Research, 1999).

INTERNATIONAL COLLABORATION

Colonial governments and foreign missions built the foundations of modern health services in most African countries. Foreign agencies continue to exert much influence on their subsequent development. WHO, UNICEF, the World Bank, and other multilateral UN agencies provide technical support, guidance, and substantial resources. Bilateral donor agencies, international nongovernmental development agencies, and other foreign donors make significant contributions to the health sector in Africa. On the whole, such external aid has been valuable both for routine services and for dealing with epidemics and other emergencies. However, the relationship of national health authorities to these external agencies is in need of review. Ministries of health often have difficulty coping with the varying demands of their foreign partners. Conflicting recommendations and competing programs sometimes tend to distort national priorities and disrupt the orderly development of the health sector. In recent years, major donors are experimenting with new mechanisms based on sectorwide programming as a means of rationalizing external aid.

External support should promote self-reliance rather than increased dependence on foreign aid. Some external agencies do not give sufficient priority to strengthening national capacity, and some of their policies undermine the advancement of national experts and institutions. The Commission on Health Research for Development (1990) recommended that 5 percent of the budget for large externally funded programs should be assigned to capacity strengthening. This approach should be the focus of external aid to Africa in the twenty-first century.

WHO's Regional Office for Africa plays an important role in coordinating regional collaboration and South-to-South technical cooperation (Monekosso, 1989, 1992). The West African Health Organization and its counterpart in East Africa also promote subregional training and other collaborative health projects. Other regional organizations such as the Organization of African Unity (OAU) and the Economic Organization of West African States (ECOWAS) should strengthen their health programs and expand mechanisms for mutual support and joint action in tackling common health problems.

CONCLUSION

The twentieth century witnessed enormous gains in the health of the populations in sub-Saharan Africa, but the region needs to alleviate the massive burden of disease that is impeding its development. The challenge in the twenty-first century will be to consolidate the gains that were made in the past century and tackle both residual and emergent problems. African countries must do more than copy methods that have worked in other countries; they must also devise creative ways to deal with their own problems. The challenge is to achieve "good health at low cost" (Halstead, Walsh, and Warren, 1985). It calls for careful objective analyses of needs and opportunities. It will be facilitated by the development and nurturing of partnerships among the key stakeholders, including the public sector, the private sector, health-related professionals, foreign partners, and credible representatives of civil society.

References

Akinkugbe, O. O. *Non-Communicable Diseases in Nigeria.* Prepared by the National Expert Committee on Non-Communicable Diseases, Lagos, Nigeria, 1992.

Commission on Health Research for Development. *Health Research: Essential Link to Equity in Development.* New York: Oxford University Press, 1990.

European Commission. *Health Research with Developing Countries.* Brussels, Belgium: European Commission, 1997.

Feacham, R. G., and Jamison, D. *Disease and Mortality in Sub-Saharan Africa.* New York: Oxford University Press, 1991.

Gilles, H. M., and Lucas, A.O. (1998). "Tropical Medicine: 100 Years of Progress." *British Medical Bulletin, 54,* 1998, 269–280.

Global Forum for Health Research. *The 10/90 Report on Health Research.* Global Forum for Health Research. Geneva, 1999.

Godal, T., Goodman, H. C., and Lucas, A. O. "Research and Training in Tropical Diseases." *World Health Forum, 19,* 1998, 377–381.

Halstead, S. B., Walsh, J. A., and Warren, K. S. *Good Health at Low Cost.* New York: Rockefeller Foundation, 1985.

Lucas, A. O. "Health Research in Africa: Priorities, Promise, and Performance." *Annals of the New York Academy of Sciences, 569,* 1989, 17–24.

Martey, J. O., and Hudson, C. N. "Training Specialists in the Developing World: Ten Years On, a Success Story for West Africa." *British Journal of Obstetrics and Gynaecology, 106,* 1992, 91–94.

Martey, J. O., and others. "Innovative Community-Based Postgraduate Training for Obstetrics and Gynecology." *Obstetrics and Gynecology, 85,* 1995, 1042–1046.

Monekosso, G. L. *Accelerating the Achievement of Health for All Africans: The Three-Phase Health Development Scenario.* Brazzaville, Congo: World Health Organization/African Regional Office, 1989.

Monekosso, G. L. *Working for Better Health in Africa.* Brazzaville, Congo: World Health Organization/AFRO, 1992.

Osuntokun, B. O., and Hashmi, J. "Issues for Research Capability Strengthening. In A. M. Davies and B. Mansourian (eds.), *Research Strategies for Health.* Lewiston, N.Y.: Horgrefe and Hubers, 1992.

Shaw, P. R., and Griffin, C. C. *Financing Health Care in Sub-Saharan Africa Through User Fees and Insurance.* Washington, D.C.: World Bank, 1995.

UNICEF. *The State of the World's Children, 1998.* Oxford, England: Oxford University Press, 1998.

World Bank. *World Development Report, 1993: Investing in Health.* Oxford, England: Oxford University Press, 1993.

World Bank. *Better Health in Africa: Experience and Lessons Learned.* Washington, D.C.: World Bank, 1994.

World Health Organization. *Investing in Health Research and Development: Report of the Ad Hoc Committee on Health Research Relating to Future Intervention Options.* Geneva: World Health Organization, 1996.

Additional Reading

Lucas, A.O. "Public Access to Health Information as a Human Right." Proceedings of the International Symposium on Public Health Surveillance. *Morbidity and Mortality Weekly Report, 41,* 1992, 77–78.

Ministry of Health. *Policy Implications of Adult Morbidity and Mortality: End of Phase 1 Report.* Dodoma, Tanzania: Ministry of Health, 1997.

World Health Organization. *The World Health Report, 1999: Making a Difference.* Geneva: World Health Organization, 1999.

CHAPTER THREE

Latin America and the Caribbean

George A. O. Alleyne

George A. O. Alleyne, MD, *is Director of the Pan American Health Organization and Regional Director for the Americas of the World Health Organization.*

All evidence points to Latin America and the Caribbean having better health indicators in the years to come. People will live longer, and the disease pattern will change significantly. The dominant concerns, at least for the makers of policy, will be both the state of health itself and the health inequity that will exist unless efforts are made to recognize it and address it. This region has the dubious distinction of being the most inequitable in the world, and that label—usually applied in an economic sense—is being used in the other social areas, including health.

The state of health and the manifestation of health inequities in any people will depend fundamentally on demographic trends and changes in the major determinants of health as we know them today. This chapter will deal with these matters and outline the current and projected health status of the region, using many of the traditional measures of health. The focus will be mainly on a population's health and less on the diseases of individuals, important though that topic may be.

One of the most notable features of the health panorama at the end of the twentieth century has been the reduction in communicable diseases. Age-adjusted mortality rates for men show that the risk of dying from a communicable disease has fallen, overall, about 50 percent in the past fifteen years, with the most marked decline of about 70 percent occurring in Central America and the Andean region, where the rates were highest initially. The same phenomenon has been observed in women, although the improvement has been somewhat greater among men.

This drop does not imply that communicable diseases are no longer a problem, as they still account for 10 percent of the risk of dying for both men and women. There were almost a quarter of a million cases of tuberculosis in the region in 1995, and some twenty-two thousand persons died from the disease. Approximately one-quarter of a million people have been diagnosed with AIDS since the epidemic began, and about half of them have died. With about twenty-five thousand cases reported in 1997, there is cause for cautious optimism, as the annual incidence seems to be falling, albeit slowly. Epidemics of dengue still occur, and one million cases of malaria were reported in 1997.

The prospects for improvement are good. We can expect to see tuberculosis brought under control in the new century. HIV/AIDS will continue to be a major problem for some time because many countries will be unable to afford the drugs that have reduced mortality rates in more developed countries. The disease is still very much an affliction of the poor, as the epidemic is concentrated among the most socially disadvantaged. I do not envisage the elimination of epidemic dengue in the near future.

In spite of the recent advances and increased attention being given to malaria, this age-old scourge will be with us for many years yet. Hope for a malaria vaccine remains high, but in the meantime we have to depend on the traditional methods of early therapy with efficacious drugs, especially in areas that have been determined through epidemiological stratification to be zones of ready transmission.

Part of the reduction in communicable diseases has been due to advances in the control of diseases preventable by the use of vaccines, particularly in children. Ours was the first region to have eliminated smallpox, and the last case of poliomyelitis occurred in 1991. In 1994, the countries agreed to eliminate measles by the year 2000, and the approximately twelve hundred cases in Latin America and the Caribbean in 1996 was the lowest figure ever recorded. Unfortunately, major outbreaks occurred in the Southern Cone countries in 1997 and 1998. These are slowly but surely being brought under control and there is every expectation that measles will be history in the twenty-first century.

The new century will undoubtedly bring new epidemics as man invades new ecological niches or the microbial dynamics change. We are hopeful that the current attention to emerging and reemerging diseases will bear fruit. Surely we will recognize the value of good surveillance systems and the need to strengthen the capacity for laboratory diagnosis. Research will be critical to the development of new and more rapid diagnostic methods. The ease of transfer of information will both facilitate and complicate the possibility of dealing with epidemics of infectious disease.

It is not far-fetched to speak of an epidemic of cardiovascular diseases, as diseases of the circulatory system already account for about one-third of the risk of dying in both sexes, and it is estimated that by the year 2020, 38 percent of all deaths will be due to these diseases. The major problems are stroke, coronary heart disease, and hypertension. Mortality from stroke seems to be decreasing, but coronary heart disease is not showing the same steady downward trend, and success will depend on a concerted approach to attenuating the risk factors in some coordinated way. Projects are already under way in Latin America and the Caribbean to address these risk factors from a community perspective.

Mortality from cancer has remained steady, but there will be a strong emphasis on the early detection and cure of cancers of the breast and cervix and prevention of cancer of the lung by reducing tobacco use. Cancers of the breast and uterine cervix account for 20 percent of all cancers reported, and the region has some of the highest incidence rates of cervical cancer in the world, especially in the Andean and Southern Cone countries.

Thus Latin America and the Caribbean can look forward to a continuing reduction of communicable diseases as a whole, as well as an increasing incidence of chronic noncommunicable diseases. These trends will determine the organization of the health services and the nature of the human resources that deal with health.

It will become more and more evident that tools for dealing with both communicable and noncommunicable diseases have much in common, as both sets of diseases are in large measure amenable to control through changes in behavior. The approach to HIV/AIDS is fundamentally based on the need to change behavior; the control and prevention of epidemics of dengue depend on the maintenance of a clean peridomestic environment. Similarly, the approaches to the control of the cardiovascular diseases are, in the main, those geared to inducing lifestyle changes. Marketing skills and social communication tools will be needed as much as those possessed by epidemiologists and cardiologists. Social engineering will become as valuable as environmental engineering for dealing with the health problems of Latin America and the Caribbean.

The demographic trends indicate that as we enter the twenty-first century, the population of Latin America and the Caribbean will be just over five hundred million, representing about 62 percent of the hemisphere's population. This will be an increase of 43 percent over the figure twenty years ago. Life expectancy at birth, currently 69.8 years on the average, is increasing, although in some countries there is the concern that a rise in young adult mortality may slow that increase. The average hides the variation that exists in the region. Whereas Costa Rica has a life expectancy at birth of 76.9 years, the figure for Haiti is only 54.5 years.

The trend is toward a decrease in total fertility and infant mortality in almost all countries. In the past fifteen years, the birthrate has decreased by 23.6 percent, although the average number of children born each year has remained about the same. There has been a steady decrease in death rates as well. Infant mortality rates are currently at 35.5 per 1,000 live births, and have fallen by 35.8 percent in the past fifteen years. The variation is wide, with Cuba showing a figure of just over 7.9, and Bolivia registering 59 infant deaths per 1,000 live births.

If these trends continue, we will see an increased graying of the population. Already we are noticing the impact of an elderly population in all countries. In Uruguay, the percentage of the population over the age of sixty is already higher than in Canada or the United States. The increased life expectancy and decreased fertility rates will inevitably lead to a greater dependency ratio, with serious consequences for social security and pension schemes. The health consequences of these changes are that chronic diseases like diabetes, hypertension, and chronic arthritis, with their increased treatment costs, will become more prevalent.

There will be changes in the major determinants of health that must, of necessity, influence the health status of individuals as well as of populations. Changes will affect both physical and social factors. If we consider first the macroenvironmental scenario, we must note the active debate on the nature and magnitude of climate changes that may occur. If they are as sweeping as some experts predict, we will see significant changes in disease patterns. An increase in ultraviolet exposure will lead to an increase in skin cancers. Global warming will produce ecological changes such that diseases formerly restricted to certain climes will invade new niches. We have already seen in Latin America outbreaks of hantavirus infection as a result of climatic changes.

But perhaps it is the change in the microenvironment that will be of most immediate significance. The outbreak of cholera after an absence of almost a century was an indication of the microenvironmental deficiencies in the region. The early epidemic phase, which was characterized by three-quarters of a million cases and over six thousand deaths in the first two years, has passed, but the disease is still endemic in some countries as a result of lack of an adequate supply of clean water. But there has been progress. Between 1980 and 1997, the population with access to drinking water and sewer systems increased by 22 percent and 63 percent, respectively. This may account in part for the fact that over the past ten to fifteen years, the percentage of deaths due to diarrheal disease in children under five years of age has declined by about 60 percent.

Disasters have had a major effect on health in the region, and we will continue to be exposed to natural hazards such as hurricanes, floods, earthquakes, and volcanic eruptions. Hurricanes Mitch and George provided stark examples of the destruction of health facilities and the loss of life that can occur. We cannot prevent natural disasters, but the new century must see a more determined effort at mitigation and preparedness to reduce the vulnerability of the countries most likely to be affected.

The social environment will of course be an important factor in determining the health status of Latin America and the Caribbean. There was hope that robust economic growth would herald the new century. The rate of economic growth in 1997 was one of the highest of the past two decades, and inflation was at its second-lowest level since the end of World War II. But the good times have not lasted, and the expectation now is the kind of modest growth that may be accompanied by increasing unemployment and increased social deprivation.

Poverty is associated with ill health, not only because basic needs are not being met but also because poverty lowers self-esteem and reduces social cohesion, both of which are essential for good health. Concern in this region is also focused on inequality, which appears to be increasing. There is evidence of widening inequality not only in income but also in terms of access to health services and hence of health outcomes. This socially unjust inequality is referred to as inequity. For example, there is a twenty-four-fold difference in maternal mortality between the countries with the best and worst indicators. Further inequities reflect differences in ethnicity, geography, and gender.

Regardless of the economic situation, the region must aggressively tackle the problem of equity in health and other areas that impinge on health, such as education. Health must figure more prominently in the political agenda of the countries. We see at various meetings that the summits of the Americas and the Ibero-American summits are devoting more attention to health, not merely for moral or humanitarian reasons but because a reduction in health inequity and an improvement of health status generally will lead to enhanced economic performance in the region.

Health will be affected both by the globalization process and by the information revolution that has spurred that process. Globalization will generate increased movement of people around the world, with the consequent internationalization of health risks. No longer will one country in the region be unaffected by the health status of the others. Globalization will also spur the development of agile mechanisms for the surveillance and reporting of communicable diseases.

The region will experience the effects of the information revolution in several ways. Telemedicine will become commonplace, and diagnostic capabilities will not be bound by space. Telemedicine will not be the exclusive province of wealthy countries; already, countries such as Costa Rica are investing in this technology, which will decrease some of the geographically determined inequities in health. The availability of scientific health information will be almost limitless, and libraries will all be virtual institutions. The ready transmission of information will also have negative effects, such as the rise in smoking we already are seeing as a result of increased advertising.

Information will also be used in more traditional ways. I see the region recovering or strengthening its capacity in the area of vital statistics, which in some cases are so fragile as to make it difficult to develop accurate measures of such things as the burden of disease. Because of technological advances, it will be feasible and desirable to present data that have been disaggregated in different ways. The development of geographical information systems will allow decision makers to identify the differences in various areas and to direct resources appropriately.

Almost every country of the region is engaged in some type of reform of its health services. In some, the process is part of a sweeping reform of the state and an examination of the essential functions to be performed by the various social actors. In many, the motive was an economic one, but in all cases increased coverage and enhanced equity have been essential goals. The process has taken many forms, but in almost all one can recognize a genuine effort to improve the organization of the services, with an attempt to define those responsibilities that fall to the state and those that can be discharged by other actors. A wide range of institutions are competing to offer services to the state and be paid for them. As the profit potential shrinks in the United States, we can envisage North American companies entering this health care market, which is sizable. It has been estimated that the overall revenues from managed care in Brazil were US$2.99 billion in 1995. The target will be the not inconsiderable social security funds. The growing income inequality in the region will also favor the growth of managed care as more and more persons reach income brackets that allow them to purchase private insurance. A major concern is the extent to which this process will be "anti-equity," with the system discriminating more and more against the poor.

In this changing scenario with multiple actors, emphasis must be placed on the steering role of the state and, in this case, the ministry of health. In the twenty-first century, ministries of health will be less and less responsible for the actual delivery of services but will ensure equity in the system and see to it that certain norms and standards are followed to guarantee the delivery of quality services. The current perception is of a modern ministry overseeing the discharge of what are being designated essential public health functions.

This chapter has attempted to give an overview of the major trends in health and the factors that will determine them. I am optimistic that there will be steady improvements in our health. Such improvements can be more rapid and have a wider reach if we address the fundamental problem of the socially unjust inequalities. The fact that health issues that go beyond those related to individual care are rising higher on the public agenda augurs well that this part of the world may slowly but surely approximate the goal of health for all, as construed by those who see it as a social desideratum.

CHAPTER FOUR

Eastern Mediterranean Region

Hussein A. Gezairy

Hussein A. Gezairy, MD, FRCS, is the World Health Organization's Regional Director for the Eastern Mediterranean, a position to which he was elected by the member states of the region. A former Minister of Health of Saudi Arabia, he was the Founding Dean of the Faculty of Medicine in Riyadh and the first President of the Supreme Council of the Arab Board of Medical Specializations. He is the recipient of a number of awards and honorary degrees.

The Eastern Mediterranean Region of the World Health Organization (WHO) includes twenty-two member states and the self-rule areas under the Palestinian Authority. It extends from Morocco to Pakistan, covering an area of 13.8 million square kilometers. The total population of the region is almost 457 million (1997–98).

By far the largest majority of people in the region are Muslim, and Arabic is the language of eighteen of the countries. However, around 50 percent of the region's population speaks other languages, such as Urdu, Farsi, Dari, and Greek. Except for religion and language, the countries in the region are markedly heterogeneous, as shown in Table 4.1. They vary in area from about 700 to 2.5 million square kilometers and in population from slightly more than half a million to more than 139 million. Some countries are quite affluent, while others are very much the opposite.

The main obstacle to economic growth in the majority of the countries continues to be the unprecedented level of external debt, amounting to billions of U.S. dollars. The cost of servicing this debt acts as a continuing brake on the economic development of these countries.

Despite the end of the cold war and the hopes raised by the Oslo Accords and the peace process in general, Palestinian, Syrian, and Lebanese territories remain under Israeli occupation, and the prospects for a just peace settlement are gloomy. Such a situation has a negative impact on the health of displaced and colonized populations in the region. Ethnic and civil strife are causing human losses and suffering for millions of people in Afghanistan, Somalia, and southern Sudan, disrupting health systems and limiting access to basic health care.

The region is committed to achieving health for all through primary health care, the long-term policy of WHO. Healthy cities and healthy villages programs and basic development needs (BDN) programs aimed at improving the quality of life have been initiated and are expanding in quite a few of the countries. In recent years, a process of health sector reforms has been initiated, aiming at improving health care financing, enhancing management and performance, and addressing population needs.

Trends indicate a clear tendency to shift the burden of health care financing from the government to households. Even high-income countries are considering relieving government budgets through adoption of user charges and risk-sharing schemes, such as health insurance.

GLOBAL CHALLENGES TO THE HEALTH SECTOR IN THE TWENTY-FIRST CENTURY

The health sector in the region faces the impact of several global changes and challenges in the twenty-first century. These challenges include (1) an unprecedented movement toward globalization, which is supported by very rapid liberalization and global free trade and capital flow, as well as huge advances in communications, technology, and transport; (2) progress in health and biomedical technology, which has widened the gap between developed and developing countries because the latter lack sufficient resources, appropriate expertise, and easy access

Table 4.1. Selected Demographic, Socioeconomic, and Health Status Indicators for the Eastern Mediterranean Region.

Country	Population		Adult Literacy Rate (Age 15 Years and Over)		Per Capita GDP		Annual Budget of Ministry of Health (Per Capita)		Mortality Rate (per 1,000 Live Births)		Infant Dying Before Fifth Birthday (per 1,000 Live Births)		Probability of Mortality at Birth (Per 10,000 Live Births)		Maternal Life Expectancy	
	000	Y	%	Y	US$	Y	US$	Y	Rate	Y	Rate	Y	R	Y	Years	Y
Afghanistan	20,452	96	27	95	n.a.	n.a.	n.a.	n.a.	165	95	250	95	170.0	96	43.5	96
Bahrain	620	97	n.a.	n.a.	9,667	97	210	96	8	97	11	96	3.9	96	72.4	96
Cyprus	855	97	n.a.	n.a.	12,892	97	250	95	8	96	10	96	3.9	96	72.4	96
Djibouti	670	97	57	96	750	97	15	96	114	93	n.a.	n.a.	n.a.	n.a.	49.0	n.a.
Egypt	61,452	97	51	95	1,220	97	10	96	25	97	n.a.	n.a.	17.4	93	64.7	96
Iran	63,800a	97	80	96	1,460	97	65	97	26	96	33	96	3.7	97	69.0	95
Iraq	21,847	97	54	95	1,027	96	n.a.	n.a.	112	94	140	94	13.0	94	58.0	94
Jordan	4,576	97	86	97	1,533	97	40	97	28	97	39	96	4.1	97	68.0	97
Kuwait	1,809	97	88	97	17,482	97	422	96	13	97	16	97	1.6	97	75.3	97
Lebanon	3,700	97	88	97	3,750	97	46	97	28	96	32	96	10.4	96	71.3	96
Libya	4,664	97	82	96	8,220	96	124	97	24	95	30	95	4.0	95	66.0	95
Morocco	27,301	97	42	95	1,178	97	13	95	37	97	46	97	22.8	97	68.8	97
Oman	2,302	98	80	95	6,995	97	147	97	18	98	25	98	2.1	96	72.2	98
Pakistan	139,020	98	39	97	467	97	4	96	86	96	137	95	30.0	95	62.5	96
Palistinian Self Rule Areas	2,893	98	84	95	1,580	96	37	96	18	95	31	95	2.9	96	71.3	96
Qatar	693	96	79	95	15,570	97	309	96	12	96	15	96	1.0	96	74.3	96
Saudi Arabia	18,885	97	75	96	7,477	97	107	96	21	95	30	96	1.8	93	71.4	95
Somalia	6,602	96	24	95	n.a.	n.a.	n.a.	n.a.	126	97	265	97	n.a.	n.a.	46.2	97
Sudan	30,326b	99	53	93	486	97	n.a.	n.a.	108	96	157	96	36.5	93	54.0	95
Syria	15,597	98	79	96	1,097	97	19	96	28	98	32	98	9.5	98	68.0	98
Tunisia	9,227	97	67	95	2,065	97	47	94	35	95	43	94	6.9	94	72.9	95
United Arab Emirates	2,624	97	86	96	17,554	97	148	97	9	97	11	97	0.2	97	73.0	96
Yemen	16,333	97	45	94	442	96	4	96	79	96	122	94	n.a.	n.a.	57.5	95

Source: WHO Regional Office for the Eastern Mediterranean. "Demographic and Health Indicators for Countries of the Eastern Mediterranean Region."

Notes: Y = last two digits of reference year for the data; n.a. = not available; aAge 10 and over; bEstimate.

to scientific databases; and (3) a communications revolution that is redefining the geographical and social boundaries for exchange of health information and health services.

The state of human development in the region is improving, but overall progress is marred by great and increasing inequalities between people and countries and is threatened by potential setbacks. Health care systems in the twenty-first century will cover a very wide technical spectrum. The most technologically advanced health systems will be based on up-to-date developments in science and technology; by contrast, other health systems will still be struggling to satisfy basic needs and will still be based primarily on traditional medicine and basic health services.

Therefore, in response to the present status and projected future of the health sector, national health policies need to be based on clear, deeply rooted values and aimed at clearly defined targets that address priority health concerns. The values and traditions of the Eastern Mediterranean Region can provide a solid basis for health-for-all policy formulation. The main values that will contribute to the successful achievement of health-for-all goals in the twenty-first century are the following:

- Recognition that the enjoyment of the highest attainable standard of health is a fundamental human right

- Implementation of equity-oriented policies and strategies that emphasize solidarity and cooperation

- Continued and strengthened application of ethics to health policy, research, and service provision

- Incorporation of a gender perspective into health policies and strategies

STRATEGIC ORIENTATION FOR THE TWENTY-FIRST CENTURY

The following are the principal strategic orientations that can promote public health interest in the region in the twenty-first century.

Health and Development

It is essential to emphasize the centrality of health in socioeconomic development. This has several components:

- Each society should identify and define its own profile of vulnerability using health status as a key indicator.

- Development strategies should act on the integral links between health status and economic well-being and productivity, especially in the case of highly vulnerable groups.

- Health-related knowledge should become accessible to people in a form that increases their self-reliance and their capacity to manage and cope with a rapidly changing health environment.

- Health-promoting activities should be linked to investments, to income-generating activities, and to economic enterprises.

Basic Development Needs: A Community-Based Approach to Development

In this time of great challenges, community action is probably the most outstanding and influential action in developing health systems and achieving health for all. The Eastern Mediterranean Region has enhanced community action through a variety of approaches, including the basic development needs approach. BDN is a process that aims at achieving a better quality of life. It is integrated socioeconomic development based on full community involvement. It promotes self-reliance through self-management and self-financing by the people. It is a people-oriented strategy that offers vital support to intersectoral collaboration.

In addressing socioeconomic development, the most important challenge for governments is to promote and improve health on the basis of equity and need. BDN provides the mechanism for meeting the obligation. It is firmly focused on people and what they feel they need rather than what they are told they need. The approach reverses the traditional roles: people become the doers, and government workers become the facilitators and supporters. The BDN concept promotes the understanding that if people are given the right collaboration and partnership, they can successfully undertake and manage a considerable proportion of their needs-based microdevelopment initiatives.

The Development of Sustainable Health Systems

The challenge of the health system in the twenty-first century is to provide sustainable health care and maintain health gains, in particular the improvement of the health status of the poor and vulnerable. Health systems have to be built that are financially, technically, and managerially sustainable. It is the responsibility of the state to guarantee equity of access to health services and to ensure that essential functions are performed at the highest level of quality for all people. In view of the changing roles of the institutions, there is a need to give greater emphasis to ensuring that essential functions are maintained and that individual health care services are made available.

Human Resources for Health

To meet the challenges of health for all in the twenty-first century, a well-educated and well-trained health workforce that is oriented to meet the needs of the communities has to be developed. A trained and motivated workforce is essential for health systems to function properly. Support by the state, WHO, and various partners in training institutions should reflect the need for ongoing and comprehensive capacity building for health.

Education of health professionals should be community-based and community-oriented and should strengthen the partnership between health care delivery and training institutions. Human resource planning should recognize the need to consider changing mixes of health care providers working in a multidisciplinary and collaborative fashion. The mix would extend to public health providers, technicians, therapists, doctors, and nurses, among others.

Response to Emergencies and Health as a Bridge for Peace

Large-scale disasters, of both natural and human origin, present serious threats in many parts of the world in general and in the Eastern Mediterranean Region in particular. Health concerns can transcend political divisions, promote dialogue, foster solidarity, and contribute to peace among people and between nations. Health can be deliberately employed in a variety of situations to prevent disputes from arising or escalating and to foster peace building and rehabilitation. Health can play a vital role during all stages of a conflict—peace, tension, hostilities, war, and aftermath. During peacetime, health interventions such as the promotion of health for all or socioeconomic development can decrease tensions and the chance of conflict, while during war, health-related activities can promote confidence-building measures, provide humanitarian assistance, and intervene as a mediator for cessation of hostilities and attainment of peace.

Promotion of Healthy Lifestyles

All human beings are in possession of a certain health potential, which they must develop if they are to enjoy complete well-being and ward off disease. The lifestyles human beings adopt have a major impact on their health and well-being. Lifestyles to be encouraged embrace numerous positive patterns promoting health and reject any behavior that is deleterious to health. Governments and voluntary and nongovernmental organizations should promote health by encouraging positive lifestyles, particularly through the following means:

- Introducing health-promoting lifestyles and advocating them through proper channels
- Providing conditions that are conducive to the promotion of health and healthy lifestyles
- Reorienting educational institutions in the health field in such a way as to give a human dimension to the health professions

Eradication, Elimination, and Control of Specific Diseases

Disease prevention across the life span is crucial to human development. Community-based population-oriented disease prevention and control and health protection services benefit everyone, and their implementation requires little individual participation. Priority should be given to endemic and commonly occurring infections, noncommunicable diseases, injuries, and violence. Maintenance and extension of the ability to promote such services should be decentralized as much as possible, recognizing that successful decentralization requires competent local authorities.

Conclusion

Global changes in many areas, such as economics, demographics, epidemiology, science and technology, and communications technology, will have a tremendous impact on the health care delivery system in the coming century. These developments should ultimately result in significant improvements to the quality of health care systems, including health promotion, health protection, and disease prevention and control. However, coupled as they are with the trend toward privatization and market economics, they will also be accompanied by a tremendous increase in the cost of health care services. It can therefore be expected that countries will experience increasing inequity in access to up-to-date health care technology and that the gap between health care systems both within and between countries will also increase. Such increases in inequity will have serious consequences for global health and stability. It is therefore important to develop national, regional, and global health policies that are based on solidarity and cooperation, adherence to ethical standards, and incorporation of a gender perspective. All these values are deeply rooted in the culture and traditions of the Eastern Mediterranean Region. However, policy objectives have to be translated into operational strategies and programs. The experience gained so far in the region with the BDN programs, using health as a bridge for peace, and promotion of healthy lifestyles is very positive. We should continue to pursue these and similar approaches to promote health for all in the new century.

CHAPTER FIVE

Europe

Jo E. Asvall and Richard Alderslade

Jo E. Asvall, MD, *a Norwegian, has had a long career in national and international health in numerous industrialized and developing countries. His experience includes clinical work and health care administration both in primary health care and in highly specialized medical fields. He served as the World Health Organization's Regional Director for Europe from 1985 to 2000.*

Richard Alderslade *is Regional Advisor for Partnerships in Health and Humanitarian Assistance at the European Regional Office of the World Health Organization in Copenhagen. He is responsible for external relations and coordination, resource mobilization, and the management of health-related humanitarian relief programs in Europe.*

What do we mean by "Europe"? Is it the territory of the European Union, with its fifteen countries? Or the Council of Europe, with its forty-one countries? Or the European Region of the World Health Organization (WHO), with its 870 million people living in fifty-one countries stretching from Greenland to the Pacific Coast of the Russian Federation? Where exactly does Europe lie?

The answer to this question remains of the profoundest importance, for Europe is more than a simple piece of territory. It is a metaphor for a set of liberal political, social, economic, and institutional ideals based around human rights, individual freedom, political pluralism, representational democracy and democratic accountability, the rule of law, and the regulated operation of free capital and commodity markets.

This chapter will deal with the situation of the fifty-one countries of WHO's European Region. The above-mentioned principles embodied in the term *Europe* have been firmly embedded into a broad yet specific and detailed policy framework, shared by all fifty-one countries. This is the European health for all policy, which together with its targets is systematically updated every six to seven years. The latest update, HEALTH21, the health policy framework for the European Region, was published in 1998.

THE HEALTH OF EUROPEAN POPULATIONS AT THE END OF THE TWENTIETH CENTURY

In the 1950s and 1960s, health status did not vary much among European countries. However, since the 1970s, the health of people in western Europe has improved steadily, while for people in central and eastern Europe it has stagnated and for those in the former Soviet Union countries it has deteriorated sharply (see Figure 5.1).

For the population of the Soviet Union, the health standard declined from 1970 until 1985, when it suddenly saw a sharp improvement following an intensive anti-alcohol campaign. However, with the collapse of the USSR in 1990, a new and sudden fall in health status ensued, a result of the political, economic, and administrative chaos that followed this dramatic change. As a consequence, the Russian Federation, for example, during the first part of the 1990s, lost forty years of improvement in health development, and WHO's European Region as a whole consequently suffered a setback of some ten years' progress.

In the newly independent states of the former Soviet Union, the rapid rise in poverty, unemployment, criminality, and social alienation, together with sharp reductions in health care budgets, brought in their wake a new diphtheria epidemic, a sudden rise in tuberculosis prevalence, a sharp rise in sexually transmitted diseases (see Figure 5.2) and HIV infection, and rises in infant and maternal mortality, accidents, suicides, homicides, drug abuse, and smoking. Even cholera epidemics reappeared and malaria returned to the southeast parts of the region, where they had been eradicated.

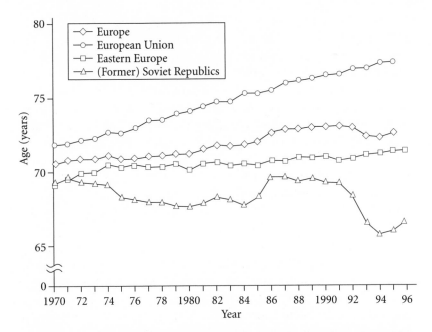

Figure 5.1.   Life Expectancy at Birth in the European Region, 1970–1996.
Source: HFA database, World Health Organization, Regional Office for Europe.

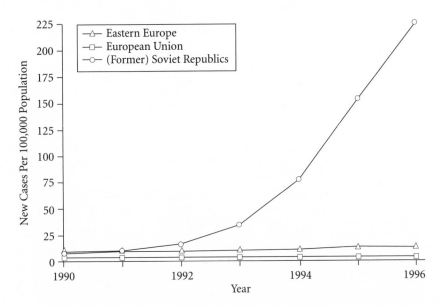

Figure 5.2.   Incidence of Syphilis in the European Region, 1990–1996.
Source: HFA database, World Health Organization, Regional Office for Europe.

These dramatic changes at the beginning of the 1990s were also associated with ethnic and other conflicts, bringing a total of ten member states of the European Region into armed conflicts. Unfortunately, potential areas of conflict remain, especially in the southeastern part of the region. Elements of socioeconomic underdevelopment, potential conflict over newfound oil resources, fundamentalist religious fervor, and the tensions associated with the transition to new democratic pluralistic societies all create a particularly difficult challenge.

Even in the western half of the region, where there has been a steady health improvement and the strengthening European Union provides increasing political stability, ensuring continuous progress with regard to health and quality of life will not be an easy task. Increasing urbanization; strong migration pressures; a global market economy with pressure for privatization (seen also in the health sector); and a rapid growth of the elderly population are all factors leading to growing inequities in health and social rights in many countries. At the same time, previously well-functioning health care systems are affected by relentless pressure for cost-cutting, as well as rising expectations from an increasingly well-informed public and the media.

How can we find a way out of these dilemmas?

EQUITY IN HEALTH THROUGH SOLIDARITY IN ACTION

No endeavor in modern society is as complex as health development. In few areas are so many experiments being undertaken, and in fewer still is it so difficult for individual countries and institutions to grasp the complexity of the issues and identify the most suitable solutions to the problems. Therefore, for Europe in the twenty-first century, it is essential that the fifty-one member states of WHO's European Region not only have, *but also use,* the concrete policy guidance that they themselves have created.

Making health for all a dynamic, living, continuously developing concept is also necessary in order to turn ideas into clearly value-based, active programs that can deal effectively with the root causes of health development problems. In no area is this more important than when we talk about equity and health. No conceivable scientific breakthrough, no new technology, can bring such a meaningful, large improvement in the health status of Europeans as would a reduction in current inequities in health, both between and within countries.

Policies need to be adopted that consistently increase the income, educational background, living conditions, and social environment of the most significantly disadvantaged groups *more* than for the rest of society. Important in this context is that financial deprivation leads to prejudice and social exclusion, with increased rates of violence and crime. Thus HEALTH21 advocates a rethinking of the fundamental social values and development policies in this particular field.

HEALTHY LIFESTYLES IN A HEALTH-PROMOTING ENVIRONMENT

The major threats to people's health in the region come from the lifestyles they follow and from the environment that surrounds them. The challenge for the twenty-first century is therefore to find a way to create a societywide movement for health that can deal with such issues in a much more systematic, synergistic, integrated way.

HEALTH21 outlines in very concrete terms how this can be done. First, it stresses our need to make the healthy choice the easy choice by strengthening two elements: the individual and society. Regarding the individual, the aim is to strengthen the ability to make more mature and healthy choices. In so doing, it points to the need for undertaking a much more systematic analysis of the values, knowledge, and skills that individuals need to acquire as they go through their life course, from infancy through childhood, adolescence, maturity, and on to old age. Second, while the ability of individuals to engage in mature decision making is extremely important, even more important is the question of whether the physical, economic, social, and cultural characteristics of the environment that surrounds individuals, groups, and societies make the healthy choice the easy choice. For example, the easy availability of safe bicycle lanes may make people choose that mode of transport instead of a private car, thus improving physical health as well as reducing air pollution in cities. A smoke-free working environment will help nonsmokers remain nonsmokers and help smokers drastically cut their daily consumption. The availability of condoms in kiosks, bars, hotels, and other appropriate areas will increase the likelihood of the practice of safe sex, and expensive alcohol will reduce its consumption by the young and excessive consumption by adults.

The third principle of health for all is that the emphasis should not only be, for example, on reducing pollution of air, water, food, and soil but also on integrating the wider aspects of human settlements, urban planning, and regionwide environmental protection. This must be done so that both the environment and lifestyle and health concerns can be integrated into holistic packages.

So as to bring all these elements together in a practical and coordinated way, HEALTH21 strongly encourages European countries to adopt a "settings" approach to organize their health-promoting actions for the new century, focusing on the family in the home, schools and universities, workplaces, prisons, and old-age homes, as well as in local and regional communities, cities, and nations.

Thus a multisectoral strategy for health is an indispensable approach, as it is obvious that the physical, economic, social, cultural, and other factors that need to be regulated to provide for healthy choices and healthy environments can be ensured only if all major sectors of society in these various settings incorporate health protection as a key component in each individual sector.

One of the many important sectors is the media, for television, radio, and newspapers have a tremendous influence on individuals, groups, and societies. Major efforts should therefore be made to reach out to journalists and others who control today's media to make them conscious of their important role as key partners in health development.

IMPROVING THE QUALITY AND EFFECTIVENESS OF HEALTH CARE

During the past ten to fifteen years, extensive developments in health care reform have taken place in the European Region and beyond. In 1996, WHO organized the biggest conference ever held on this theme in Ljubljana, Slovenia, as a result of which several principles emerged. First, it was agreed that health care reform could not take place in a vacuum; it had to be based on the Health for All values, as this was the best way to guide alternative decisions in a very complex field. Second, primary health care was felt to be the most important part of the health care system and the highest priority for further development in the European Region. Third, there had to be a much clearer focus on the outcomes of the activities of the health care system. Fourth, the market principle could not be applied without clear controls, as the health care system could not follow the same rules as many other parts of social developments.

In primary health care, HEALTH21 promotes the role of the family health nurse and family health physician as key elements for future health development in Europe. The work of these care providers should be based on clearly defined family health epidemiology and information systems. Furthermore, this family health team must work intimately with the community mobilization mechanism that completes the primary health care concept.

Local primary health care must incorporate a series of programs that address the main problems and client groups at the local level: water, sanitation and food, immunization, mental health, the elderly, child and adolescent health, and so on. In the twenty-first century, programs dealing with socioeconomic-related problems (depression, drug abuse, alcoholism, violence), as well as the elderly, will have to be given much higher prominence than in the past.

In the hospital sector, it is clear that the rapid development of medical science and communication technology will have major implications for the services that hospitals can offer; their organization, staffing, and costs; and many other matters. These issues will pose major management challenges.

Here a key issue relates to improving the quality of clinical care. One of the main problems in the current situation is that no country has a nationwide system whereby the outcomes of daily clinical practice are systematically recorded and fed back to the individual clinical providers. Extensive work over the past fifteen years has clearly indicated that developing a minimum data set of quality indicators for different health conditions and providing information systems and data registers that make possible their feedback are important elements in improving the quality of patient care. The further development and routine use of such approaches throughout all health services in the European member states must be one of the top priorities for development as we enter the twenty-first century.

The same concept should be applied with regard to management of public health programs at population-based levels. Research and development efforts need to be undertaken to identify suitable indicators and information systems that can compare the relative effectiveness and efficiency of health promotion, disease prevention, curative, and rehabilitative and care policies and interventions in dealing with given health problems so that overall health program development can be managed in a more purposeful, focused way and so that resources can be distributed accordingly.

MANAGING OVERALL HEALTH DEVELOPMENT

In the pluralistic, democratic societies of Europe in the twenty-first century, the detailed long-term, all-encompassing health planning systems of the past will no longer suffice and are no longer politically acceptable. The European Health for All policy offers a way forward here. There is a need for the formulation of national policy frameworks of the health-for-all type. Such policies should identify major health and health development problems, identify "aspirational targets" in the medium term (ten to twenty years), incorporate multisectoral action and health services in integrative strategies to reach the targets set, institute a systematic monitoring of progress through clearly identified indicators, and outline an evaluation system.

Inspired by these national policies, similar ones should be developed in other settings (at the level of the city, the local school, the work site, and so on) where the choice of targets and target levels, strategies, and participating organizations would reflect the local situation. In this way, the partners responsible for implementation at national, intermediate, and local levels would themselves have been part of developing, implementing, monitoring, and evaluating the policies—a simple principle to follow if one wants to stimulate people for active follow-up.

Such developments must, however, be supported by the requisite professional expertise. Therefore, an important element for the twenty-first century is to stimulate the creation of more effective infrastructures and better training for public health management. The health-for-all policy identifies four main categories in this context: (1) broadly trained public health experts, (2) technical experts (such as epidemiologists and sanitary engineers), (3) hospital and health center managers, and (4) schoolteachers, social workers, architects, engineers, economists, and other professionals.

THE EUROPEAN PARTNERSHIPS FOR THE TWENTY-FIRST CENTURY

The fifty-one member states of the European Region have asked the WHO Regional Office for Europe to act as the region's "health conscience," to be a center for information on health, to advocate health-for-all policies, to provide evidence-based tools and guidance to turn those policies into action, and to work as a catalyst for action throughout the region.

The European Union will develop its health competence further during the twenty-first century. This will make a much more concerted action possible to deal with lifestyles and environmental health issues—a tremendously important element for the fifteen current member states and the ten others who are expected to join in the near future.

The Council of Europe, the World Bank, other UN organizations, and the many nongovernmental organizations in the European Region complete the wide array of institutions and organizations that together represent a formidable potential for health development.

Although HEALTH21 provides a framework of the best strategies that have emerged from Europe's collective experience during the past ten to fifteen years, Europe needs stronger partnerships among its many institutions and organizations that have an interest in and commitment to health. The experience, the know-how, and many of the tools for influencing the determinants of health are all there. What is needed now is strong leadership and the political will to pick the tools up and use them.

Additional Reading

Asvall, J. E. "WHO's Vision of Health for All: 2000 and Then?" *Eurohealth*, 1998, 4, 5.

Commission of the European Communities, Brussels. (15 April 1998). *Communication from the Commission to the Council, the European Parliament, the Economic and Social Committee and the Committee of the Regions on the development of public health policy in the European Community.* (COM(1998)230final). Brussels.

HEALTH21. *The Health for All Policy Framework for the WHO European Region.* European Health for All Series, No. 6. Copenhagen: WHO Regional Office for Europe, 1998.

Precker, A. S., and Feachem, R.G.A. *Market Mechanisms and the Health Sector in Central and Eastern Europe.* World Bank Technical Paper number 293, 20–21, 1995.

Staehr, J. K. *The Evolution from Health Technology Assessment to Quality of Care Development. Government and Health Systems Implications of Differing Involvements.* West Sussex: John Wiley and Sons, Ltd., 1998.

Walberg, P., and others. "Economic Change, Crime, and Mortality Crisis in Russia: Regional Analysis." *British Medical Journal,* 1998, *317,* 312–318.

World Health Organization. *The Charter Against Tobacco. It Can be Done: A Smoke-Free Europe: Report of the First European Conference on Tobacco Policy.* WHO Regional Publications: European Series: No. 30, Copenhagen: WHO Regional Office for Europe, 1988.

World Health Organization. *European Charter on Alcohol.* Copenhagen: WHO Regional Office for Europe, 1995.

World Health Organization. Healthy Cities Office. *Twenty Steps for Developing a Healthy Cities Project* (2nd ed.). Copenhagen: WHO Regional Office for Europe, 1995.

World Health Organization. *Protocol and Guidelines. Countrywide Integrated Non-Communicable Diseases Intervention (CINDI) Program.* Copenhagen: WHO Regional Office for Europe, 1996.

World Health Organization. *European Network of Health Promoting Schools (ENHPS).* Technical Secretariat. Copenhagen: WHO Regional Office for Europe, 1997.

World Health Organization. *Proceedings of the WHO Conference on European Health Care Reforms, Ljubljana, June 1996.* Copenhagen: WHO Regional Office for Europe, 1997.

The World Health Organization. *Health for All in the Twenty-First Century.* Geneva: World Health Organization, 1998.

World Health Organization. *Health in Europe.* Copenhagen: WHO Regional Office for Europe, 1998.

The World Health Organization. *Social Determinants of Health: The Solid Facts.* Copenhagen: WHO Regional Office for Europe, 1998.

World Health Organization. *Framework for Professional and Administrative Development of General Practice/Family Medicine in Europe.* Copenhagen: WHO Regional Office for Europe, 1998.

CHAPTER SIX

Western Pacific

Shigeru Omi

Shigeru Omi, MD, PhD, *became Regional Director of the Western Pacific Region of the World Health Organization on February 1, 1999. Born in Tokyo in 1949, he earned his medical degree in 1978 and his doctorate in molecular biology of the hepatitis B virus in 1989. Before taking up his appointment with WHO, Dr. Omi was a professor of public health at Jichi Medical School in Japan and a technical adviser at the Ministry of Health in Tokyo.*

The past half century has witnessed a continuous and steady improvement in the overall health status of practically all populations in the Western Pacific Region.[1] Although it is impossible to predict with any certainty that this will continue throughout the next century, some projections can be made, particularly for the first twenty years of the century. This article outlines some scenarios for a diverse region that contains both the most populous nation in the world and some of the smallest.

EPIDEMIOLOGY

The Western Pacific Region will continue to progress through the epidemiological transition. The region has always been very diverse; even today it contains countries such as Cambodia and some Pacific island nations that have disease profiles dominated by communicable diseases and nutritional, perinatal, and maternal conditions. Over the course of the early part of the twenty-first century, this diversity will decrease as more countries proceed through the "epidemiological transition" to join the ranks of Australia, Japan, New Zealand, and Singapore. By 2020, noncommunicable diseases and injuries will dominate the disease profile in almost all countries of the region (see Figure 6.1).

Considerable progress has been made in countering some of the diseases that have plagued the populations of the region for centuries. The region has been free of poliomyelitis since March 1997. Leprosy cases have decreased by 90 percent in ten years, while in the same period the number of malaria cases has decreased by more than 60 percent. However, even for these diseases, progress has been uneven (for example, malaria remains a significant public health problem in nine countries of the region), while for other communicable diseases, such as tuberculosis and some sexually transmitted infections, progress in some countries has been slight.

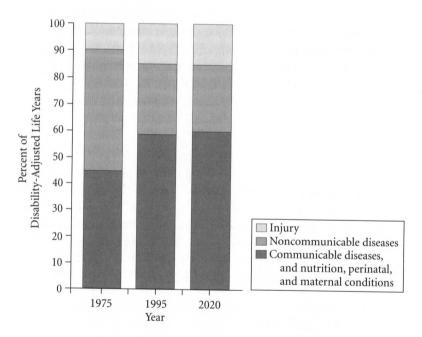

Figure 6.1.   Disease Profile in the Western Pacific Region, 1975–2020.
Source: Disease Burdens in the Countries of the Western Pacific Region. WHO, Manila, 1998 (p. 467).

As demonstrated by the emergence of AIDS in the last quarter of the twentieth century, it is probable that even as some diseases such as leprosy and poliomyelitis are eliminated or eradicated, new threats will arise during the twenty-first century. For example, recent years have witnessed the first human cases of the H5N1 influenza virus, or avian flu, in Hong Kong and a new encephalitis virus in Malaysia. In our increasingly interconnected and fast-moving world, accurate surveillance and rapid responses to outbreaks will be essential.

The emergence of new threats, coupled with the reemergence of diseases such as tuberculosis, means that for the early decades of the twenty-first century, developing countries in the region will still need to devote considerable resources to communicable disease prevention and control.

With regard to noncommunicable diseases, it seems probable that morbidity and mortality from cancer, cardiovascular diseases, and diabetes will continue to rise. Noncommunicable diseases already impose an enormous burden: approximately 3.5 million cancer cases occur in the region every year, and there are 1.3 million deaths from cancer in China alone. Projected increases in smoking in the region (the Western Pacific is the only WHO region where smoking rates are increasing) are a considerable concern, especially as a significant proportion of the increase in cancer mortality is due to a rise in the prevalence of lung cancer. Cardiovascular diseases also exact a heavy and rising toll on the population of the region; no fewer than 3 million deaths a year are due to these diseases.

Injuries will increase in number, particularly injuries associated with road traffic.

DEMOGRAPHY

The population of the region will continue to increase in the first two decades of the century by approximately 1 percent a year. (When examining demographic and other trends in the Western Pacific Region, it is important to recognize that China makes up 76 percent of the total population of the region.)

In some countries, overpopulation constitutes one of the major threats to public health. If current population growth rates continue, the population of fourteen countries in the region will double in less than thirty years (see Table 6.1). Such growth rates will put an enormous strain on both the environments and the economies of many

Country or Area	Years
Mariana Islands	17
Solomon Islands	21
Brunei Darussalam	23
American Samoa	23
Marshall Islands	23
Lao People's Democratic Republic	24
Federated States of Micronesia	24
Cambodia	25
Nauru	26
Vanuatu	28
Hong Kong	29
Palau	29
Philippines	29
Malaysia	30
Papua New Guinea	31
Viet Nam	32
French Polynesia	34
Guam	34
Mongolia	35
Singapore	36
Kiribati	36
Fiji	46
New Caledonia	46
Tuvalu	46
Samoa	49

Table 6.1.   Population Doubling Time in the Western Pacific Region at Current Rates.

Source: The Work of WHO in the Western, Report of the Regional Director, 1 July 1998–30 June 1999. Manila (p. 151).

developing countries. If governments of the region are to guide rather than simply react to population growth rates, they will have to formulate and implement policies to meet their own particular circumstances. No one policy can be applied throughout the region.

For example, facing a rapidly growing population and finite land and other resources, the government of China has since the late 1970s pursued policies intended to lower the country's fertility rate. The effect that this will have on the population of China in the new century can be seen in Table 6.2.

In Singapore, by contrast, population policy is to an extent governed by the dramatic projected increase in the number of older persons. By 2025, the population aged sixty-five years and over will grow from 7 percent to 19.8 percent. The prospect of such an increase in dependency rates has led the government to take measures to reverse the falling

Year	Population	Year	Population	Period	Growth Rate
1950	562,580	1996	1,214,988	1950–1960	1.5
1960	650,661	1997	1,226,275	1960–1970	2.3
1970	820,403	1998	1,236,915	1970–1980	1.8
1980	984,736	1999	1,246,872	1980–1990	1.5
1990	1,138,895	2000	1,256,168	1990–2000	1.0
1991	1,153,472	2010	1,334,486	2000–2010	0.6
1992	1,166,661	2020	1,397,434	2010–2020	0.5
1993	1,179,149	2030	1,406,655	2020–2030	0.1
1994	1,191,486	2040	1,384,560	2030–2040	−0.2
1995	1,203,383	2050	1,322,435	2040–2050	−0.5

Table 6.2.   Midyear Population Estimates and Average Annual Period Growth Rates in China: 1950–2050.

Source: U.S. Census Bureau (http://www.census.gov/cgi-bin/ipc/idbsum).

birthrate to ensure that the population structure does not become too top heavy. The age distribution of the region is described in Table 6.3.

Although it is an extreme case, Singapore is not alone in facing the problem of a growing number of older persons supported by a dwindling number of people in the economically productive years. The population of the region is aging. Of all the trends described in this chapter, this may exert the greatest influence on health services in the region. We know from the experience of Western countries that older persons have special needs and that curative care for older persons is expensive. Much more needs to be done in developing sound evidence-based strategies for health for older persons as well as ensuring that these are accessible and affordable.

One of the major social developments of the twentieth century that will play an even greater role in the next hundred years is migration,

Age Group	1995	2020
0–14	26.9	20.6
15–64	66.6	69.7
65+	6.5	9.7
Total	100.0	100.0

Table 6.3.   Age Distribution of Population in the Western Pacific Region.

Source: United Nations Population Division World Population Prospects. 1996 Revision. (United Nations, New York).

both internal and external. In many newly developing countries, huge disparities already exist between the income levels in rural areas and in the major cities. Urbanization is projected to increase steadily throughout the early years of the new century (see Figure 6.2).

How governments manage the migration of large numbers of people in search of better living conditions will have a critical effect on public health. If their response is inadequate or housing, employment, and transport policies are inappropriate, we can expect rising levels of communicable diseases, diseases associated with pollution (such as acute respiratory infections), food- and water-borne diseases, injuries, and mental illness. However, the consequences of urbanization are by no means wholly negative; the economic growth of the region in the last half century has been largely an urban phenomenon. If adequate and appropriate policies are put in place to mitigate the negative effects of urbanization, it is possible that the spectacular public health gains of the twentieth century will continue in the twenty-first. WHO has promoted the Healthy City initiative as a way of ensuring that urban development benefits from an integrated approach from all sectors.

Many of the same issues apply with regard to international migration. The Western Pacific Region contains many small Pacific island states that are very vulnerable to out-migration, particularly of people of working age. In Tokelau, for example, population growth is negative, despite a fertility rate of 4.8. In-migration has its own set of

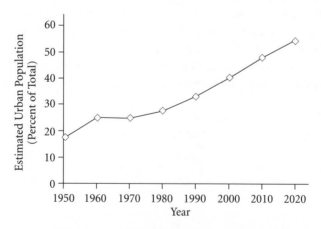

Figure 6.2.   Increase in Urban Population in the Western Pacific Region, 1950–2020.

Source: Disease Burdens in the Countries of the Western Pacific Region. WHO, Manila, 1998 (p. 467).

problems, as immigrants may bring with them diseases that were either unknown or controlled or eliminated in the receiving country.

We should not, however, assume that all the demographic trends that have characterized the past two centuries will necessarily continue throughout the whole of the next. Although the move to the city will continue in the short and medium term, it is quite possible that technological and social developments may eventually lead to a flight back to the countryside, or at least to the suburbs, as has already happened in North America. Delivery of health services to these new migrants to the countryside, carrying with them expectations of urban levels of health services, will be a particular challenge, both for policymakers and for the scientific community.

ENVIRONMENT

The environmental impact on health is particularly difficult to predict, being determined in part by unknown factors, such as the effect of global warming, and in part by governmental policies that are equally difficult to anticipate. Advocating health-promoting environments will be an increasingly important mission for international and national public health organizations in the twenty-first century.

Though the threats to health from environmental degradation should not be underestimated, there are encouraging signs that an important attitude shift has taken place in the past decade. Most governments in the Western Pacific Region now acknowledge that unrestrained economic growth often carries with it unacceptable environmental costs. More important, many are working with WHO to implement policies to improve the environment, ranging from small-scale healthy workplace activities to much more ambitious citywide or even national projects.

The environmental movement has been one of the most influential additions to the global political culture of the late twentieth century. How the movement develops in the new century and is incorporated into mainstream political ideologies and practices will define the extent to which the environment promotes health rather than threatens it.

TECHNOLOGY

It is almost impossible to predict the technological advances that will affect health care in the next hundred years. However, it should be noted that the management of technology will be as important as discoveries in the laboratory, particularly in view of the anticipated demographic changes in the region. For example, some estimates from developed countries suggest that 50 percent of technology expenditure in the health sector is for the over-sixty-five age group. Reducing the morbidity of this age group by promoting healthy lifestyles among younger age groups will be a major goal of public health bodies, including WHO, in the twenty-first century.

Progress in cloning and genome studies will greatly affect the existing pattern of health service provision. Developing health care systems that incorporate these new technologies will be another challenge.

New vaccines will completely change our ability to respond to outbreaks of communicable diseases. So too will improvements to surveillance capacity.

The unique geography of the Western Pacific, with its large number of remote island states, means that developments in telehealth could have very significant impacts on health. Small island countries often cannot justify spending large sums of money on medical technology that will benefit only a small percentage of their small populations. At some stage in the twenty-first century, and the indications are that it will be nearer the beginning than the end, selected health services will be delivered electronically to some of the more remote islands of the region, opening up a whole range of health options that are currently not available. These services will range from health education and promotion to disease management.

PERSONAL RESPONSIBILITY

One concept that unites all of our concerns—epidemiological, demographic, environmental, and technological—is the notion of individual responsibility for health. Particularly in countries that have passed through the epidemiological transition, there is a limit to the extent to which the provision of curative care, however sophisticated, can affect morbidity and mortality. It seems inevitable that health care in the twenty-first century will move from the avoidance of illness to the promotion of wellness.

CONCLUSION

It must be stressed that the tentative scenarios outlined here may reveal more about the status of our knowledge and attitudes at the end of one very eventful century than about health futures in the next. The unanticipated played an enormous role in determining public health in the Western Pacific Region in the twentieth century and will continue to do so. We cannot predict the role that wars, economic crises, revolutions, and disasters of natural and human origin will play, nor can we foresee the medical and scientific advances, economic improvements, and social changes that will ultimately improve the health of the people of the region beyond all recognition.

Nevertheless, public policy can influence many of the determinants of health. As the leading global agency for health, WHO will continue to work with countries in the region to ensure that the spectacular improvements of the second half of the twentieth century are continued into the twenty-first.

Note

1. The Western Pacific is one of six regions of the World Health Organization. It is composed of the following countries and areas: American Samoa, Australia, Brunei Darussalam, Cambodia, China, the Cook Islands, Fiji, French Polynesia, Guam, Hong Kong (China), Kiribati, the Republic of Korea, the Lao People's Democratic Republic, Macao (China), Malaysia, the Northern Mariana Islands, the Marshall Islands, the Federated States of Micronesia, Mongolia, Nauru, New Caledonia, New Zealand, Niue, Palau, Papua New Guinea, the Philippines, the Pitcairn Islands, Samoa, Singapore, the Solomon Islands, Tokelau, Tonga, Tuvalu, Vanuatu, Viet Nam, and Wallis and Futuna.

CHAPTER SEVEN

People's Republic of China

Zhang Wenkang and M. Roy Schwarz

Zhang Wenkang, MD, graduated from Shanghai Medical University and became a professor and Vice President of the Shanghai Second Military Medical University. In 1998, he was appointed Minister of Health of the People's Republic of China, after serving as Vice-Minister for five years.

M. Roy Schwarz, MD, is President of the China Medical Board of New York, Inc. The CMB supports faculty training, research, and medical, nursing, and public health education programs in China and Asia as well as infrastructure development in health institutions in the region. It founded the first Western science-based medical school in China in 1913 when the CMB was still part of the Rockefeller Foundation.

The authors would like to thank Dr. Ba Denian, President of the Chinese Academy of Medical Sciences and Peking Union Medical College, and Dr. Liu Xiaocheng, Vice President of these institutions, for sharing their opinions about this chapter. We also thank Dr. Wang Rukuan, who provided information and data.

The Chinese Communist Party and the central government have always attached great importance to the health of the people. From the extremely difficult state of "poverty and blankness" at the beginning of the People's Republic, China has endeavored to change the health status of the people of China by gradually establishing the efficient health service structures and health secure systems that conform to various economic development levels and needs of the people. Dramatic developments have taken place in China's health services, especially since China's reform and opening to the outside world. Using the limited funds available and taking measures suited to China's local conditions, the government has made impressive strides in improving the health of the Chinese people.

China has built up medical and health preventive care systems for both urban and rural areas of the country. This includes over three hundred thousand medical and health institutions, six million medical staff, around eight hundred scientific research institutions, and four major medical scientific academies covering Western science-based medicine, traditional Chinese medicine, preventive medicine, and military medicine. The scientific enterprises employ more than one hundred thousand scientific and research staff members. As a result, significant achievements have been made in such areas as the trachomatous virus, synthetic proteins, RNA, tumors, plague, epidemiological pathogenesis of Keshan disease, chorioepithelioma, liver cancer, cancer of the esophagus, prevention and treatment of Keshan disease, burn treatment, replantation of severed limbs, and studies of harringtonine and arteannuin.

The output of medical products has also been greatly enhanced, and traditional Chinese medical undertakings have been carried forward. Health system reform has continued uninterrupted, and its impact is being widely felt. As a result of a national health campaign, diseases such as smallpox, plague, cholera, and schistosomiasis, which once seriously harmed the health of the people, have been largely brought under control or eliminated altogether. In addition, significant achievements have been made in the prevention and treatment of various chronic diseases.

As a result of these efforts, the health conditions of the Chinese people have been greatly improved. The average life expectancy has increased from thirty-five years before the founding of the People's Republic in 1949 to seventy years today. Infant mortality has declined from 31.4 per thousand live births to 20, and maternal mortality has been reduced from 1,500 per hundred thousand live births to 61.9.

THE CHALLENGES AHEAD

Although China has significantly improved the health care of 22 percent of the world's population with less than 1 percent of the world's health funds, the nation is still a developing country with a poor economic foundation and a large population to care for. As such, there is still a big gap between China and the developed countries in terms of the health care provided. Today, China faces the following major challenges:

- The development of the health system cannot keep up with the demands brought about by economic and social developments.

- There is a great disparity in the economic development of the eastern and the western regions of the country and between urban and rural areas. This is reflected in all parts of society in the affected regions.

- The health care available in rural areas is much poorer than in urban centers, and a comprehensive system providing equal services has not been realized.

- Insufficient investment in the health system is exacerbated by the system's illogical and complex structures.

- The distribution and utilization of health resources is not as efficient as it might be, in part reflecting the complex structure of the system.

- Total health costs are growing too rapidly for the economy to sustain.

- The needs of the population exceed the quality of care available.

- Major pressures are being imposed on the health care system by the growing population, a deteriorating environment, and the ever-increasing demand for medical care.

GUIDELINES FOR THE FUTURE

To maximize the likelihood of success of its efforts and to make optimum use of its resources, China has adopted a limited number of guidelines for activities in the immediate future. Among these are the following:

First, the goals of each human being should include being of good mental and physical health and living harmoniously with the environment. If this is achieved, each person will realize his or her desire for a peaceful existence, the opportunity to develop physically and mentally, and the time for personal enjoyment. The pursuit of these desires is a basic right of all humanity, not just the Chinese people.

Second, the main objective of China's modernization efforts is to achieve sustained economic and social growth and development. This can be done only if the Chinese people are in good health and if basic health care is available to all citizens. Science and education, economic development, politics, prevention, and health promotion are major keys to achieving good physical and mental health. Implemented properly, these five efforts can reduce health expenditures, improve the efficiency of the workforce, and protect the future workers of China. As such, any public welfare benefits should be designed to achieve "good health for all." If the nation is to be healthy, all sectors of Chinese society must assume their respective roles and fulfill their responsibilities.

Third, a long-term plan must be developed that takes full advantage of traditional Chinese medicine and focuses first on rural health care. The latter is essential because 80 percent of Chinese people live in rural areas, and these people represent the bedrock of China's strength.

THIRTY-YEAR HEALTH OBJECTIVES AND ACTIONS

Since the general goal of the government of China is to create a supportive environment in which all citizens enjoy health care such that they are physically and mentally healthy, it follows there must be specific health targets for increments of time in the new century. China has chosen to divide these into thirty-year periods.

For the first thirty years of the twenty-first century (2000–2030), China has established three general objectives, as follows:

- Focus on rural health problems and reduce or eliminate as rapidly as possible any differences with respect to "health care for all."

- Speed the transition from a cure-oriented system to a prevention- and care-oriented system.
- Control and, if possible, eliminate the major diseases affecting the Chinese people.

For the second thirty years of the twenty-first century (2031–2060), three additional aggressive objectives have been defined:

- Complete the transition from a cure-oriented system to a prevention- and care-oriented system with a greater emphasis on health promotion.
- Raise the quality of physical and mental health care for all people and improve the health conditions of the people.
- Control and eliminate, if possible, the emerging major diseases.

For the final thirty to forty years of the century, the objectives are to solidify the gains that have been made, respond to new challenges that have emerged, and continue to work toward the general goal of good mental and physical health for all Chinese citizens.

To achieve these aggressive objectives, various actions must be taken, including the following:

- Deepen and broaden health reform in order to strengthen health services and establish the necessary health legislation to achieve this reform while recognizing the extreme importance of pertinent moral principles.
- Increase government's investment in health services.
- Allocate resources in an optimal fashion, and use the resources wisely to reduce the imbalances that exist between regions and populations.
- Give highest priority to prevention and direct the appropriate human, material, and financial resources toward this activity.
- Adopt health-for-all standards as the reference for China's activities.
- Combine traditional Chinese medicine and Western science-based medicine.
- Place an emphasis on rural areas, especially in regions that have a shortage of physicians or medicine.

- Pay special attention to the frail, teenagers, the elderly, mothers, and children.
- Strengthen health education in order to acquaint all people with knowledge of environmental protection and health care.
- Mobilize all sectors of the population to achieve these goals.
- Speed the development of the health sciences and technology.
- Coordinate all efforts to reduce the health risk factors found in nature, the economy, and the social environment.
- Perfect, develop, and implement supervision of the environment; set up measures for monitoring the prevention and rescue responses to disasters; set up systems of environmental supervision and protection that will have a rapid response time and a significant impact.
- After appropriate study, establish methods and measures to eliminate factors that are harmful to psychological health in modern society; carry out extensive psychological counseling, and strive to improve psychological health.
- Strengthen international exchange and cooperation. This must include attempting to eliminate factors harmful to health, such as environmental pollutants and disease, circulation of all kinds of contraband goods, and detrimental trade. This must be approached on a global basis.

If the methods are implemented fully, the welfare and health of the Chinese people will be markedly enhanced. Health status is a fundamental concern for a developing country such as China.

CHAPTER EIGHT

India

V. Ramalingaswami

V. Ramalingaswami, MD, ScD, *is National Research Professor at the All India Institute of Medical Sciences, New Delhi. Formerly, he served as Professor of Pathology and Director of the All India Institute, Director-General of the Indian Council of Medical Research in New Delhi, and Chairman of the Global Advisory Committee of Medical Research for the World Health Organization in Geneva. He completed his undergraduate studies at Andhra University in India and his postgraduate studies at Oxford University.*

Areasonable forecast of the shape of things to come in the health field during the twenty-first century would include a number of themes, many of them identified by Hunter (1997). The broad thrust of the health movement in the new century would be from health care to health and from life expectancy to health expectancy. Some of the elements of this movement would be the following:

- Advances in medical technology with associated issues of rising costs of care, equity, and access
- The double burden of disease exemplified by the restless tide of newly emerging and reemerging infectious diseases and an upsurge of chronic noncommunicable diseases

- Ensuring the quality of services in the context of constrained resources
- Increased practice of evidence-based medicine and public health
- Balancing public and private inputs leading to a mixed economy of health care
- Integrated care pathways
- A changing role and shape for the hospital
- A shift to primary health care and supportive use of higher levels of care
- Involvement of the public as active coproducers of their health
- Increased awareness of the political, organizational, and managerial context of health care
- Fostering an attitude of humility, tolerance, open-mindedness, and shared responsibility in the health care system

THE CHANGING PARADIGM OF INDIA'S HEALTH

India's health history is a mixture of successes and failures. The successes have been largely in the area of communicable diseases, but even there, sustaining the momentum and overcoming the complacency that followed initial success can be considered among India's major failures. The conquest of diseases such as malaria, leishmaniasis, and most recently plague had lulled the country into a dangerous complacency.

Table 8.1 gives an idea of the brighter side of India's health history, depicting the behavior of three key health indices between 1947, when India became independent, and 1995. Substantial improvements in

Indicator	1947	1995
Crude death rate	27.4	9
Infant mortality rate (per 1,000 live births)	146.0	74
Life expectancy at birth (years)	32.7	62

Table 8.1. **Selected Health Indicators for India, 1947–1995.**
Source: Voluntary Health Association of India, 1997, pp. 3–5.

the three indices—crude death rate, infant mortality rate, and life expectancy at birth—are obvious. But they are in reality only improvements on the average. When the averages are disaggregated, regional diversity, disparities, and tragedy of India become obvious. For example, the infant mortality rate ranges from a low of 17 in the state of Kerala to a high of 115 in Orissa. The other health indices behave similarly.

Real progress should be measured in terms of reducing inequity, in addition to improving the averages. The less well-off segments of the population have to be targeted for provision of better services. Improvement of health on the average may have no impact on inequities in health and may even increase inequity (Acheson, 1999). We should also conduct a health inequities impact assessment. For example, the answer to the elimination of protein-calorie malnutrition lies in ensuring a targeted public food distribution system that reaches the poor. We need to ensure that people have the socioeconomic access to adequate food. This is a direction to pursue.

Infectious diseases continue to be the leading cause of mortality in India and will be so well into the twenty-first century. HIV/AIDS is darkening horizons in India, with four to five million persons already believed to be infected. Although there is no vaccine yet in sight against AIDS, and effective treatment with a cocktail of drugs is out of reach of the vast majority of Indians, much can be done to prevent transmission through the combined use of education, condoms, and effective treatment of sexually-transmitted diseases. The lesson of the AIDS experience is that there need no longer be a conflict between technological solutions and sociocultural, behavioral, and educational approaches to human health. Policy issues in health must encompass this broad spectrum with an emphasis on intersectoral approaches for health improvement (Ramalingaswami, 1997). Tuberculosis is now a leading infectious disease in India, threatening to get worse owing to the concurrent AIDS epidemic. The control program in India has now been modified to include improved program management, directly observed treatment, attention to behavioral components.

The golden age of malaria control in the subcontinent was in the early 1960s, when India was a showpiece of success in the eyes of the rest of the world. Since then, however, there has been a resurgence that continues to this day. Having peaked at the level of 6.47 million cases in 1976, the annual incidence now ranges between 2 and 3 million, along with rising incidence of *Plasmodium falciparum,* rising mortality, and biological resistance of the parasite. India has now embarked on a revised strategy for malaria control consisting of active surveillance, early detection, and prompt and effective treatment; prevention of mosquitogenic conditions relating to so-called developmental activities; reduction of human-mosquito contact through cost-effective, user-friendly protective methods; and sustained bioenvironmental control methods. Indian scientists are working on developing antimalarial drugs from traditional systems of medicine with a focus on development of resistance-reversal agents from plant sources (Kamboj and Dutta, 1998). A multistage multivalent vaccine against malaria is under development through collaborative efforts between Indian and American scientists (Shi and others, 1999). Another approach, using as vaccine candidates conserved sequences of the genome of malarial parasites that do not undergo changes when under immunological pressure, is under development in India (Chauhan, 1998).

THE UPSURGE OF NONCOMMUNICABLE DISEASES

The overall burden of noninfectious diseases in India, including cardiovascular diseases, cancer, diabetes, chronic respiratory disease, and hereditary disorders, is on the increase. India is thus confronting a double burden—high rates of infectious diseases with rising rates of chronic noncommunicable diseases. Indeed, many developing countries are experiencing a hidden epidemic of cardiovascular disease ("Hidden Epidemic," 1998). Cardiovascular risk factor reduction and low-cost management are feasible and expected to be used increasingly in India in the coming decades. The use of hepatitis B vaccination as a part of the Expanded Programme of Immunization to prevent liver cancer is on the agenda.

HEALTH AND ENVIRONMENT

India is facing an environmental crisis of vast proportions, and economic liberalization is a major factor, because a healthy economy can only exist in symbiosis with a healthy ecology. Experts agree that economic growth leads to health improvement. But unless it is reconciled with disparity reduction and environmentally sustainable development, it will have failed in its social mission.

Water and Sanitation

While the rivers of rich countries are steadily becoming cleaner, those of poor countries are continuing to be sources of pathogenic microbial and microchemical contamination ("Survey of Development," 1998). At present, approximately 85 percent of the rural and urban population in India has a safe water supply, but when it comes to sanitation, the gap is very large. At present, only 20 percent of the population has toilet facilities. In India, community toilet facilities are generally provided by the government. There are signs of increasing private initiative in this regard and now nongovernmental organizarions are providing community toilet facilities in towns and villages. Provision of clean water and sanitation does not assure disease control unless there are appropriate changes in human behavior leading to hygienic use of water.

Arsenic, Fluoride, and Lead

Apart from microbiological pollution of water supplies, microchemical intoxication is an area of great concern to India. A calamity of major proportions has exposed an estimated thirty-eight million people in West Bengal (and fifty million more in neighboring Bangladesh) to the health consequences of prolonged exposure to unsafe levels of arsenic contained in groundwater. The tragic tale of endemic fluorosis is being enacted in several geographical areas of India. Efforts need to be intensified to protect people's health from waterborne infections and excessive consumption of arsenic and fluoride (Ramalingaswami, 1997). Added to this burden are the results of recent surveys in six Indian cities in which more than 12 percent of the children tested had blood lead concentrations of 20 μg/dL or more. The use of lead-free gasoline is now mandatory in Delhi, and ambient air lead concentrations have fallen by 17 percent since the use of unleaded fuel was enforced (Sharma, 1999).

Air Pollution

The levels of fine particulate matter, less than 10 μm in the air samples of Delhi, are higher than the prescribed standards. Diesel vehicles emit in their exhaust fine particulate matter of less than 2.5 μm, believed to be damaging to lungs. The proposed increase in the dieselization of motorized transport in India is an ominous sign unless proactive measures are taken. The Supreme Court of India prescribed that Euro I emission norms be applicable to gasoline- and diesel-powered vehicles in Delhi starting in June 1999 and Euro II norms as of April 2000; it also restricted the number of motor vehicles that can be registered in Delhi. We also need to popularize a new business and industrial ethic wherein profit helps promote the public good and not widen the rich-poor divide.

POPULATION

Population growth can be limited if people have a duty toward those who are not yet born; that duty is not to give them existence but to give them happiness.

—Marquis de Condorcet, 1795

India has the highest annual net increase in population in the world; its population, currently 990 million people, may reach 1.26 billion by the year 2016 (see Figure 8.1). Total fertility rates vary greatly from state to state, from 1.7 in Kerala to 3.5 in Uttar Pradesh. The decline in the sex ratio is most worrying (see Figure 8.2).

India's current strategy is to regard population as a developmental issue rather than as a technological one. India has embraced reproductive health and child survival in line with the Cairo Declaration of

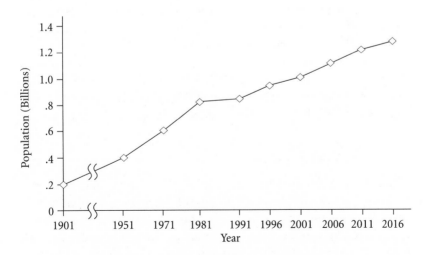

Figure 8.1. India's Burgeoning Population.

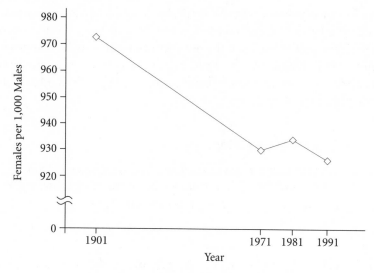

Figure 8.2.   India's Declining Sex Ratio.
Source: Swaminathan, 1999.

1994 issued by the United Nations Conference on Population and Development held in Cairo that year. The declaration recommended the concept of reproductive health and child survival as the key strategy for limiting excessive population growth.

By any standards, maternal mortality rate ought to receive the most urgent attention in India. The rate had not declined over the years, remaining at a national average of around 400 deaths per 10,000 live births. Policies to improve the health of mothers and reduce early adverse influences on children should be the focus. In terms of nutrition, South Asia has the poorest record in the world, even worse than that of sub-Saharan Africa, especially as reflected in low birth weights. The nutrition of girls and women in anticipation of pregnancy is a key concept in public health nutrition today and must guide future policy.

CONCLUSION

Medical education in India today focuses increasingly on clinical specialization and superspecialization, to the detriment of public health specialization and general practice. Too many physicians are being produced, and too few other members of the health team. Performance-based policies of professional advancement have yet to take root. One suspects that the medical colleges in India are in danger of gradually transforming into commercial high-tech institutes, replacing the older image of a medical college as a place of teaching and learning, of research and development, of healing and caring, and of apprenticeship and scholastic achievement. Prominent in the new public health paradigm for India should be public participation in health matters by individuals, families, and communities. Decentralization, local control, and building on local wisdom are strategies of the utmost importance in harmony with the devolution of power and responsibility to *panchayats* (village councils), as reflected in the recently approved Amendments Seventy-Three and Seventy-Four to the Indian Constitution.

The problem everywhere is one of limited resources and rising expectations. If the limited resources are not managed optimally and effectively, the situation becomes serious. A better outcome at less cost is a good dictum, but the resources made available should be reasonably adequate to produce the desired results. Concerns about funding for defense in India may be well-placed, but of equal importance should be concern about better funding of health, education, and social development, which hold the key for the future.

References

Acheson, D. "Equality of Health: Dream or Reality?" *Journal of the Royal College of Physicians,* 1999, *33,* 70–77.

Chauhan, V. S. "Antigenic Variation and Immune Evasion in Malaria Vaccine Development." In *The Changing Face of Malaria.* Round Table Conference Series no. 4. New Delhi: Ranbaxy Science Foundation, 1998.

"The Hidden Epidemic of Cardiovascular Disease." *Lancet,* 1998, *352,* 1795.

Hunter, D. "Session 4. Fitness to Practice in the 21st Century: What Will Doctors Be Doing in the 21st Century?" *Medical Education,* 1997, *31*(suppl. 1), 71–74.

Kamboj, V. P., and Dutta, G. P. "Newer Antimalarial Drugs, Including Indigenous Drugs." In *The Changing Face of Malaria.* Round Table Conference Series no. 4. New Delhi: Ranbaxy Science Foundation, 1998.

Ramalingaswami, V. "Welcome and Introductory Address." In *Water-Borne Diseases: The Continuing Challenge.* Round Table Conference Series no. 2. New Delhi: Ranbaxy Science Foundation, 1997.

Sharma, D. C. "Alarming Amounts of Lead Found in Indian Children." *Lancet,* 1999, *353,* 647.

Shi, Y. P., and others. "Immunogenicity and In Vitro Protective Efficacy of a Novel Recombinant *Plasmodium falciparum* Candidate Vaccine." *Proceedings of the National Academy of Sciences of the United States of America,* 1999, *96,* 1615–1620.

"A Survey of Development and the Environment: Dirt Poor." *Economist,* Mar. 21, 1998, 1–16.

Swaminathan, M. S. "Population and Human Security." Third Dr. Veda Prakash Memorial Lecture, given at the National Institute of Health and Family Welfare, New Delhi, May 1999.

Voluntary Health Association of India. *Report of the Independent Commission on Health in India.* New Delhi: Voluntary Health Association of India, 1997.

CHAPTER NINE

Russian Federation

John W. LeSar, Yuri M. Komarov,
Rafael G. Oganov, and Robert W. Porter

John W. LeSar, MD, MPH, *is the Senior Vice President for Health, Nutrition, and Population at the Academy for Educational Development, Washington, D.C., and played a major role in developing USAID's initial health program in the Russian Federation.*

Yuri M. Komarov, MD, PhD, ScD, *is the Director General of the Public Health Research Institute MedSocEconomInform and is also Vice President of the Russian Independent Association of Social Medicine and Health Care Organizations. He is recognized as one of the Russian Federation's foremost leaders in public health.*

Rafael G. Oganov, MD, *is the Director of the National Research Center for Preventive Medicine, Moscow, and is one of the Russian Federation's leading experts in the prevention and management of cardiovascular and other chronic diseases.*

Robert W. Porter, PhD, *is a Senior Program Officer in Health, Nutrition, and Population at the Academy for Educational Development. A specialist in social marketing and health communications, he is currently leading a project on the policy implications of USAID-Russian collaborative work in public health.*

Note: Complete references to the research and data sources underlying our discussion are available at http://www.aed.org.

As the third millennium opens, the everyday lives of ordinary Russians are still insecure, unpredictable, and filled with hardship. A decadelong economic depression continues. Gross domestic product has declined by nearly 50 percent since 1989, and the monthly income of an estimated fifty-five million Russians, or 38 percent of the population, is now below the subsistence level.

For decades, health conditions in Russia have also been deteriorating. It is tempting to characterize the current situation in catastrophic terms. Certainly conditions are critical. Life expectancy, a good overall indicator of a country's health, is lower today in Russia than it was thirty-five years ago. Death rates for working-age men and women are unusually high. The Russian population is both shrinking in numbers and aging rapidly, a trend that will accelerate over the next two decades.

The current health crisis has been building for several decades. It is the culmination of: (1) long-term economic stagnation and decline; (2) a population increasingly exposed to a growing number of health risks; and (3), a health care system that has never given priority to the leading cause of adult mortality, chronic illness, though it did successfully control infectious diseases. Social and economic stress in the early 1990s, coupled with severe financial constraints in the health sector (affecting the availability of vaccines, pharmaceuticals, medical equipment, and health personnel), has now made an already grave situation worse.

The current crisis, then, results from an interplay of shorter-term socioeconomic shocks and more deeply rooted and longer-term problems. Although recent economic, political, and social turbulence has exacerbated Russia's health problems, the underlying foundation for good health is also uncertain.

LIFE EXPECTANCY AND CAUSES OF DEATH

Mortality patterns and leading causes of death over the past few decades tell much of the story. Death rates among the most vulnerable population groups—children and pensioners—have remained fairly stable, while mortality in the working-age population has increased dramatically. Cardiovascular mortality and, to a lesser extent, cancer deaths (gradually rising since the early 1980s) are primarily responsible for the *longer-term,* overall decline in life expectancy. Suicide, homicide, deaths from alcohol poisoning, and other traumas are primarily responsible for *shorter-term* fluctuations, especially during the 1990s. In addition, mortality from tuberculosis and HIV/AIDS is now increasing exponentially (although it is not yet affecting overall mortality in a significant way).

Outbreaks of other communicable diseases such as diphtheria, typhoid, typhus, and cholera occurred in the 1990s as health system capability deteriorated, yet they do not explain Russia's health decline. In 1995, for example, infectious and parasitic diseases accounted for only about 2 percent of Russia's overall age-standardized death rate. Deteriorating environmental conditions—radioactive and chemical contamination, lead emissions, and polluted water—are creating significant health problems in specific regions. But again, they do not appear to be measurably contributing to the country's overall mortality.

Of course, cause-of-death data do not fully capture the growing burden of ill health and disability. Accurate measurement of morbidity (as opposed to mortality) presents serious conceptual and technical problems in Russia, as it does elsewhere. Still, it is likely that disability from injuries and chronic illness among working-age adults represent a double cost to society—in both lost productivity and the increased costs of supporting a disabled population.

The policy and planning implications of this health profile are clear. To improve the overall health of the Russian population, reduction of cardiovascular disease, injuries, and cancer are top priorities.

RISK FACTORS

In Russia, as in other industrialized countries, smoking, drinking, obesity, hypertension, high cholesterol, consumption of fatty foods, sedentary lifestyles, and genetic predisposition are the underlying determinants of cardiovascular disease and many cancers. Tobacco use is a major public health concern: Nearly seven out of ten Russian men smoke cigarettes, and average daily consumption has risen. Age-adjusted death rates from lung cancer are correspondingly high, yet smoking also plays an important role in fatalities from coronary heart disease, stroke, and other cancers. Alan Lopez of WHO estimates that smoking in Russia may already be implicated in 30 percent of all deaths among men.

Russia is historically known to have a very high level of alcohol consumption, which contributes to both cardiovascular disease and injuries. The psychosocial stress that has accompanied the social and economic turbulence of the early 1990s also contributed to higher rates of cardiovascular mortality, suicide, homicide, and fatal accidents. Here alcohol has played an important mediating role. The unusually high death rates among working men and women (especially those in their early forties) during this period were paralleled by a steep rise in alcohol consumption. Many fatal injuries were clearly related to alcohol abuse.

Prevalence of other risk factors, such as hypertension, elevated cholesterol, obesity, and lack of physical exercise, generally fall within ranges characteristic of European countries. Yet a large proportion of the Russian population suffers from a combination of two or more of these major health risks, and the accumulation of multiple risks over a lifetime dramatically increases the probability of premature death and disability.

HEALTH SERVICES

It is difficult to assess how the deterioration in health services may have contributed to the mortality crisis of the early 1990s. Child health has not seemed to suffer, suggesting that child health services have been maintained and that parents continue to care for their children. The major problem is with chronic diseases affecting the working-age adult population, a group that the Russian health system has seldom viewed as a priority. Health services still follow the Soviet model in their excessive orientation to hospital-based curative care. Seventy percent of health sector spending is for inpatient treatment, and the vast majority of physicians (also 70 percent in a recent World Bank estimate) are specialists. The underfunded, underutilized primary health care system remains primarily focused on infectious diseases. Managers in some regional and local health systems are taking steps to strengthen screening, diagnosis, and care for cardiovascular and other chronic diseases. Others are continuing to experiment with new evidence-based clinical guidelines and more cost-efficient approaches to service delivery. But everywhere, health care systems are under extraordinary stress, and the overwhelming preoccupation is to maintain basic services.

TOMORROW'S TRENDS

Will the health crisis continue? Public health is very much a matter of political economy, and Russia's political and economic future is uncertain. Rather than offer a simple forecast, we describe three alternative scenarios. In the first, current trends remain largely unchanged. In the second, the crisis deepens. In the third, conditions gradually improve.

Scenario 1: Muddling Through

In this scenario, current health trends continue. Life expectancy fluctuates over the next several decades but generally remains close to the somewhat improved levels of the late 1990s. Cardiovascular diseases continue to be the leading cause of excess mortality. Smoking prevalence, particularly high among younger adults today, results in rising rates of lung cancer around the year 2020. Russians continue their historical pattern of alcohol use, contributing to high rates of fatal and disabling injuries among working-age men, but HIV/AIDS will emerge as a significant cause of death among younger, sexually active women. Outbreaks of other infectious diseases will be more or less contained. Infant and child mortality remains at current, moderate levels. As Russia's fertility decline continues, fewer working-age adults are supporting a growing population of the elderly. Women continue to outlive men by about twelve years—meaning that they bear the burden of caring for the sick and dying, as they have in the past. Yet basic medical services are still widely available, although disparities in access to care, across regions and socioeconomic classes, has become considerably more pronounced.

Scenario 2: From Crisis to Catastrophe

Deteriorating socioeconomic conditions and a collapsing public health system result in a triple burden of ill health and a new kind of mortality crisis. Infectious and parasitic diseases spread unchecked, environmental health problems proliferate, and the epidemics of cardiovascular disease and fatal injuries worsen while tobacco use rises in all age groups. As drug-resistant strains of tuberculosis spread beyond the reservoir of Russian prisons, death rates attributable to TB approach those of cardiovascular disease. The incidence of HIV and AIDS also skyrockets, following trends already seen in other, less lethal sexually transmitted infections. The public health consequences of long-standing environmental problems become evident: Polluted water leads to the reemergence of bacterial dysentery and cholera. Cancers resulting from radioactive and chemical contamination increase. Alcoholism grows worse, and the increasing consumption of home-brewed spirits leads to higher death rates from alcohol poisoning. Fertility continues to fall, though it is driven now more by reproductive health problems and less by couples' fertility preferences.

Scenario 3: Improvement Thanks to Public Health Investments

As Russia begins to lift itself out of acute economic depression and as structural changes lead to long-term economic improvements, the health crisis moves squarely onto the government's agenda. Investments in public health, long given low priority as "nonproductive," are now regarded as essential to economic recovery and national security. With significant support from the international health community, progress is being made against tuberculosis, and other infectious diseases are being contained. Now the attention of central and regional governments turns to the leading causes of premature death and disability—cardiovascular diseases, cancers, and fatal injuries—and their two main risk factors, smoking and excessive alcohol consumption.

Discussion

Which of these scenarios is most plausible? In our view, scenarios 1 and 3.

The first scenario assumes that socioeconomic stability will arrive, but only slowly, and that the current economic contraction will take several decades to reverse. In the short term, significant investments in public health will continue to be crowded out by other priorities. Yet the health system will not collapse, and a new onslaught of infectious diseases, successfully controlled in the past, will not lead to a new kind of mortality crisis.

The second scenario, of growing catastrophe, describes the public health consequences of an industrial power undergoing an extreme process of social and economic "demodernization"—an event without historical precedent. This doomsday scenario has received considerable attention in both Russian and Western media. It has its uses as a tool for mobilizing public and governmental attention to the health crisis. But we believe that a public health catastrophe can still be prevented.

Our third scenario is guardedly optimistic. The resilience of the Russian people has been tested by yet another "time of troubles," but as social and economic stability returns, the country's health profile gradually comes to resemble those of its neighbors to the west. This scenario assumes that the Russian Federation will pull itself out of its decadelong economic depression and that central and regional governments will gradually begin to rebuild their health systems. It also assumes that innovative strategies in health promotion and disease prevention, currently confined to pilot or demonstration areas, will expand to many more communities.

Though more positive than the others, this scenario does not necessarily predict a rapid turnaround in adult mortality. Cardiovascular diseases and cancers will continue as leading causes of death. Both diseases are typically the culmination of many incremental insults to the cardiovascular and immune systems. Improvements in disease trends and death rates resulting from dietary changes, reductions in tobacco use, and other lifestyle improvements typically do not become evident for many years.

Nevertheless, the striking rise in excess mortality among working adults in the early 1990s—due primarily to alcohol-related injuries, heart attacks, and strokes—suggests that psychosocial factors have also played an important contributory role in triggering many of these premature deaths. As individuals and families develop more adaptive coping skills and learn to manage everyday stress more successfully, injury-related and cardiovascular death rates may return rather quickly to "precrisis" levels.

PROMOTING HEALTH IMPROVEMENT

Since health improvement depends primarily on preventing and reducing cardiovascular disease, injuries, and cancer, public health strategies in Russia need to be multifaceted, systematic, and long-term.

Injury prevention strategies can, in theory, reduce mortality most quickly. There is strong evidence, for example, that Gorbachev's anti-alcohol campaign of the late 1980s had a rather immediate impact on injury-related deaths. But the high costs of the campaign, in both widespread public opposition and lost state revenues, led to its quick demise, and alcohol consumption soon returned to its former levels. Alcoholism clearly remains a key public health priority, and there is much that can also be done to improve occupational and public safety. These health problems do not call for strictly medical solutions, but given the current state of the health care system, they may prove more feasible to address—and injury prevention is clearly cost effective.

Cardiovascular disease and cancer prevention strategies require changes in living and working conditions, lifestyles, and health behaviors. In most industrialized countries, these underlying determinants of disease are dealt with in the home, at the workplace, and in the community. Government takes the lead only when individual and local efforts are ineffective or when the instruments of state policy can play a clear and effective role in reducing widespread and involuntary exposure to health hazards—as in the areas of tobacco control, public order, occupational safety, sanitation, hygiene, and environmental health.

Public health communication and community-based behavior change interventions hold considerable potential in this context. Adult literacy is nearly universal, much of Russian society is urbanized, and there is widespread access to media. Lifestyle change in twenty-first-century Russia is likely to come about, as it has in the West, through health-conscious social movements, amplified by popular media and other forms of social communication. Health information, whether delivered through media vehicles (print or broadcast) or through health care providers, is necessary to the prevention and management of chronic illness, but so are viable networks of social support. New forms of association and community are gradually beginning to fill the vacuum left by the collapse of the Soviet state. And there are signs that health improvement can itself become a motivating force, leading to new forms of organization and action and new approaches to primary prevention and care.

CONCLUSION

The wealth of nations in the twenty-first century will rest increasingly on their human resources—healthy, educated, and productive people. Russia's natural resources are without parallel. But Russia's human resources are at risk. In an increasingly technological and competitive global economy, a debilitated population is itself a barrier to economic growth. If Russia's decades-old decline in public health is not reversed, the nation's prospects for economic recovery will continue to dim. The Russian medical community is coming to recognize that investing in programs that promote lifestyles that prevent chronic disease is the key to Russia's future health. Political leaders and policy managers must also come to understand that the health of the Russian people is crucial to national prosperity—and they need to act on that understanding.

United States

J. Michael McGinnis

J. Michael McGinnis, MD, became Senior Vice President at the Robert Wood Johnson Foundation in 1999, after a four-year appointment as Scholar in Residence at the National Academy of Sciences in Washington, D.C. Prior to that, he was Assistant Surgeon General and Deputy Assistant Secretary for Health in the U.S. Department of Health and Human Services through four administrations. Dr. McGinnis founded, among other important initiatives, the Healthy People *process to establish and implement national health goals and objectives.*

Stunning opportunity is in the offing in the United States for health innovation and gain of a nature heretofore resident only in our dreams and myths. Many of the changes will come as a result of scientific discoveries and technological advances that will allow novel approaches to the treatment and prevention of disease and disability. Others will derive from new levels of personal control over health management. Some will even yield revised notions for our understanding of the boundaries for health and disease. But these changes will also have a measure of dependence on new social norms concerning our concepts of the rights of each individual with respect to health.

No aspect of life is more fundamental than health, both as a defining quality of personal and national vitality and, for the United States, as a vehicle for the dreams of liberty and opportunity codified in our founding documents. Mindful of health's centrality, Thomas Jefferson, author in 1776 of the Declaration of Independence and later our third president, in observing that without health there is no happiness, called for government to give highest priority to the health of the citizenry. In those days, government's responsibilities as guarantor of both the freedom to act and choose, on the one hand, and of health and safety, on the other, tended to be characterized as parallel responsibilities, related primarily by their association on the register of matters defining the human condition. But today, at the dawn of a new century, our choices—and rights—take on new meanings as foundation stones of the bridge to a healthier future.

THE PAST: LEADING CAUSES OF DEATH AND DISEASE

The twentieth century witnessed a remarkable transition related to the primary influences on human disease, disability, and death (see Table 10.1). In 1900, at the century's start, the major killers of Americans were pneumonia, tuberculosis, diarrhea, and enteritis. Infectious diseases, often nurtured by poor sanitation, nutritional deficiencies, and crowding, have been the primary contributors to early death among Americans throughout much of our relatively short history. The profile began to change—and rapidly—with the advent of public health departments and stronger sanitary initiatives, immunization, improved food distribution systems, and the introduction of antibiotic therapy at midcentury. Life expectancy for Americans was forty-seven years in 1900 but increased to fifty-eight years in 1925, sixty-eight years in 1950, seventy-five years in 1975, and nearly eighty years in the year 2000. By the 1920s, with heart disease ascending to the top spot among the causes of deaths for Americans, chronic diseases of older age had become our leading health challenges. At 2000, the major killers of Americans are heart disease, cancer, and stroke.

As impressive as the changes in health status have been, our gains in knowledge about the determinants of health, and hence the potential controllability of disease and disability, have been simply astonishing. In the United States, an analysis of the literature assessing the

1900	Percentage of Total Deaths	2000 (estimate)	Percentage of Total Deaths
1. Pneumonia	13	1. Heart disease	32
2. Tuberculosis	12	2. Cancer	23
3. Diarrhea, enteritis	8	3. Stroke	7
4. Heart disease	7	4. Lung disease	5
5. Stroke	6	5. Unintentional injuries	4
6. Liver disease	5	6. Pneumonia	4
7. Unintentional injuries	4	7. Diabetes	4
8. Cancer	3	8. Suicide	2
9. Senility	2	9. Kidney disease	2
10. Diphtheria	2	10. Liver disease	2

Table 10.1.   Ten Leading Causes of Death in the U.S., 1900 and 2000.
Source: "Achievements," 1999, p. 623.

contributors to the leading causes of death for Americans indicates that the actual causes of death are not those commonly listed on death certificates but rather tobacco, diet, physical activity patterns, alcohol, microbial agents, toxic agents, firearms, sexual activity, motor vehicles, and illicit use of drugs (see Table 10.2).

THE FUTURE:
LEADING DETERMINANTS OF HEALTH

Drawing on the extensive studies of the past generation, we can now speak about our health prospects as being shaped by our experiences in five domains: our genetic and gestational predispositions, our social circumstances, our environmental conditions, our behavioral choices, and the medical care we receive. Exciting developments are in the offing for each of these domains.

Genetic Predispositions

Our predispositions to health or disease begin to take form genetically at the moment of conception and developmentally throughout our exposures during gestation. The future will bring extraordinary developments in our genetic understanding and capacity. The 30,000 to 60,000 genes of the human genome were completely sequenced by the year 2001, opening possibilities for new interventions ranging from

Source	Number of Deaths (000)	Percentage of Total Deaths
1. Tobacco	400	19
2. Diet and physical activity patterns	300	14
3. Alcohol	100	5
4. Microbial agents	90	4
5. Toxic agents	60	3
6. Firearms	35	2
7. Sexual behavior	30	1
8. Motor vehicles	25	1
9. Illicit drug use	20	<1
Total	1,060	50

Table 10.2.   Actual Causes of Death in the U. S.

Source: McGinnis and Foege, 1993, p. 2208.

education with greater precision and specificity about individual vulnerabilities to environmental and behavioral factors to alteration of genetic determinants of disease and disability. Similarly, new insights will be gained on the impact of exposures during gestation once we have the results from long-term observational studies now getting under way to assess the consequences of maternal social, environmental, behavioral, and medical care factors on the health of offspring.

Social Circumstances

At birth, our first encounter is with our social circumstances, about which a great deal more has been learned in recent years. We now know that health is powerfully influenced by education, employment, income disparities, poverty, housing, crime, and the social cohesion of our communities. From cradle to grave, our interpersonal linkages matter. As a result of enhanced capacity for epidemiological analysis of large databases, as well as new insights in immunology and the neurosciences, we can anticipate in the years ahead a broader base of information on the social factors that put people at risk, on the characteristics of those at greatest risk, on the power of the influence of various factors for those at greatest risk, and on the biological pathways through which those influences take their toll. Even now, we see a strong mandate for efforts to reach out more effectively to those who are social outliers in our communities.

Environmental Conditions

To some extent, as part of our social circumstances, we find our conditions also affected in important ways by the nature of our physical environments. The places we seek to shape as nurturing and sheltering—home, work, and community environments—sometimes present hazards in the form of toxic agents, microbial agents, and structural flaws. In the coming years, we will see progress in the ability to detect and measure the physiological impact of various discrete toxic, microbial, and structural environmental factors and even their interactions with other factors, as well as improvement in our ability to take action at the local level to address these factors. Less clear is the extent of our capacity, or our resolve, to identify in a timely fashion the nature or the impact of large-scale environmental change, most notably global climate change, or to take coordinated, sustained, effective action once identified. In terms of the potential for developments to alter the human condition dramatically throughout the world, it may be in the area of environmental exposures that both the uncertainties and the consequences pose the greatest health challenges for the new century.

Behavioral Choices

In the United States, our behavior patterns represent the single most controllable domain of influence over our health prospects. The daily choices we make with respect to diet, physical activity, and sex, the substance abuse and addictions to which we fall prey, our approach to safety, and our coping strategies in confronting stress are all important determinants of health. Overall, various behavioral choices we make account for nearly half the deaths among Americans—all of them by definition early deaths—along with a compelling burden of associated illness. As people have learned more about the impact of behavioral factors, they have begun to make changes—in tobacco use, in fat consumption, in seat belt use, and in the use of preventive services, but the gap remains substantial between current practices and potential gains. With increasing discoveries from gene studies on the specific and varied susceptibilities of individuals to health problems deriving from their behavioral choices, with more work to develop social signals that support patterns of behavior more conducive to health, and with enhanced understanding of neurochemical factors that shape outlooks, attitudes, tendencies, and dependencies, the potential is great for progress. The twenty-first century may see people's behaviors transformed from a force of significant challenge to one of significant advantage in shaping the national health profile.

Medical Care

Despite the preponderant influence of nonmedical factors on the health profile of Americans, when we fall ill, our access to high-quality medical care is of vital, and increasing, importance. And as the prevalence of chronic conditions increases due to greater survival rates at both ends of the life spectrum, the importance of medical care to population health will surely grow. As a result, we can anticipate that the new century will see medical care both expanding its capacity for a more nurturing and supportive approach to the psychological and emotional needs of patients and drawing on advances in immunology, the neurosciences, molecular biology and recombinant DNA technologies, and even the engineering sciences for the application of new technologies in orthopedics, organ and tissue repair and replacement, vaccine development, pharmaceuticals and pharmaceutical delivery systems, human reproduction, and mood and memory function. New developments in communications technologies will ensure that patients will have a much more direct and sustained role in managing their own conditions.

THE POSSIBILITY: HEALTHY PEOPLE IN HEALTHY COMMUNITIES

More than two decades ago, as the Public Health Service began looking to the end of the twentieth century, it established measurable targets for health improvement: to reduce infant mortality by 35 percent, death rates among children by 20 percent, death rates for adolescents and young adults by 20 percent, adult death rates by 25 percent, and the age-adjusted occurrence of sick days among older adults by about 20 percent (U.S. Department of Health, Education, and Welfare, 1979). These targets were based on the evidence at hand about the controllability of disease and injury at various stages of life, and though ambitious, they were expected to be accomplished in a decade's time. Despite the size of these anticipated gains, the goals were largely reached, with infant mortality having declined just under 35 percent by the end of the 1980s, childhood death rate declines substantially exceeding the target, with a decline of about 29 percent, adolescent and young adult deaths falling short of the mark with a 9 percent decline, adult death rates declining by 25 percent, and the age-adjusted sick days for older adults declining by about 14 percent. Among the various component targets established, the most glaring shortfalls related to the inability to close the access and health status gaps that existed among population groups. As a result, when the decision was made to extend the activity another decade with the *Healthy People 2000* initiative, the goals established were broadened to include issues of functional status and quality of life and placed particular emphasis on reducing disparities among groups (U.S. Department of Health and Human Services, 1990). Similar priorities are found in the current work toward *Healthy People 2010*, which expresses the vision of healthy people in healthy communities (U.S. Department of Health and Human Services, 1998).

Although the notion of quantifying centurylong gains to be anticipated for the health of Americans is so daunting as to be prohibitive, it seems reasonable to project that for the United States, the primary paradigm shift for the twenty-first century will be the move from a primary focus on length of life to a primary focus on quality of life. To be sure, there will be impressive reductions in death rates. Improvements in prenatal and neonatal care ought to continue to drive down infant death rates, to less than one death per thousand live births, given the likely developments in diagnostic and intervention technologies. Death rates for children will also decline with improvements in the treatments for childhood cancers, although declines in injury death rates will inevitably begin to level out for this active population. Clearly, the death rates for adults will continue to decline as we attend more closely to our personal control over health and as new treatments are applied. By the middle of the century, the number of people over age sixty-five will likely have more than doubled to approximately seventy-five million people, representing some 20 percent of the U.S. population. It does not seem unreasonable to anticipate that by century's end, we will see life expectancies of ninety years and beyond.

Of course, the real gains will come with our ability to improve the quality of life at each of its major stages. We should be able to anticipate a life course better characterized by a healthy beginning, a long period of sustained vitality, and a gentle ending. With the gains anticipated in each of the domains of influence, we can expect dramatic opportunities to push and even redefine the boundaries of our vigor and vitality to our full biological limits. Even the ends of our lives may find us with a greater measure of control in the years ahead. The combination of demographic imperatives prompting social innovation, technologic advances affording greater capacity for comfort under circumstances of decline, and cultural change encouraging partnership in decision making ought to make for a final passage characterized by a greater measure of sensitivity and humanity.

The role of the community will be key at each stage. Whether considering the challenge of assuring the availability of necessary health and social services, of forging supportive links that afford a sense of security and hope to those at risk of isolation and estrangement, of fostering physical environments that reinforce lifestyles of vigor and vitality, or of supporting microperspectives that contribute to productive engagement of macroenvironmental challenges, the culture of our communities will be key. The interwoven fates of healthy people cannot be separated from the health of their communities.

A HEALTH BILL OF RIGHTS FOR THE TWENTY-FIRST CENTURY

Given the resources with which the United States has been blessed, the true measure of the success of the twenty-first century for our nation will reside in the extent to which all citizens are afforded the opportunity to reach their full health potential. Against the backdrop of potentially exciting prospects for health gains among Americans in the twenty-first century is the need to ensure that the advances extend throughout the population. Despite the impressive record of overall improvement in the health of Americans, the health access and health status of poor Americans continue to lag. Bridging this gap will be quite a challenge: the poor have more risk factors and suffer higher rates of disease and disability than the rest of the population, more than one of every six Americans lacks health insurance coverage, and the chasm between rich and poor in American society is widening— the income of the wealthiest 1 percent of Americans is equivalent to the income of the bottom 40 percent. Increases in the costs of medical care anticipated with the introduction of new breakthrough technologies in the coming century will raise compelling challenges to our responsibility to define and address the basic needs of the poor here and abroad.

Shortly after the U.S. Constitution was ratified, the nation's founders sought to protect the rights of individuals from potential abuse by an insensitive majority by proposing several amendments that upon ratification became known as the Bill of Rights. Were we, as a nation, to take to heart Thomas Jefferson's admonition that attention to health should "take the place of every other object," we might set about to fashion a twenty-first-century Bill of Rights focused on matters important to health, such as the following:

- *Right to a well-attended birth and infancy.* Every newborn deserves the full advantage of a healthy pregnancy, a birth attended by a skilled practitioner, and the attention and resources of the community in support of a nurturing infancy.

- *Right to a safe childhood.* The early years may have lifelong impact. Every child should anticipate a childhood that is as safe, secure, and free of fear as possible.

- *Right to essential food and shelter.* Food and shelter are the factors of most direct physiologic necessity to human survival. They should not merely be a presumption amid our plenty but a guarantee.

- *Right to an effective education.* The most powerful predictor of good health is found in educational attainment, which provides the opportunity, choice, and understanding essential to full attainment of one's health potential.

- *Right to a safe and supportive environment.* We who live today deserve environments free of overt hazards to our safety and sense of well-being; moreover, those who will live tomorrow have the right to a legacy free from harm.

- *Right to information about identifiable risks.* Whether our risks are endogenous and genetic or exogenous and environmental, we deserve full access to rapidly emerging information to help us make decisions that will shape our health.

- *Right to privacy.* Except for matters of direct and immediate concern to the health of others, we have the right to keep our health and medical profiles personal and private.

- *Right to proven preventive services.* Advances in genetics, immunology, the neuro- and behavioral sciences, and early diagnostics will redefine our capacity to prevent disease, and that capacity should be available to every citizen.

- *Right to freedom from unusual barriers to care.* No one should be presented with undue economic, social, or geographical barriers to care.

- *Right to compassion and control at the end of life.* Just as we encourage control throughout life's course, people have the right to as peaceful and painless an exit as possible.

Although full acceptance and application of these rights would not even then allow us to realize our dream of health for all, the net result of our democracy's acknowledgment of these basic health rights would move us closer and would represent the kind of progress toward the promotion of the general welfare envisioned by our Constitution. While it is true that, as President John Kennedy noted, a rising tide raises all boats, we must keep in mind that the heaviest buffeting occurs at the level of the rowboats and dinghies. As the tides of the economy, knowledge, and science rise to the challenges of the new century, it is fundamental that we not leave the disadvantaged swamped in their wake. That is the first obligation of our nation as we move forward to what, if we are able to reach our full potential, will be a century remarkable both for our gains and for our enlightenment.

References

"Achievements in Public Health, 1900–1999: Control of Infectious Diseases." *Morbidity and Mortality Weekly Report,* 1999, *48,* 621–629.

McGinnis, J. M., and Foege, W. H. "Actual Causes of Death in the United States." *Journal of the American Medical Association,* 1993, *270,* 2207–2212.

U.S. Department of Health, Education and Welfare. *Healthy People: The Surgeon General's Report on Health Promotion and Disease Prevention.* Washington, D.C.: U.S. Department of Health, Education and Welfare, 1979.

U.S. Department of Health and Human Services. *Healthy People 2000: National Health Promotion and Disease Prevention Objectives.* Washington, D.C.: U.S. Department of Health and Human Services, 1990.

U.S. Department of Health and Human Services. *Healthy People 2010 Objectives: Draft for Public Comment.* Washington, D.C.: U.S. Department of Health and Human Services/Office of Public Health and Science, 1998.

CHAPTER ELEVEN

Mexico

Juan Ramón de la Fuente, Fernando Alvarez del Rio,
Roberto Tapia-Conyer, and A. Rodrigo Ares de Parga

Juan Ramón de la Fuente, MD, *is the Health Minister of*
Mexico. He was previously Dean of the Medical School of the
National University of Mexico, where he graduated before
training in psychiatry at the Mayo Clinic in Rochester, Minnesota.
Dr. de la Fuente has written more than 150 original papers
published in leading medical journals and has edited ten books
on subjects related to health, medical education,
and scientific research.

Fernando Alvarez del Rio, *is Chief of Staff for the Health*
Minister of Mexico. He earned his degree in economics at McMaster
University, Canada. In the Ministry of Health, he has also served
as General Director of Health Economic Studies.

Roberto Tapia-Conyer, MD, *is a professor in the Faculty*
of Medicine of the National University of Mexico. He is Vice
Minister for the Prevention and Control of Diseases at Mexico's
Federal Ministry of Health. He is a member of the National
Academy of Medicine and the Mexican Academy of Science and
a consultant to the American States Organization–CICAD, the
United Nations, and the Pan American Health Organization.

A. Rodrigo Ares de Parga, *is General Director of Program-*
ming, Organization, and Budgeting at Mexico's Federal Ministry of
Health, where he previously served as Chief of Staff to the minister.
After graduating as an economist in Mexico, he earned master's
degrees in international affairs and public administration at
Columbia University, New York.

Health is universally recognized as of crucial importance to the well-being of individuals and societies, and so it seems unnecessary to define it as a concept. Nevertheless, several particular aspects may be relevant when setting public policy and anticipating the results of current and future actions.

First, health must be pursued not only because it is an indispensable component of well-being but also because it is both a prerequisite and a catalyst for basically every other activity at the individual and societal levels, including economic performance (World Bank, 1993). This perspective will inevitably force issues of health care and health-generating activities onto the political agenda of every country.

Second, health is a basic life component that allows individuals to enjoy the benefits of education, nutrition, employment, and cultural and political participation (Pan American Health Organization/World Health Organization, 1995). People in poverty lack the wherewithal to take advantage of these opportunities—a situation that inhibits the very principle of a democratic society. Thus the right of access to health care is and will remain one of the tenets of every nation's underpinnings.

Third, notwithstanding that health care delivery services are needed, they are not the exclusive vehicle for achieving better health. New and innovative mechanisms must be adopted to promote healthy lifestyles and prevent diseases, given that social and environmental factors and individuals' knowledge, attitudes, and behavior determine the health of communities and populations (Adams and Hirschfeld, 1998).

The foregoing considerations are clear evidence of the importance and value that all societies will place on health in the coming years, and we can expect that health policies around the world will become more and more similar in the future. With regard to health care systems, every society will face constraints that may be tackled differently, reflecting core values and principles.

One of these core principles is *solidarity of coverage.* Each society will strive for universal access to a comprehensive health care package independent of people's willingness and capacity to pay. This implies that states will enforce mechanisms for the financing and provision of services regardless of individuals' desires and views. Nevertheless, the very definition of this "comprehensive" package will depend on each society's epidemiological profile as well as on the society's views of the role of the individual in terms of responsibility, capacity to pay, and social obligation to others.

A second core principle involves *quality and costs*. Each society will expect the most humane care of the best possible quality; however, achieving this goal will depend on resource constraints. Thus issues surrounding the operation of cost-effective health systems, with their corresponding repercussions in macroeconomic areas such as financing, insurance, and provider incentives, will have an impact, as will microeconomic considerations such as the identification and funding of cost-effective programs and interventions.

THE MEXICAN HEALTH CARE SYSTEM

There is no health care blueprint applicable to all countries, only elements common to people and communities. Any strategy must be in accordance with the history, development, and idiosyncrasies of a country. In Mexico, policies are and will continue to be oriented toward achieving social justice, democracy, and economic efficiency.

Since 1994, Mexico has had a segmented health care system, divided into several vertically integrated institutions, each covering a different population group. There are various social security schemes, the largest being the Mexican Social Security Institute (IMSS), which provides coverage to private-sector workers (nearly half the employed population); the Federal Ministry of Health (SSA), which provides medical care and public health services to the so-called open population (without social security); and a heterogeneous private sector operating on a fee-for-service basis, financed by out-of-pocket payments and indemnity insurance plans.

A set of comprehensive and specific strategies was outlined in 1995 in the Program for Health Sector Reform, 1995–2000. The reform of the system centered on four objectives: to increase coverage; to promote quality and efficiency in the delivery process; to decentralize resources and responsibilities to states, and to introduce initiatives and modifications for a more efficient operation of health care markets and other economic activities (Federal Ministry of Health, 1994b).

In terms of coverage, the main priority has been to guarantee access for every Mexican at least to a basic bundle of health care services (Federal Executive Office, 1994). For this, a special expanded-coverage program was created, Programa de Ampliación de Cobertura (PAC), making accessible by the year 2000 a basic health care package to more than ten million people who lacked or had very limited access to health services, particularly in geographically remote and economically deprived areas. This strategy has been adopted by PROGRESA, an important initiative that aims for a permanent solution to extreme poverty by exploiting the interrelations with other components of poverty alleviation like education and nutrition.

To increase affiliation with the social security system, which had stagnated during the first half of the 1990s, a major financial reform was introduced in IMSS, shifting the financing toward general taxation and reducing the burden on employer and employee contributions. This strategy has allowed the stabilization of the Mexican economy, facilitating economic growth and job creation and opening the possibility of offering voluntary participation in the social security system (Organization for Economic Cooperation and Development, 1998). In the second half of the 1990s, around eight million persons, including workers and their families, joined IMSS.

Decentralization is a basic tool for more efficient operation of the state health systems by forging a closer link between health needs and resources and between responsibility and the capacity to respond (Federal Ministry of Health, 1994a). To make the state ministries accountable, decentralization required the introduction of a clearly defined and equitable resource allocation mechanism, gradually approximating an adjusted capitated payment whereby the federal government guarantees a minimum capacity of response in all states. Simultaneously, flexibility in the use of resources was introduced by evaluating the performance of the state health systems by focusing on health outcomes rather than on a historically rigid evaluation of budget items (Federal Ministry of Health, 1998). Decentralization has been consolidated in all thirty-two states, and local participation has been strongly encouraged.

Target programs for specific groups have been developed, including vaccination campaigns reaching almost 100 percent of the children between one and four years of age, preventive health programs designed for women, and life-prolonging treatment for AIDS patients free of charge. Health quality has been boosted through a wide variety of initiatives. To compensate for the lack of incentives for doctors and nurses in the past, salaries for these professionals have been increased (more than 50 percent in real terms), and extra bonuses have been granted for individuals working in rural areas. Other measures implemented to increase quality standards have been the accreditation of hospitals and specialists by an independent body (with public and private representation) when they comply with quality standards exceeding what is required by law and the creation in 1996 of the National Commission for Medical Arbitrage (CONAMED), a new organization that protects the rights of the consumers of health services and issues recommendations to providers.

Acknowledging that tomorrow's health challenges will not be met unless all the participants are involved, several initiatives were introduced for more effective participation of the private sector both in the health care market and in the overall functioning of markets in the country. In the first case, generic drugs have been introduced, generating a new market for the pharmaceutical industry and making high-quality drugs accessible to consumers who need them at affordable prices. Managed care regulation is being introduced to guarantee its finding a durable niche in the private sector, with a special emphasis on disease prevention and health promotion programs. In the second case, a process of deregulation and modernization of sanitary surveillance has facilitated economic activity while strengthening supervision in sectors with health risks.

FUTURE OF THE MEXICAN HEALTH CARE SYSTEM

Before attempting to explore the results of our current efforts for the next century, it is possible to identify three types of constraining factors: demographic, epidemiological, and scientific.

According to recent demographic projections, Mexico's population will reach around 129 million people by the year 2030—a 50 percent increase in just forty years (National Commission on Population, 1996). And because the population as a whole is aging, a dramatic change is expected in the demographic structure of the Mexican population, with more than seventeen million people (13.2 percent) categorized as elderly.

Epidemiological changes are taking place in Mexican society partly as a result of the new demographic structure. The increasing prevalence of chronic degenerative diseases fundamentally changes the risk factors associated with health and the interventions required.

Impressive advances were made in the public health field, including molecular epidemiology, during the final decades of the twentieth century. These improvements are clearly offering us both the challenges that we anticipate and the tools to overcome them—for instance, the development of methods to assess health conditions and risk factors beyond the reductionism of a one-cause, one-disease vision, in parallel with the application of modern statistical models, which show a higher goodness of fit with complex phenomena. Better and timely decisions are now feasible mainly at the local level, thanks to the deployment of health information systems based on the latest information technology available.

The future of the Mexican health system will be the result of the significant advances of the twentieth century, continuous efforts by all actors, and the interaction of principles, actions, and constraining factors mentioned earlier. Taking all this into account, it is possible to expect a number of specific outcomes, subject of course to the obvious limitations of this type of exercise.

Objectives

The goal of current and future efforts will be, first and foremost, to attain a universal health system rooted in the principle that all Mexicans will have access to a comprehensive and integral health package irrespective of their capacity to pay. That is, equity and universal access will continue to be the guiding principles. Second, a goal will be to guarantee the conditions and incentives for the most cost-effective and quality-oriented delivery of services with the greatest impact on health outcomes. Finally, a goal will be to honor as much as possible the informed decisions of individuals with regard to access, choice of providers, and healthy lifestyles.

Given these objectives, we expect the following characteristics, which for ease of exposition we divide according to the functions performed at different levels of the health care system.

Financing

The health care system will be for the most part a publicly financed system in which it is compulsory for all citizens with the capacity to contribute to do so on an honest income-related basis in order to provide a clearly defined comprehensive health care package to all. Think of this as a universal health insurance fund where all these resources are gathered for their distribution according to the health needs of various population groups. This fund will reflect the social solidarity inherent in the Mexican health care system. Direct private financing will supply services outside the comprehensive health care package.

Current reforms are leading in that direction. While maintaining compulsory social security affiliation, the government has shifted toward a general taxation approach that uses a progressive income-related contribution scheme applied to all individuals. Also, the introduction of a voluntary social insurance plan for those in the informal economic sector is expanding the pool of contributors to encompass all citizens who have the economic capacity to contribute.

The federal budget for the population without social security and, particularly, citizens covered by the federal and state health ministries has increased since 1995 more than 70 percent in real terms, far more than the numbers in social security. This commitment, if continued, coupled with the enrollments in social security, will permit a homogenization of per capita spending by all institutions and hence the attainment of a universal insurance fund. As stated before, a similar process is taking place in the Federal Ministry of Health with regard to resource allocation to the states.

Administration and Delivery of Services

State health authorities will become the main administrative bodies in charge of contracting health care services for their respective populations. These bodies may be viewed as a blend between current social security and non–social security institutions that receive funds on a capitated basis adjusted by health risk factors. In this manner, they will all be on an equal footing and have a similar capacity of response to provide for health care coverage. Contrary to present arrangements, under which the population is divided by employment status, it is expected that eventually everyone will have equal access.

Considering the current health care infrastructure in Mexico, it is expected that care will be delivered mostly by public institutions organized in autonomous bodies either separately or in networks integrating primary care and hospital services. These bodies, derived primarily from IMSS, ISSSTE (the social security system for public-sector workers), or SSA, will be placed under contract by the state authorities on behalf of geographically defined populations, on the basis of cost effectiveness, quality of care, and the informed decisions of the population.

It is important to note that if Mexico were to continue its present arrangement indefinitely, duplication of services would increase because the population is spread throughout the country, irrespective of employment status, and each public institution would be required to have sufficient physical and human capacity everywhere.

The main objective would be to guarantee an accountable health care system. As such, certain elements of competition will be introduced to reinforce this accountability by linking reimbursement to performance, as well as introducing choice for patients. Thus individuals will be able to choose their networks of providers and their family physicians. With strong and autonomous public providers, it is expected that private ones will also play a role, albeit, given the present situation and magnitude, a complementary one.

Current reforms point in this direction. Decentralization of the Federal Ministry of Health has been completed and will be consolidated in the years to come as state ministries find new and innovative ways of providing coverage and care delivery. In social security, a project is under way for the establishment of medical zones, encompassing a hospital and a network of primary care providers who sign performance agreements with their regional authority. Pilot projects have begun which allow beneficiaries to choose their family practitioners, who serve as gatekeepers, and who are paid a base salary plus bonuses based on the number of beneficiaries who chose them as providers. From a different perspective, a similar situation is beginning in the private sector, where regulation is being introduced to guarantee well-established networks of providers and adopting the best aspects of managed care.

Public Health and Regulation

The new shape of the Federal Ministry of Health will be centered around its normative and regulatory functions, with a special focus on information collection and processing (Federal Ministry of Health, 1998). One key aspect will be to coordinate the epidemiological surveillance required in the future with a unique automated system that will integrate currently dispersed databases and make use of geographical information systems. This will allow the authorities, both central and local, to respond to health challenges effectively and in a timely manner.

There will also be a constant effort in health promotion, and public health programs, such as those for immunization, reproductive health, and family care, will continue to be priorities in the Mexican system. Finally, the Federal Ministry of Health will continue to have a key role in coordinating and fostering education and research. While generating new knowledge and developing better links with our education system and our universities, we can ensure better clinical practice and a better distribution of our human resources to the regions in greatest need.

Biomedical research will facilitate the improvement of health status and the abatement of costs. Strategies such as evidence-based medicine, which are already gaining importance, will support the integration of individual clinical expertise with the best available external evidence from research (Sackett and Richardson, 1997). Furthermore, a better-informed population will contribute to the popularization of preventive actions and the adoption of healthy lifestyles.

References

Adams, O.B. and Hirschfeld, M. "Human resources for Health: Challenges for the 21st Century." *World Health Statistics Quarterly.* (*Rapport Trimestriel de Statistiques Sanitaires Mondiales*). 1998. Geneva: World Health Organization, *51,* 28–32.

Federal Executive Branch. *Health Sector Reform Program, 1995–2000.* Mexico City: Federal Executive Branch, 1995.

Federal Ministry of Health. "Decentralization of the Health Services: The Challenge of Diversity." *Cuadernos de Salud, 4,* 1994.

Federal Ministry of Health. "Reform of the Health Sector: Improving the Health of Mexicans". *Cuadernos de Salud.* 5, 1994.

Federal Ministry of Health. *Activity Report 1997–1998.* Mexico City: Federal Ministry of Health, 1998.

National Population Council. *Population Projections for Mexico, 1996–2050.* Mexico City: National Population Council, 1996.

Organization for Economic Cooperation and Development. "Special Chapter: Health Sector Reform in Mexico." *OECD Economic Surveys, Mexico, 1997–1998.* Paris: OECD Publications, 1998.

Pan American Health Organization. *Health in Social Development: Position Paper of the World Health Organization.* Document Reproduction Series no. 51. Washington, D.C.: Public Policy and Health Program, Health and Human Development Division, 1995.

Sackett, D. L., Richardson, W. S., Rosenberg, W. and Haynes, R. B. *Evidence-Based Medicine: How to Practice and Teach.* New York: Churchill Livingstone, 1997.

World Bank. *World Development Report, 1993: Investing in Health.* Washington, D.C.: World Bank, 1993.

CHAPTER TWELVE

Canada

Irving Rootman, Trevor Hancock

*Irving Rootman, PhD, is Director of the Centre for Health
Promotion, a WHO collaborating center, and a professor in the
Department of Public Health Sciences at the University of
Toronto. Prior to joining the University of Toronto in 1990, he
worked for the Canadian Department of Health and Welfare
and as a consultant and senior scientist for the World Health
Organization.*

    *Trevor Hancock, MB, BS, MHSc, is an independent public
health physician and health promotion consultant. As a pioneer
of the healthy cities and communities movement, he has a long-
standing interest in the relationship between health, environment, and economy and in sustainable development.*

According to a recently released report on the health of
Canadians, *Toward a Healthy Future* (Federal, Provincial and Territorial Advisory Committee, 1999), we are by and large
healthy and are becoming healthier. For example, almost two-thirds
of adult Canadians say that their health is excellent or very good, and
fewer than 10 percent consider their health fair or poor. Life
expectancy in Canada is among the highest in the world, and infant
mortality has dropped below 6 per 1,000 live births, the lowest level
ever. In addition, Canada was ranked number one among more than

170 countries in the two last reports on the United Nations Index of Human Development.

However, *Toward a Healthy Future* also makes clear that this overall high standard of health is not shared equally by all Canadians. There are significant disparities in health status, depending on gender, age, socioeconomic status, place of residence, and other dimensions. In particular, Canada's aboriginal people usually experience the worst conditions and hence have the worst health status (Royal Commission on Aboriginal People, 1996). Recognizing these disparities, the United Nations report on human development took Canada to task for failing to ensure that every resident of Canada has a chance to enjoy the enviable living standards in the country. So although overall, the Canadian population tends to be healthy, there are important exceptions or areas for improvement.

WHAT MAKES CANADIANS HEALTHY OR UNHEALTHY?

Toward a Healthy Future used the health field concept (Lalonde, 1974) to analyze the determinants of the health of Canadians. It examined Canadian's health in relation to four key factors, or fields: *environment, lifestyle, health care organization,* and *human biology.*

Environment was divided into two categories—socioeconomic and physical. In relation to the former, the report noted that Canadians with low incomes were more likely to suffer illnesses and die early than those with high incomes and that the proportion with low-income status increased from 16 percent to 20 percent between 1990 and 1995. In addition, disparities in income between the wealthiest and poorest families in Canada seem to have grown over the past two decades. On the other hand, levels of schooling have risen for all population groups in Canada over the past fifteen years. The unemployment rate has also recently eased in Canada, although satisfaction with work has declined recently, especially among females. Canadians also report high levels of social support, caring for others, volunteerism, and civic participation. Thus there appear to be both positive and negative trends in aspects of the socioeconomic environment that affect the health of the people of Canada.

Similarly, from a global perspective, the quality of the *physical environment* in Canada is relatively good. Canada has one of the safest food supplies in the world, the quality of our air and drinking water is generally good, and the built environment is generally clean and healthy. However, there is a growing concern that some of the pollutants that we release into our environment will persist and pose a risk to human health. In addition, environmental tobacco smoke continues to be a health hazard. Access to affordable housing has become a major concern for many low-income Canadians, with as many as two hundred thousand estimated to be homeless or living in substandard housing.

With regard to *lifestyle,* generally, Canadians are making impressive efforts to improve their health. For example, almost half of Canadians reported changing some behavior to do so, and there has been a substantial decline in fatal motor vehicle accidents over the past twenty years, due in part to increased use of seat belts and reductions in impaired driving. On the other hand, rates of smoking among adolescents and youth, particularly young women, have increased in recent years, as has multiple drug use among high school students. Similarly, the proportion of overweight Canadians has increased steadily since 1985. So once again, there are mixed trends in relation to the lifestyle practices of Canadians.

As for *health care organization,* Canadians continue to enjoy and value universal access to publicly insured health services, although in the 1990s all of the provinces and territories underwent health care reform to varying degrees. Government efforts to improve their fiscal health, which resulted in significant cuts to health care expenditures in the 1990s, have taken their toll on the health care system, as well as on the public's confidence in it. Nevertheless, despite slowdowns in health care spending, most major measures of population health in Canada have continued to improve, and increases in health transfer payments from the federal government to the provinces have recently been announced.

Finally, with regard to *human biology,* Canadians have contributed to, learned from, and benefited from recent advances in biotechnology and genetic research. At the same time, the development of new reproductive and genetic technologies designed to overcome infertility or manipulate the conventional conception process have raised profound ethical, legal, social, and health issues that likely will become more important as science progresses. Increasingly, however, this new knowledge is being put into practice in our programs and policies.

HOW HEALTHY WILL CANADIANS BE IN THE FUTURE?

One way of considering the health of Canadians in the new century is simply to make projections based on recent information on our health status and trends. If we did this using the information presented here so far, we would reach the conclusion that even though some discrepancies between various groups in the population will probably still exist in twenty-five years, Canadians would generally still be relatively healthy in comparison to residents of other countries and to Canadians in the late twentieth century. Canada will also probably still be ranked relatively high on the UN Index of Human Development, although it may no longer be ranked first, perhaps as a result of improvements in other countries or a change in the index to take actions to address poverty into account. Such predictions are plausible and may well be borne out. However, the basis for making them would be shaky, in that they do not take into account the *trends* and possible *changes* in the determinants of health in the early twenty-first century.

So another approach to considering our health status in the twenty-first century would be to project *trends* in the determinants of health. If this were done, we might anticipate increasing discrepancies in income between rich and poor, increasing pollution, increasing heart disease and cancer related to general obesity and smoking among young women, and declining quality of care related to funding cutbacks, all of which might contribute to the decline in the health status of the population as a whole. On the other hand, positive trends that we have noted might counter the decline. Nevertheless, projecting trends in the determinants of health would probably lead us to predict that there may be an overall decline in the health of Canadians over the next twenty-five years.

However, this approach is also unsatisfactory because it does not take into consideration possible *changes* in the determinants of health or possible unpredictable events.

POSSIBLE CHANGES IN THE DETERMINANTS OF HEALTH

It is difficult to predict *changes* in the *socioeconomic environment* in Canada, or in any country for that matter, because there are so many factors that must be taken into consideration, many of them affecting the world as a whole. However, Canada's economic environment has been and is increasingly linked most strongly to that of the United States. Hence our economic fate in the twenty-first century is likely to hinge in large measure on the economic fate of the United States, and this will affect many of the social changes that will take place in Canada. Already we are seeing the influence of American approaches to welfare on our Canadian system, resulting in much less support for the poor and increasing hunger and homelessness. At the same time, Canada's own economic performance and infrastructure are likely to be key factors in our future prosperity, which is in turn linked to the health of the population. In the latter regard, the Conference Board of Canada recently expressed concern about Canada's innovation performance, labor productivity, adult training programs, and unemployment rate. If the Canadian economy does deteriorate, this will likely lead to widening gaps between rich and poor and negative impacts on the health of Canadians.

Similarly, if we consider possible changes in the *physical environment* in the twenty-first century, we would also predict a more substantial decline in health status. One important and often overlooked point is that the built environment is now our most important environment. We are 80 percent urbanized and spend 90 percent of our time indoors—and 5 percent in our cars! Thus how we design, build, and operate our cities, suburbs, neighborhoods, schools, workplaces, and homes will have an enormous impact on health. For example, continued urban sprawl and the resultant car-based society will increase air pollution, foster a sedentary lifestyle, and have many other significant health effects.

Turning to the *natural* environment, it has been suggested that there are four main aspects of global environmental change that will have an impact on human health: climate and atmospheric change, ecotoxicity, resource depletion, and reduced biodiversity (Hancock and Davies, 1997). With regard to the first, it is now widely accepted that human activity is contributing to global warming. The health impacts of global warming include increased mortality and morbidity from heat waves and severe weather events;, increases in a variety of infectious diseases, disruptions to food supplies, and rising sea levels that will displace large populations and create large numbers of "ecorefugees."

As for ecotoxicity, since the 1950s, people have been born with a body burden of persistent organic pollutants such as DDT and PCBs and have continued to be exposed throughout their lives to a multitude of toxic chemicals at very low levels. Thus we are nearly five decades into a major experiment to find out what happens when an entire cohort is exposed to such ecotoxicity throughout its life. While we do know that the average age of death for those born before 1930 is still increasing, we have absolutely no way of knowing what will be the average age of death of those born in the 1950s and thereafter. So we will just have to wait and see whether ecotoxicity shortens life, although there is already concern with respect to sexual and child development.

Among the key forms of resource depletion that we are beginning to experience in Canada and that are likely to increase in the new century are loss of topsoil and grasslands and the depletion of fisheries, resulting in the loss of livelihood of farmers and fishers and, in the worst case, malnutrition or famine; deforestation and depletion of aquifers and pollution of ground and surface waters, with an impact on agriculture and the provision of clean, safe water; and depletion of the fossil energy resources that power our industrial society. Finally, we are likely to continue to experience a loss of species diversity, leading to a fracturing of the web of life and threatening ecosystem stability and consequent effects on the health of Canadians.

The implications of all these major environmental changes for human health is significant, particularly on a global scale. The impacts in Canada will depend on a number of factors, including our ability to adapt to and cope with such changes, but it would not be unreasonable to expect that there will be some significant negative effects on the health of Canadians.

With regard to possible changes in *lifestyle* practices in the twenty-first century, it is possible that the serious economic and environmental changes that we have mentioned could lead to the adoption of practices that are more harmful to health. For example, they may lead to more drug use and other health-compromising attempts to cope with an increasingly unpleasant reality. In addition, the five-hundred-channel TV universe and telematics may contribute to an increasingly sedentary lifestyle. It is also possible that increasing global mobility will lead to the acceptance of more immigrants and refugees from other countries who may bring unhealthy lifestyles with them. Thus there is some reason to predict a deterioration of the health of Canadians on the basis of changes in lifestyle in the twenty-first century.

Similarly, it is possible that changes in *health care organization* in Canada will lead to a drop in the quality of services. For example, it is possible that with the increased influence of the United States on the Canadian economy and with increased pressures from globalization will come substantial pressure to abandon our current universal health system. This will certainly affect access to health services for Canadians with less financial resources but may also mean less coverage for the middle classes. Thus we have another reason to predict a deterioration in the health of Canadians in the twenty-first century.

On the other hand, it is possible that the advances in biotechnology, genetics, and information and communications technology that will undoubtedly take place in the twenty-first century will improve the health of Canadians. However, unless these new treatments are accessible to citizens with fewer resources, their impact on the health of the population may be marginal or may further widen the gap between rich and poor.

Overall, when we consider possible changes in the determinants of health in the twenty-first century, we come away with a much less optimistic assessment of the future health of Canadians than we made using the first two forecasting approaches. What, then, can Canada do to increase the likelihood of a more positive outcome?

WHAT CAN BE DONE TO IMPROVE THE HEALTH OF CANADIANS?

Toward a Healthy Future made a number of recommendations for action. Specifically, it recommended adopting three priorities: renewing and reorienting the health sector, investing in the health and well-being of key population groups, and reducing inequities in income distribution and in literacy and education. These recommendations are sensible and should, if properly implemented, increase the probability that Canadians will be healthy in the twenty-first century. However, aside from wondering whether governments, the business community, and other actors are committed to implementing these recommendations, we wonder whether the recommended actions are sufficient to address the changes in the determinants of health we anticipate. There is reason to believe that the predicted environmental changes will *not* be addressed adequately by these recommendations.

In the final analysis, given the potential threat to the environment and to our social capital and human resources posed by old-style economic growth, we believe that one of the fundamental challenges for the promotion of population health in the twenty-first century will be to *reinvent capitalism* so that we simultaneously increase all four forms of capital—ecological, social, economic, and human. Indeed, the true measure of progress in the new century will be an increase in human development, human potential, and human capital. At the same time, we will need to increase social and ecological capital and maintain an adequate level of prosperity to ensure health for all. How well we succeed will determine the health of the Canadian and global population in the twenty-first century.

References

Federal, Provincial and Territorial Advisory Committee on Population Health. *Toward a Healthy Future: Second Report on the Health of Canadians,* Ottawa: Health Canada, 1999.

Hancock, T., and Davies, K. *The Health Implications of Global Change: A Canadian Perspective.* Ottawa: Royal Society of Canada, Canadian Global Change Program, 1997.

Lalonde, M. *A New Perspective on the Health of Canadians.* Ottawa: Information Canada, 1974.

Royal Commission on Aboriginal People. *Gathering Strength.* Ottawa: Government of Canada, 1996.

PART TWO

The Organizational Landscape in Global Health

CHAPTER THIRTEEN

Infectious Diseases

William H. Foege

William H. Foege, MD, MPH, *is a professor of international health at the Rollins School of Public Health, Emory University. He served as Director for the Centers for Disease Control (CDC) from 1977 to 1983 and then as the Executive Director of the Carter Center and the Executive Director of the Task Force for Child Survival and Development.*

It is difficult to capture the feelings of people who lived through the terror of the great plagues of the past. In our time, AIDS comes closest to allowing us to identify with our ancestors, and yet within a few years of recognizing AIDS, there was an understanding of the means of transmission. In the past, epidemics were simply inexplicable. The apparent random selection of victims mixed with rumors and inaccurate information made every day a trial. Even as recently as the experience of our grandparents, children were lost to diphtheria, measles, and polio, and spouses succumbed to tuberculosis before they had seen their children grown. Young adults could leave for work in the morning and develop the symptoms of fatal influenza before their work shift had ended.

Someone has said that it is fine to predict the future if you don't actually believe what you have said. To predict the picture of infectious diseases in the next century is to realize that predictions of what the twentieth century would present in the area of infectious diseases, made in 1900, did not foresee antibiotics, the digital revolution, electron microscopes, or virus fingerprinting. Likewise, the twenty-first century cannot be mapped out with clarity. Yet some improvements appear almost certain, a few problems are already foreordained, while most things are simply unknowable.

Four improvements seem assured, despite the dynamism of infectious disease adaptability.

First is the primacy of immunization. Vaccines will continue to be the foundation of infectious disease control. Vaccines will improve in quality and specificity, and they will continue to get safer, with a continuing decline in adverse reactions. They will also increase in numbers. By midcentury, it seems likely that literally dozens of vaccines will be routinely given to children and increasingly to adults. The complicated schedules necessary at the end of the twentieth century will be simplified as vaccines are combined and the need for booster doses eliminated. The fears of the immunization process, engendered by needles and syringes, will be but a memory as vaccines are given by mouth, in food, or by transdermal application.

Smallpox was the only disease to be eliminated in the twentieth century. The first decade of the twenty-first century will add poliomyelitis and guinea worm. Measles will likely be next, and then, as tools, confidence, and global organization improve, the trickle will increase until dozens of infectious diseases have been vanquished. Why will this happen? Because the global public health world will learn to do two things at once: focus on a specific disease problem while strengthening the entire infrastructure for the delivery of health. It will become clear that eradication need be done only once in the history of the world, and therefore the benefit-cost ratio is the best available over the long term. It is an investment by current generations in the future health of everyone.

Second, while the miracle of vaccines will be the foundation of infectious disease control, treatment will also improve. The new century will usher in new chemotherapeutic agents, precise and specific in their antibacterial and antiviral activity. Understanding the genetic composition of organisms and the physiology of their growth and reproduction will suggest elegant ways of thwarting their fight for reproduction.

Third, diagnostic agents will become fast, specific, and reliable. Rapid saliva tests will make it possible to identify susceptible children who would benefit from immunization. Differences between the immunity engendered by measles vaccine versus measles disease, for example, will allow rapid evaluation of immunization coverage. Computer profiles of organisms or special reagents will permit immediate identification of organisms recovered from saliva, throat swabs, urine, or other body fluids, eliminating the need for awaiting laboratory growth of the organism. Distance diagnosis will be possible from the home of the patient.

Fourth, the digital revolution will not only improve diagnosis, tracking, and treatment but will also provide for early detection of outbreaks. Intelligent surveillance systems will detect unusual organisms or patterns of infectious organisms. Virtual systems will make it possible to assemble the necessary expertise to respond to and protect individuals or groups anyplace in the world.

The improvement in tools will be matched by improvements in organization. Smallpox eradication demonstrated the ability of the world, even during the cold war, to select a global objective, work in a concerted fashion to reach the objective, and share expertise, people, and resources across national boundaries. Why did the United States become involved in smallpox eradication at a time when there had not been a case of smallpox in this country for many years? Because no country is safe from infectious diseases unless all countries are safe, and the price to keep smallpox from this country finally became prohibitive compared to the cost of freeing the world of the disease. The desire to protect our own citizens forced a global approach.

At the start of the new century, the same global approach is being pursued with AIDS, polio, guinea worm, river blindness, lymphatic filariasis, and a handful of other health problems. But the lesson is apparently learned reluctantly and selectively.

Only recently, because of HIV/AIDS, emerging infections, and the fear of bioterrorism, has there been a concerted effort to organize the world in a more systematic manner. Protecting the world will require a comprehensive global surveillance system, capable of detecting and sharing information on the occurrence of all infectious diseases. It will also require a global approach to analyzing and predicting the course of disease, as well as a global approach to selecting the most appropriate interventions. Finally, it will require coordinated and unified programs in every country. A major lesson of recent decades has been that health advances are the result of coalitions, and the health leaders of the twenty-first century will be identified by their ability to assemble and motivate coalitions rather than by their title or identification with an agency.

The need for health successes is forcing the world to improve its global health agencies. In our frustration for progress, it is common to denigrate global health agencies. The truth is that we have only fifty years of experience with effective global health governance. The League of Nations experience was too fragmented, too short, and too political to draw firm lessons. Since World War II, the experiences of the World Health Organization, UNICEF, UNFPA, the World Bank, and the United Nations Development Program are actually very encouraging. We are learning how to improve the effectiveness of their work and the efficiency of their working together. Einstein reminded us that nationalism is an infantile disease. He called it the "measles of mankind." That provides a fitting mental picture for why infectious disease control will supersede nationalism in the twenty-first century and in so doing will strengthen the entire UN system.

The infectious diseases will do more than improve health or the agencies of global government: they will also provide a positive impetus for peace. The fear of infectious diseases is a common fear that requires a cooperative approach from opponents and even from combatants. Smallpox eradication workers found that they were allowed to work on both sides of coups, conflicts, and civil wars because both sides feared uncontrolled outbreaks. Later the same fears were tapped, even when the combatants themselves were not at risk, to arrange cease-fires or "days of tranquillity," in order to immunize children. In many cases, the combatants would use their vehicles to move vaccines and supplies for the immunization effort. In the 1990s, former U.S. President Jimmy Carter arranged for a cease-fire in the Sudan civil war to permit work on guinea worm, onchocerciasis, and polio eradication on both sides of the conflict. Experience has demonstrated the power of this concept. Countries and opposition groups, who work together because they have a common enemy in a microorganism, take a major step in learning how to work together for other objectives.

Globalism has developed of necessity in infectious disease control. The new century will see improvements in everything from scientific tools to organizational tools. Computer programs, for example, will assist in all aspects of immunization programs, from planning, logistics, and maintenance of supplies to tracking of children immunized and evaluation of programs. Creative combinations of public and private collaboration and incentive systems for health workers will provide and maintain successful infectious disease programs. Just as the current development of the integrated management of childhood illness (IMCI) was built on earlier models for diarrheal diseases, followed by the addition of acute respiratory infections and finally malaria, so will this in turn be replaced by computer-assisted approaches to the integrated management of childhood health (IMCH) and finally by the combining of all infectious disease problems, regardless of geography or age, into an integrated management of global health (IMGH).

On the negative side, what can we expect with some certainty? We can expect the continued evolution of microorganisms as they fulfill their Darwinian destiny to counter advances in control. The recent experiences with Lassa fever, Legionnaires' disease, Ebola virus, green monkey virus, toxic shock, Nipah virus, and HIV/AIDS lead to one conclusion: newly discovered infectious diseases will be the norm. Add the experience of multidrug-resistant tuberculosis (MDRTB), and we see the predictable outcome of organisms adapting, ecology changing, human lifestyles in transition, urbanization, and an aging population. The only mystery is where each new agent will first be identified, what the agent will be, what clinical syndrome will be involved and how prepared we will be to intervene.

The new century will also provide surprises regarding the role of infectious diseases in the pathogenesis of other diseases. The medical world was reluctant to believe a microorganism was involved as an etiologic agent for ulcers. The twenty-first century will disclose infectious diseases to be involved in a variety of cancers in addition to liver and cervical cancer. Explorations on the role of chlamydia in coronary heart disease will lead to many other investigations, and some will demonstrate infectious disease connections to everything from arthritis to mental illness.

The new century will have to deal with the problem of the marketplace and infectious diseases. Developing new antibiotics or antiparasitic agents leads quite naturally to marketing: drugs have to be sold to be profitable. Yet it is widespread use that leads to misuse and the development of resistance. The world will need to balance market needs and social needs. One company, GlaxoWellcome, is attempting such a balance with a new antimalarial drug, Malarone. The drug is being used under controlled conditions for selected patients who have either demonstrated resistance to first-line drugs or have such a high risk of mortality that one cannot wait for a trial with another drug. Those selected are treated for the required three days under direct observation. This greatly increases the complexity of infectious disease treatment in Africa and makes the effort more labor intensive. Yet it may be the most efficient approach in the long run. If the demonstrations show it is possible to have a major impact on health without risking rapid development of resistance, it could change the way new antimicrobials are introduced in the future.

Many infectious disease challenges will have to be met even if we cannot be certain of the methods that will be employed. How will the world respond to providing safe water and food? What impact will population pressures have on infectious disease transmission? What success will be achieved in modifying behavior that increases the risk of acquiring infectious diseases? What success will be achieved in improving nutritional status to reduce the impact of infectious diseases that will develop? Great mysteries exist regarding the type of new infectious diseases that will develop. The HIV virus literally disarmed us by taking a new evolutionary step, attacking the very system designed to provide us protection. What if a new agent with a similar ability also had the ability to spread with the rapidity of influenza and overwhelm the immune system in hours rather than years? The nuclear arms race convinced many people that no scenario is unthinkable. Could the nuclear fears be replaced by bioterrorism fears where the ingenuity of scientists and the increasingly powerful tools of science combine to create epidemics that cannot be controlled?

Richard Feynman, in a 1963 lecture at the University of Washington on the uncertainty of science, quoted from an inscription that he credited to a Buddhist temple. "To every man is given the key to the gates of heaven. The same key opens the gates of hell." This is the uncertainty of the twenty-first century. Will our abilities in science turn against us?

In 1265, Pope Clement asked Roger Bacon for a summary of science. Roger Bacon was no ordinary scientist. He predicted the use of automobiles and airplanes and had an uncanny ability to anticipate the future. In his summary, he spoke of the beauty and power of science, but he concluded that science lacked a moral compass, and then, at some risk, in a day when the church had such power, he attacked the papal court for having failed to provide such guidance. If Roger Bacon would return today to anticipate the interplay of science and infectious diseases in the twenty-first century, it is likely that his fear would still be that science lacks a moral compass and always will. But even more important, would he still be disappointed to find a society where governments, both global and local, faith groups, universities, service agencies, political parties and others fail to provide the necessary guidance to ensure that *all* share in the benefits of science and are protected from its misuse?

CHAPTER FOURTEEN

Chronic Disease

James S. Marks, David V. McQueen

James S. Marks, MD, MPH, *became Director of the National Center for Chronic Disease Prevention and Health Promotion (NCCDPHP) at the Centers for Disease Control and Prevention in Atlanta in 1995. The following year, he was sworn in as an Assistant Surgeon General of the United States. He plays a major role in shaping the direction of research and practice in chronic disease prevention in the United States.*
David V. McQueen, ScD, is Associate Director for Global Health Promotion at the NCCDPHP. He has been active in health promotion and health behavior research in the United States and Europe for more than thirty years.

Historically a burden for industrialized nations, chronic diseases had dramatically altered the health of the global population by the start of the twenty-first century. It is not simply that infectious, communicable disease has declined but also that the success of public health has allowed populations to survive, age, and, alas, acquire the diseases of privilege, including the privilege of age. At the dawn of the new century, deaths from chronic diseases outpaced deaths from communicable diseases in every part of the world except sub-Saharan Africa and the Middle East and now account for 60 percent of all deaths globally. Of course, deaths explain only a fraction of the impact of chronic disease; individuals with chronic diseases live for long periods, with the concomitant suffering and financial impact.

Recently, the World Bank and the World Health Organization (WHO) engaged a large team of experts to produce a systematic and comprehensive estimate of the relative impact of the major diseases affecting populations around the world. Titled *The Global Burden of Disease* (Murray and Lopez, 1996), this work presents a picture of mortality and morbidity for the major regions of the world. Using an index called a disability-adjusted life year (DALY) that combines the number of years of life lost from premature death with the loss of health from disease and disability, the DALY provides a way to assess both suffering and death on a worldwide basis. At the beginning of the new century, heart disease, diabetes, depression, and injuries have become the major global health problems. This is the inherited burden awaiting the twenty-first-century solutions.

The improvement in the length of life has resulted from two main factors. First, socioeconomic conditions improved throughout much of the world during the twentieth century. Second, major public health achievements of the past century, including vaccination, the control of infectious diseases, and general sanitary improvement, have led to longer life spans and lower mortality worldwide. Statistical projections are that this transition from acute to chronic conditions will accelerate in the next fifty years, leading to radically different disease patterns across the globe.

A plethora of terms is used to delineate chronic diseases internationally. Whatever terminology is used, chronic diseases are generally characterized by long duration, unlikelihood of cure, noncontagion, and complex causality. Internationally, many health organizations, such as the World Health Organization, refer to these as *noncommunicable diseases* (NCDs). Nevertheless, many communicable or infectious diseases have chronic sequelae. Furthermore, although risk behaviors may not be contagious, they spread among populations through the media, popular entertainment, and advertising in a manner that mimics an epidemic.

For a person with a chronic disease, it is the experience that counts; it takes little definitional artistry for one to distinguish when one is afflicted by a long, sometimes painful, and sometimes debilitating illness in the course of life. Beyond the individual level, what distinguishes most chronic diseases is that they are often the product of a combination of socioenvironmental and behavioral factors. Thus in contrast to infectious diseases, the causal agents are complex and multilevel. Importantly, many sociocultural factors influencing the development, spread, and persistence of chronic disease are tied to macro-level factors such as poverty, race, social status, education, work, and income.

The United Nations classifies countries by level of development based on (1) gross domestic product (GDP) per capita; (2) augmented physical quality of life (APQL), a measure that includes life expectancy, per capita calorie supply, school enrollment, and adult literacy; and (3) an index of economic diversification. Countries of the world are classified into least developed countries (LDC), developing countries (excluding LDCs), economies in transition, and developed market economies. In 1994, forty-eight countries were classified as LDCs.

The World Bank classifies countries chiefly by income into four categories: low-income (for example, Afghanistan), lower-middle-income (Algeria), upper-middle-income (Argentina), and high-income (Australia). Of the ten countries that together contain more than 60 percent of the global population, four are in the low-income group (Bangladesh, India, Nigeria, Pakistan), three are in the lower-middle-income group (China, Indonesia, Russia), one is in the upper-middle-income group (Brazil), and two are in the high-income group (Japan, United States). Despite this variation in wealth, very few countries have life expectancies below sixty years, and many have life expectancies in the seventies and even eighties.

TRENDS

The most visible demographic trend affecting chronic disease is the aging of the world population. Whereas improvements in the control of diseases early in life led to the health transition in the twentieth century, aging of the population in the first quarter of the twenty-first century will be the major force in the further tremendous increase in the burden of chronic diseases. The statistics are consequential: at the end of the twentieth century, more than half the elderly, defined as persons aged sixty-five years or older, lived in the developing world; by 2025, this will increase to nearly 70 percent. Absolute numbers of elderly in the world will grow from around four hundred million now to around a billion and a half by 2050. In addition, if present trends continue, the proportion of the oldest old, defined as having reached the age of eighty, will also increase dramatically. At the close of the twentieth century, in Scandinavia, the oldest old accounted for nearly 5 percent of the population.

There are many notable effects of this drastic population transition. Economic impacts are pronounced and exacerbated by the phenomenon of labor force participation rates declining in most of the developing world. In seemingly direct contradiction to the increase in life span has been a lowering of retirement age. This picture places heavy burdens on old-age economic security programs and on the shrinking proportion of the population that is working. Related to this economic impact is the effect on health care expenditures.

World Bank estimates are that by 2050, most developed countries will be consuming a quarter of public funding on pension and health costs. Further, many developing economies will be having very similar age structures and, by intuition, similar chronic disease impacts. Unfortunately, the developing countries are growing old faster than they are growing rich.

The implications for medical care, quality of life, burden of disease, and suffering because of this massive health transition to chronic disease in the elderly are profound. The Western solutions to health care in older populations are probably inappropriate for most of the globe, but feasible alternative models have not yet appeared.

IMPACT ON CHRONIC DISEASES THROUGH THE LIFE COURSE

Careful research in chronic disease epidemiology has linked lifestyle— personal behaviors and their associated risk to health—with morbidity and mortality. This research has been largely repeated worldwide with a significant emphasis on the three principal lifestyle behaviors relative to chronic diseases: smoking, diet, and physical activity. Of note is the relationship of these lifestyle behaviors with aging. Lifestyle practices are not consistent in magnitude and pattern over the life course, and many chronic diseases manifest themselves very late in relationship to the putative lifestyle causes.

Although the research literature on lifestyle and health is extensive, it is largely limited to North America, Europe, and Australia. However, it is likely that many observed relationships between behavior and illness would hold for the less developed world. This assertion is already well manifested with regard to tobacco, although most countries are still in the epidemic phase of the health consequences of this behavior. As surely as night follows day, this presages increases in cardiovascular disease (CVD), cancer, and lung diseases. In fact, the *Global Burden of Disease* project estimates that tobacco will be the leading cause of DALYs by 2020. It is also reasonable to assume that other lifestyle practices will lead to chronic disease patterns reflecting those in the West.

One thing is certain—lifestyle plays a critical role in CVD. In the developed world, it has long been the leading cause of death and disability. At the end of the twentieth century, CVD accounted for around 20 percent of all deaths globally. A great emerging cause of death and disability in the developing economies, it is already the leading cause of death in countries from Argentina to Russia. Despite economic growth, we anticipate that CVD, barring startling preventive interventions, will be the leading cause of death and disability throughout the world for the foreseeable future.

The pattern of CVD mortality is extraordinarily diverse throughout the world, and even within countries there is considerable variation by age, race, and gender. For example, in the United States, the age-adjusted mortality rate for men in 1995 was 55 percent higher than for women, and age-adjusted mortality rates were considerably less for white men and women than for blacks. Ethnic variation is considerable, with Asian and Hispanic Americans displaying considerable variation from the Northern European–derived white population. It is notable that the United States is about in the middle of the industrialized nations (sixteenth out of thirty-five) in CVD mortality rates, although the country has experienced a substantial decline in mortality over the past three decades. The U.S. experience illustrates the difficulties of making any simple generalizations about country comparisons at the global level.

The global situation for CVD was captured well in a recent Institute of Medicine Report titled *Control of Cardiovascular Diseases in Developing Countries* (1998):

> It is surprising that CVD ranked second as a cause of death in all developing countries in 1990. . . . Given the falling rates of infectious and parasitic diseases and the increasing rates of CVD in developing countries, CVD was most likely the developing world's leading cause of death by the mid-1990s. If ignored, this epidemic will increase drastically in the coming years. . . . Evidence shows that in 1990, CVD

contributed to three times as many deaths worldwide in 30- to 69-year-old men and women as did infectious and parasitic diseases. This is true for all regions of the world except Sub-Saharan Africa. This burden of disease and death in the economically most productive age stratum has important consequences for health care resources and for the economy in general [p. 77].

Although we have discussed CVD in this chapter, similar scenarios fit other chronic diseases such as cancer and diabetes, where projections are for large increases in burden over the next several decades.

THE DESPAIR

There is reason for concern when considering the worldwide chronic disease picture in the new century. The Western experience during industrialization may be repeated, although more rapidly. Already this is occurring in the middle-income countries with the rapid adoption of tobacco use, less physical activity, and a higher-fat diet. In fact, the wide penetration of mass media and advertising messages means that in a very real sense, the chronic conditions may now be the most communicable of diseases, with rates being influenced by exposures generated thousands of miles away from the victims.

Another reason for despair is the overwhelming threat of the cost of care for chronic diseases even at the most basic level. The aging of the population worldwide means that the increasing burden of disease threatens to bankrupt countries if they attempt anything resembling Western case practices. Nonetheless, there is a seeming lack of strong political concern with chronic disease in developing countries. The mortality caused by infectious diseases is still highly visible and extensive in much of the developing world. This demands immediate attention and uses the scant health resources available for control and elimination. Furthermore, years of building public health systems around infectious disease control has resulted in few health professionals with expertise in chronic diseases as part of the public health infrastructure. The Western-based public health professionals and epidemiologists who have witnessed the great transition in the developed countries have themselves only recently begun to grasp the global significance of the prevention, care, and treatment of chronic disease in the developing world. Finally, the main levers for prevention often are policy changes that affect powerful commercial interests and hence are resisted by those interests.

THE HOPE

Given the projected global trends, it is easy to be pessimistic about the prospects for lessening the burden of chronic disease. However, when one looks back at the achievements in public health in the twentieth century, an optimistic picture emerges. Life expectancies in the past century increased by more than thirty years in many countries, yet at the beginning of the century, there was ample reason for concern. The etiology for the leading causes of death, such as tuberculosis, was just becoming known, and our understanding of the role of sanitation in combating diarrhea was in its early stages. A century later, much is known about the leading causes of chronic disease and its burden; this understanding will surely lead to developments in treatment and prevention.

The success of global public health will be met if certain challenges are addressed. First, there is a worldwide need for better information and surveillance systems to track the emergence and patterns of the major risk factors for chronic disease, particularly those behavioral risk factors that public health programs should address. It can be asserted that the understanding of risk factor trends and patterns will lead to an informed public health practice that addresses determinants of these risks and thus to the amelioration of chronic diseases. Second, we must harness the global developments in information technology to develop health promotion strategies that address the diverse needs of population groups and deprived groups and to help us identify rapidly and reach groups in need. Just as media and information technology have been used to encourage tobacco use, they can become a powerful force for health.

We can also be optimistic because of the quickly occurring transition in information dissemination. Evidence of best practices in public health intervention can be made electronically available everywhere in the world in an instant. Limited resources in developing countries may be offset by more accurate and more useful information on what works to address chronic disease. The developing countries may be able to avoid a large part of the epidemic and more rapidly embrace the solutions.

CONCLUSION

In the twenty-first century, the chronic diseases will be the principal global health problems. The rapidly aging world population exacerbates this trend. The costly medical care that accompanies many chronic diseases will continue to have an economic impact on all countries and present tremendous challenges to the poorer countries. Behavioral and lifestyle risks increasingly imported from developed countries foreshadow continued growth of these problems.

Over this seemingly gloomy picture of chronic disease and illness in the twenty-first century must be laid the hope of public health efforts. In truth, public health has produced remarkable achievements for most of the world. Indeed, the rise and dominance of chronic diseases by the end of the twentieth century could be viewed as the consequence of success. Because we were so successful at conquering communicable diseases and extending life expectancy in the past century, we must now grapple with the increased incidence of chronic diseases. We must also seek to eliminate disparities between populations in a world that is increasingly tied together socially and economically and in supporting the quality of our now longer lives.

References

Institute of Medicine, Board on International Health. *Control of Cardiovascular Diseases in Developing Countries.* Washington, D.C.: National Academy Press, 1998.

Murray, C.J.L., and Lopez, A. D. *The Global Burden of Disease: A Comprehensive Assessment of Mortality and Disability from Diseases, Injuries, and Risk Factors in 1990 and Projected to 2020.* Cambridge, Mass.: Harvard University Press, 1996.

Additional Reading

Anand, S., and Hanson, K. "Disability-Adjusted Life Years: A Critical Review." *Journal of Health Economics,* 1997, 685–702.

Beaglehole, R., and Bonita, R. *Public Health at the Crossroads: Achievements and Prospects.* Cambridge University Press, 1997.

Belloc, N. B. "Relationship of Health Practices and Mortality." *Preventive Medicine,* 1973, 67–81.

Berkman, L. F., and Breslow, L. *Health and Ways of Living: The Alameda County Study.* Oxford: Oxford University Press, 1983.

Brownson, R. C., Remington, P. L., Davis, J. R. (Eds.). *Chronic Disease Epidemiology and Control,* (Second Edition). American Public Health Association, 1998.

Caldwell, J. C. "Health Transition: The Cultural, Social, and Behavioural Determinants of Health in the Third World. *Social Science Medicine,* 1993, *36,* 125–135.

Centers for Disease Control and Prevention. "Ten great public health achievements—United States, 1900–1999." *Mortality and Morbidity Weekly Report,* 1999, *48*(12), 241–243.

Epstein, F. H. "The Relationship of Lifestyle to International Trends in C.H.D." *International Journal of Epidemiology,* 1989, *18*(3 Suppl. 1), S203–S209.

Foege, W. H. "Preventive Medicine and Public Health." *Journal of the American MediCal Association,* 1993, *270,* 251–252.

Fries, J. F. "Aging, Natural Death, and the Compression of Morbidity." *New England Journal of Medicine,* 1980, *303,* 130–135.

Institute of Medicine. Board on International Health. *America's Vital Interest in Global Health.* Washington, D.C.: National Academy Press, 1997.

Labarthe, D. R. *Epidemiology and Prevention of Cardiovascular Diseases: A Global Challenge.* Gaithersburg, Maryland: Aspen Publishers, Inc., 1998.

Mackay, J. *The State of Health Atlas.* New York: Simon and Schuster, 1998.

Murray, C.J.L., and Lopez, A. D. "Regional Patterns of Disability-Free Life Expectancy and Disability-Adjusted Life Expectancy: Global Burden of Disease Study." *Lancet,* 1997, *349,* 1347–1352.

Murray, C.J.L., and Lopez, A. D. *Global Health Statistics: A Compendium of Incidence, Prevalence, and Mortality Estimates for Over 200 Conditions.* Harvard School of Public Health, World Health Organization and the World Bank, 1996.

Murray, C.J.L., and Lopez, A. D. *The Global Burden of Disease: A Comprehensive Assessment of Mortality and Disability from Diseases, Injuries, and Risk Factors in 1990 and Projected to 2020.* Harvard School of Public Health, World Health Organization and the World Bank, 1996.

Orman, A. R. (1971). The Epidemiologic Transition: A Theory of the Epidemiology of Population Change. *Milbank Memorial Fund Quarterly,* 1971, *49,* 509–538.

Report of a Conference on Trends and Determinants of Coronary Heart Disease Mortality: International Comparisons. *International Journal of Epidemiology,* 1989, *18*(suppl1), S1-S232.

Rose, G. "Causes of the Trends and Variations in C.H.D. Mortality in Different Countries." *International Journal of Epidemiology*, 1989, *18*(3, Suppl. 1), S174–S179.

Thom, T. J., and Epstein, F. H. "Heart Disease, Cancer, and Stroke Mortality Trends and Their Interrelationships. An International Perspective." *Circulation*, 1994, *90*, 574–582.

Vita, A. J., Terry, R. B., Hubert, H. B., and Fries, J. F. "Aging, Health Risks, and Cumulative Disability." *New England Journal of Medicine*, 1998, *338*, 1035–1041.

World Bank. *World Development Report 1993: Investing in Health*. New York: Oxford University Press, 1993.

World Health Organization. *The World Health Report 1997: Conquering Suffering Enriching Humanity*. Geneva: World Health Organization, 1998.

World Health Organization. *The World Health Report: Life in the 21st Century, a Vision for All*. Geneva: World Health Organization, 1998.

World Health Organization. *The World Health Report: Making a Difference*. Geneva: World Health Organization, 1999.

World Health Organization. *Tobacco or Health: First Global Status Report*. Geneva: World Health Organization, 1996.

CHAPTER FIFTEEN

Mental Health

Eugene B. Brody

Eugene B. Brody, MD, *Professor and Chairman Emeritus of psychiatry at the University of Maryland, is currently on the faculties of the Harvard Medical School and the Johns Hopkins University School of Public Health and is Editor in Chief of the* Journal of Nervous and Mental Disease. *He is the Senior Consultant to the World Federation for Mental Health and served as its President from 1981 to 1983 and its Secretary General from 1983 to 1999.*

The leading contemporary perspective on global mental health is that of the World Federation for Mental Health (WFMH), the oldest citizen-based nongovernmental mental health organization in official relations with UN agencies. Its August 1948 founding document, *Mental Health and World Citizenship,* defined mental health as a condition that permits the "optimal" physical, intellectual, and emotional development of the individual, "insofar as this is compatible with that of other individuals" (p. 277). The goal of mental health was to help people "live with their fellows in one world" (p. 304). This perspective foreshadowed the UN's Universal Declaration of Human Rights, approved by the General Assembly in December 1948. Both implied that contexts that respect human rights, including those for self-expression and self-determination, permit the realization of individual potential, contribute to the availability of personal opportunity, and foster health and well-being. Conversely, violating human rights can result in serious emotional distress and impaired mental health. As the twenty-first century begins, WFMH's concern has become more focused on the prevention of mental illness and the well-being and rights of people defined as mentally ill.

The concept of a normal state called "health" arose in the middle-class cultures of industrial societies. Prior to World War II, Sigmund Freud described mentally healthy middle-class Viennese as those with the capacity to work, love, and play. Contemporary scientists in the developed world include optimal functioning (within the limits of one's capacities) and resilience, the ability to adapt, cope, and rally in the face of stress or adversity.

The mental health of both individuals and populations varies with age, gender, ethnicity, nationality, geographical locality, cultural context, and socioeconomic status. It is impaired by conditions that degrade the quality of life and create acute or chronic stress. Among them are collective violence (including war and its consequences), poverty, illiteracy, lack of access to health care, forced dislocation from home and community, and chronic restrictions of freedom or violations of human rights. Impairment may be revealed in failed capacities or in psychological and emotional symptoms, sometimes sufficient to result in a diagnosis of mental illness.

The mental health of communities in the industrial democracies has been estimated by social scientists on the basis of indices of social disorganization. These are rates of divorce, unmarried or adolescent pregnancies, single-parent families, high school dropouts, arrests, and unemployment, as well as social isolation indicated by lack of membership in such institutions as churches, labor unions, and social clubs. They also include behaviors corollary to the presence of mental illness or a disordered personality: violent acts including spouse and child abuse, hospitalizations for alcoholism, substance abuse, and mental disease.

MENTAL HEALTH IN THE TWENTY-FIRST CENTURY

Most trends of the late twentieth century will probably continue, at least for the near term.

Poverty

It has been estimated that one-fifth of the world's population lives in abject poverty, with 80 percent of these people in rural areas. Children who grow up in the least advantaged socioeconomic stratum of any society are less likely to develop optimally, physically or mentally, than those in the more advantaged socioeconomic strata. Contributing factors include malnutrition, inadequate shelter and sanitation, lack of education, and lack of access to medical care, as well as physical and emotional stress, disturbed socialization, abuse, and frustration. However, there is no incontrovertible evidence that poverty, as such, increases the likelihood of psychotic disease.

Women's Mental Health and Well-Being

In most of the world's societies, women and girls are in the position of a functional minority. However, with encouragement both from the United Nations and nongovernmental organizations (NGOs), the last two decades of the twentieth century witnessed a slow rise in women's social and economic status, freedom, and literacy worldwide. This has been accompanied by an increased ability to control their own fertility, reflected in longer intervals between births and increased acceptance of careers for women beyond that of motherhood. The practice of ritual genital mutilation, traditional in some societies, is being outlawed and progressively abandoned. These trends should continue. On the other hand, perhaps related to the speed of social change, there has been a marked increase in the reported incidence of violence against women.

Children

Child survival improved in the last decades of the twentieth century. However, the impact of poverty persists. Children in economically marginal areas are three to five times more likely than those from more affluent families to suffer from epilepsy or mental retardation. The adult capacities and behaviors of the millions of homeless "street children" in Latin America and Asia are difficult to predict. The children of the rural poor, who are disproportionately represented in the populations displaced by civil war, are most apt to be drafted by warring groups and injured by armed conflict. In many of these societies, young children must also engage in exhausting labor that is physically and mentally harmful. In others, they are subject to commercial sexual exploitation. NGOs, individual governments, UNICEF, and the International Labor Organization (ILO) are trying to correct these conditions and to reduce the impact of neglect and abuse. The immediate outcome is uncertain, but it is hoped that these conditions will improve rather than worsen as the twenty-first century wears on. Hopeful signs for the future are the increased use of family planning and perinatal care, leading to smaller and healthier families.

The Aging Population

WHO sources indicate that the average life expectancy of human beings increased by thirty years during the twentieth century. The overall population is becoming older, with a corresponding reduction in the numbers of people of prime working age. By 2020, the number of persons aged sixty years or more is expected to exceed one billion. This will require changes in insurance, health systems, social services, and employment practices, all of which will have an impact on the well-being of this population. Anecdotal evidence indicates that people, especially in the industrial democracies, are in fact continuing to be socially and productively engaged with others at considerably older ages than before. It seems likely that this trend will continue in the new century. Whether it will be true for the still developing countries is unclear.

Refugees

Perhaps the greatest global mental health problem of the late twentieth century was posed by the millions of people forcibly dislocated from their homes and communities by war or political oppression, who were often separated from their families, subject to assault, and sometimes tortured. Their impaired mental health has been documented in terms of not only posttraumatic stress syndromes but also the full range of diagnosable psychiatric afflictions. Refugees are typically thought of as crossing national borders, but large numbers have been "internally displaced," living as refugees in their own countries and sometimes actively persecuted by their own governments. Available data indicate a reduction from a peak of 17.6 million refugees and asylum seekers worldwide in 1992 to 13.6 million in 1997—prior to the Balkan wars of 1998 and 1999. Some are in camps of temporary asylum in other countries. Some have already been repatriated—occasionally on an involuntary basis. Others are being permanently settled in third countries. The treatment of torture survivors has become a specialty in itself. Centers in many countries specialize in the study and treatment of traumatized refugees. In this sense, it is possible to see some advances in dealing with the impaired mental health of these traumatized people. There may also be some reason to hope that as the United Nations and its regional organizations become more effective, the circumstances that produce refugees will gradually diminish. In its 1998 report, however, the office of the UN High Commissioner for Refugees (UNHCR) expressed deep concern about what it perceived as the continuing erosion of respect for human rights, especially in regard to governmental dealings with refugees, including the granting of asylum.

MENTAL DISEASE AND ITS BURDEN IN THE TWENTY-FIRST CENTURY

The nature and frequency of diagnosable mental disease will be determined by demographic changes in the world's population and by environmental stresses.

Increasing Population and Diseases of Old Age

The World Bank estimates that there will be as many as 8.4 billion people in the world by 2025, compared to 5.4 billion in 1995. With the increasing proportion of elderly people, the risk of disease will be reflected in both increasing rates of illness and greater absolute numbers of sick people. This will be especially marked for degenerative brain disease reflected in dementia of various forms. It has been estimated that the number of demented elderly in Africa, Asia, and Latin America may exceed 80 million by 2025. Old age also increases the risk of suffering from depression of varying intensity. It seems probable that these trends will continue well into the twenty-first century. At the same time, more attention is being paid to the problems of caregivers, and it is probable that changes in social organization will develop to deal with this increasing burden.

Diagnosable Mental Illness

As the population of people aged fifteen to forty-five increases, greater absolute numbers will suffer from diseases that characteristically appear in young adulthood, such as schizophrenia. Its prevalence is estimated as relatively stable, between 1.0 and 1.5 percent worldwide. The total number of people ill with schizophrenia is estimated to have increased from 16.7 million to 24.4 million between 1985 and 2000.

Affective disorders, mainly psychotic depression or mania, appear to be increasing in frequency as well as absolute numbers and appearing at younger ages. It is estimated that half or more suicide victims in the United States suffer from major depression. But although suicide is among the top ten causes of death in countries that report rates, most observers believe that it is a seriously underreported event. Some informed guesses about the future of suicide suggest that it will not be less than in the twentieth century and that due to changes in the perceived meaning of life, it may increase in prevalence.

The syndromes known as posttraumatic stress disorders are ubiquitous in populations of refugees and other traumatized individuals. Other nonpsychotic disorders such as anxiety, panic attacks, phobias, and mild depressive states are also responses to stress. They are present in approximately 5 to 20 percent of the world's populations, with regional variations. These prevalence rates may be expected to continue into the foreseeable future. Understanding and treating such disorders requires a knowledge of how they are conceived in particular cultural settings.

It seems likely that in the twenty-first century, the increasing burden of chronic or recurrent psychotic illness may be alleviated by increased facilities for dealing with afflicted individuals in community settings. If the twentieth-century speed of medical innovation is maintained, it is possible that new pharmacological and other treatments will stem the increases. Meanwhile, hopeful developments include a gradual diminution in the stigma attached to mental or emotional illness, an increased willingness to involve ex-patients themselves in the treatment or management process, and increased interest by Western psychiatrists in approaches used elsewhere in the world. These include using extended family members in supportive roles and nonpharmacological relaxation techniques. Since so many depressed people present themselves with medical symptoms, it is essential to train primary health care personnel to recognize and treat depression.

Major trends in the treatment of nonpsychotic disorders include the combination of pharmacotherapy with psychotherapy and the increased psychotherapeutic sophistication of nonmedical personnel such as psychologists and social workers. A major obstacle to be overcome is the reluctance of some third-party payers to support such treatment.

Substance Abuse

The late twentieth century witnessed both absolute and relative increases in the pathologies associated with all forms of substance abuse, including alcoholism. The absolute increase can be attributed to population growth, but the relative increase has been attributed to rapid social change (including urbanization, weakened family structures, and the loosening of cultural standards), lack of employment and other opportunities, and repressive social institutions. Public education has been effective only in limited areas for short periods of time. Substance supply reduction strategies, such as crop destruction and interdiction, have not been effective. However, there are some suggestions that reducing demand through treatment and education and reducing supply by fostering more economically rewarding work for growers may have potential. The decriminalization of narcotic use as a means of reducing its incidence continues to be debated.

Violence

Individual as well as collective violence has increased in recent decades. This reflects in part the absolute increases in population and in part the same factors that influence substance abuse. Gun control has been relatively effective in reducing murder rates in some parts of the world. The violent behavior of individuals, as well as substance abuse, will increasingly be regarded as public health problems.

CONCLUSION

In the early twenty-first century, increasing population density, with an increased proportion of older people worldwide, will continue the trend toward greater absolute numbers and proportions of people suffering from nervous and mental disease of all kinds. Similarly, the persistent poverty of large segments of the world population will continue its adverse impact on mental health. These continuing trends may be offset to some degree by improvements in the socioeconomic status and literacy of women, permitting more effective family planning and perinatal care. The trends are also being met by improved systems of community-based rehabilitation for mentally ill persons, increased mental health training for primary health workers, efforts to upgrade the quality of mental health services in the less developed world, and increasing public education leading to the destigmatization of mental illness. Research on the etiology and primary and secondary prevention of mental disorders and on their psychosocial and pharmacological treatment will accelerate in the new century, and some problems currently viewed as intractable may be solved.

References

U.S. Committee for Refugees. *World Refugee Survey 1998. An Annual Assessment of Conditions Affecting Refugees, Asylum Seekers and Internally Displaced Persons.* Washington, D.C.: Immigration and Refugee Services of America, 1998.

Additional Reading

Brody, E. B. *Mental Health and World Citizenship: The View from an International, Nongovernmental Organization.* Austin, Texas: Hogg Foundation for Mental Health, 1987.

Brody, E. B. *The Search for Mental Health. A History and Memoir of WFMH 1948–1998.* Baltimore: Williams and Wilkins Co., 1998.

Desjarlais, R., Eisenberg, L., Good, and B., Kleinman, A. *World Mental Health. Problems and Priorities in Low-Income Countries.* New York: Oxford University Press, 1995.

CHAPTER SIXTEEN

Tropical Diseases

Joseph A. Cook

Joseph A. Cook, MD, is Executive Director of the International Trachoma Initiative, an organization founded by Pfizer Inc. and the Edna McConnell Clark Foundation to eliminate the world's leading cause of preventable blindness. Director of tropical disease research for the Edna McConnell Clark Foundation for more than two decades, Dr. Cook is a past president of the American Society of Tropical Medicine and Hygiene.

In this era of globalization, it may seem anachronistic to think about "tropical diseases" and, moreover, what a discipline related to that concept entails in modern times. Many of the diseases that are traditionally classified under this rubric, such as malaria and trachoma, were once familiar to the now industrialized world. However, because these diseases faded or were brought under control in industrialized countries during the early part of the twentieth century, tropical diseases became largely defined as the endemic and epidemic infections causing disease and disability for residents and visitors in the warmer climates of the world.

Although these diseases continue to account for significant rates of death and disability in the developing world, it is important to recognize that tropical diseases, despite their name, are not necessarily *caused* by climate or geography. To some extent, these diseases exist because poor and disadvantaged people do not have access to the public health infrastructure that is available to people in the industrialized world. Therefore, tropical diseases are better understood as diseases of the poor in the developing world while keeping in mind that these diseases have the potential for spreading beyond the boundaries of the warmer climates. For example, tuberculosis and HIV/AIDS inflict the greatest burden on the poor in the tropical developing world but are public health threats in the industrialized world as well.

The study of tropical diseases focuses on how to make the new tools of medical science and disease control accessible to large population groups in areas where both trained health personnel and economic support are scarce. Scientific advances based on new technologies and a growing knowledge of host-parasite relationships suggest that the enormous burden inflicted by these diseases, particularly in developing countries, can be considerably lightened. Some of the progress will result from a slow improvement of economic conditions in these countries, and consequently, social conditions and standards of hygiene and nutrition will get better. On the other hand, the following pages will describe the current impact and the progress that can be expected if both new technologies and deliberate economic improvement are applied for the control of some common tropical diseases. Actual eradication of an organism or disease may be rare, but several diseases, including guinea worm, onchocerciasis, Chagas' disease, lymphatic filariasis, leprosy, and trachoma, can be eliminated as public health problems early in the twenty-first century. Other common tropical diseases, however, including malaria, cholera, and dengue, require more caution, continued vigilance, and additional research if elimination is to be possible.

TROPICAL DISEASES
SLATED FOR EXTINCTION

Most of the diseases on the verge of extinction are currently being conquered by pharmacological means, though the elimination of poverty during the twentieth century has restricted many of them to smaller and hence more successfully treatable areas.

Dracunculiasis

Commonly known as guinea worm, *Dracunculus medinensis* is a parasite, transmitted to humans by drinking water contaminated with tiny crustaceans (copepods) that contain immature forms of the parasite. One year after the ingestion of contaminated water, adult female worms up to one meter long emerge through the skin in the lower part of the body. This causes a painful sore that prevents children from attending school and adults from working—incapacitation for two to three months is not unusual. Water sources are contaminated when an infected human immerses the body part with the emerging adult worm in that water source. Each adult worm ejects hundreds of thousands of larvae into the water.

Dracunculiasis can be prevented by providing safe sources of drinking water, filtering contaminated water through cloth filters to remove the copepods, or using a harmless chemical, temephos (Abate), to kill the crustacean host of the parasite in open ponds and sources of drinking water. Efforts to eradicate guinea worm began in 1980, and within sixteen years, the total number of world cases had been reduced by 48 percent. The dracunculiasis campaign promises success early in the new century.

Leprosy

Leprosy is one of the world's most dreaded diseases, and its disfiguring characteristics in the later stages of infection have caused social ostracism of its victims for centuries. Caused by infection by the bacterium *Mycobacterium leprae,* the use of multidrug therapy (MDT) has cured more than nine million leprosy patients since 1985. Three drugs (dapsone, rifampicin, and clofazimine) are used in various combinations, depending on the severity of the disease. Although as many as two million patients need to be detected and treated in the next three years, 90 percent live in just thirteen countries. An international collaboration, the Leprosy Elimination Advisory Group (LEAG) will focus its program of detection on treatment at the community level and expects that leprosy will vanish as a public health problem in the first years of the twenty-first century.

Onchocerciasis

Widely known as "river blindness," onchocerciasis is caused by the filariid worm *Onchocerca volvulus.* The worm causes a severe pruritic skin disease, as well as sclerosing keratitis that can result in blindness. The disease is endemic primarily in Africa, with smaller pockets in Latin America.

In 1974, the Onchocerciasis Control Program (OCP) was launched by the World Bank and other bilateral supporters in eleven West

African countries. The OCP's initial strategy depended on aerial spraying of the disease-transmitting black fly's breeding sites in rivers. However, two-thirds of oncho-endemic areas of Africa were left out of the OCP. In 1988, ivermectin (Mectizan®), a drug used primarily for veterinary applications and found to be successful for treating onchocerciasis in humans, became widely available through a donation program from the U.S. pharmaceutical producer Merck & Company. The availability of the drug completely changed the strategy for controlling the disease. Annual treatment began in the OCP countries in 1987, and elimination is expected in those countries by 2002. Moreover, through a second effort, the African Program on Oncho Control (APOC), the annual treatments have expanded to include most endemic countries of Africa where active onchocerciasis control programs are under way in conjunction with local ministries of health and nongovernmental organizations. The Onchocerciasis Elimination Program in the Americas (OEPA) serves six endemic countries in the Western Hemisphere (Brazil, Colombia, Ecuador, Guatemala, Mexico, and Venezuela). With the use of Mectizan, onchocerciasis is likely to be eliminated in the Americas by 2007.

Lymphatic Filariasis

Lymphatic filariasis is one of the most prevalent parasitic infections and is endemic in at least seventy-three countries, with a total of at least 120 million people infected. Although acute manifestations of lymphangitis do occur, this mosquito-transmitted filariid worm is most commonly recognized by elephantiasis, the disfiguring enlargement of lower limbs, breasts, and genitalia.

Lymphatic filariasis is one of the very few diseases considered entirely eradicable by tropical disease experts. As with onchocerciasis and other diseases, drug companies stepped forward to donate essential products for the control of this particular disease. Recent research has shown that a combination of two of three active drugs quickly reduces the microfilaria circulated in the body and reduces transmission of the disease in a community for at least one year.

The drugs available are, first of all, diethylcarbamazine, a drug developed over fifty years ago that is inexpensive (2 cents per person per year). Second, through the World Health Organization, SmithKline Beecham has donated albendazole for use in elimination programs. In areas where onchocerciasis exists, Merck & Company has again donated ivermectin (Mectizan), to be used in conjunction with albendazole for treatment of lymphatic filariasis. If control programs can be applied to the areas where the poor suffer from lymphatic filariasis, the disease could cease to be a public health problem between 2010 and 2020.

Chagas' Disease

Chagas' disease, caused by the protozoan *Trypanasoma cruzi,* is endemic only in South America. Transmission occurs through the bite of the triatomine bug and less frequently through blood transfusion. Sixteen to eighteen million persons are infected, and an additional one hundred million people live in areas where they are at risk of infection. Primary infections may be mild and escape detection; however, chronic infection in some cases results in fatal cardiomyopathy or mega disease of the colon or esophagus as the protozoan attacks muscle cells.

Although there is no effective treatment unless the disease is caught early, interruption of transmission is possible. The Southern Cone Initiative, involving Argentina, Bolivia, Brazil, Chile, Paraguay, Uruguay, and southern Peru, was formally launched in 1991. In 1997, Uruguay had brought the insect vector that causes the disease under control, demonstrating that elimination of transmission vectors is indeed a feasible goal. A similar initiative has been organized for the Andean countries of Colombia, Ecuador, Peru, and Venezuela and another for Central America. Based on the earlier results achieved in the Southern Cone Initiative, it is estimated that transmission can be interrupted in these countries by the year 2005.

Trachoma

Of the thirty-eight million blind people in the world today, six million (15.5 percent) are thought to be blind from trachoma, the world's leading preventable cause of blindness. Common in Europe and North America in the early twentieth century, trachoma vanished as economic conditions improved—particularly conditions that affected water and sanitation. However, it remains a major cause of blindness in areas of poverty and poor sanitation in the developing world.

The disease, caused by a bacterium that infects the eyes, causing the eyelids to turn inward and the lashes to scratch and scar the cornea, requires different treatment at different stages. Approximately eleven million people around the world need simple eyelid surgery for trichiasis and entropion, the later forms of the disease, and 150 million children have the active infectious form of trachoma that can be controlled by antibiotics. WHO has organized an alliance for Global Elimination of Trachoma by the Year 2020 (GET 2020), a consortium of nongovernmental donor organizations, technical experts, and WHO staff. Control programs are based on the SAFE strategy: *surgery* using a simplified procedure that can be done by paramedical personnel for the lid deformity; *antibiotic treatment* (either oral azithromycin or topical tetracycline); *face washing* and improved hygiene, particularly of young children; and *environmental improvements* that would include better use of water and disposal of animal and human feces.

The recent development a single-dose long-acting oral antibiotic equivalent to six weeks of tetracycline ointment offers great promise of interrupting transmission before the target date of 2020. In 1998, the Edna McConnell Clark Foundation and the research-based pharmaceutical company Pfizer Inc. launched the International Trachoma Initiative (ITI) to promote the elimination of blinding trachoma using Pfizer-donated Zithromax® (the brand name for azithromycin). The ITI has been working in five high-priority countries designated by the GET 2020 group.

PERSISTENT TROPICAL DISEASES

Although control of all the diseases discussed so far has benefited from breakthroughs in treatment, technologies, and a marshaling of resources from various organizations, including WHO, nongovernmental organizations, and drug companies, other tropical diseases will require significantly greater investments in research and continued vigilance about prevalence and spread. Let us look at three examples: a protozoan, a bacterium, and a virus.

Malaria

Malaria is the most important parasitic disease in the world today, but its impact is disproportionately felt in tropical Africa, where approximately 10 percent of the world's population suffers more than 90 percent of the world's malaria infections. Although the disease occurs mainly in developing countries, it still poses a great risk of spreading to industrialized countries, as it did a century ago. Five hundred thousand to two million people die of malaria each year, and approximately one million deaths occurring in children under five years of age are attributed to malaria either alone or in combination with other diseases. Malaria is caused by the protozoan species of plasmodia and is transmitted by anopheline mosquitoes. Risk of malaria infections exists in as many as one hundred countries and territories. Malaria's ability to spread beyond the tropics was demonstrated in August 1999 when two Boy Scouts on Long Island, New York, were found to be infected.

As a result of the availability of the drug chloroquine for treatment and DDT to prevent insect spread, eradication was thought possible as early as 1953. The effort proved a dismal failure, however. Chloroquine resistance is now widespread in Africa, and Southeast Asia continues to be the center of multidrug-resistant malaria. No new methods of controlling the mosquito vector have been devised.

All of this would suggest no reason for optimism as the century begins. However, perhaps the very desperate nature of the situation gives rise to optimism—that perhaps malaria will finally receive the attention it deserves. Programs involving WHO, national governments, the pharmaceutical industry, and the research community will seek to increase the use of insecticide-impregnated bed nets and improve early diagnosis and treatment as well as search existing compounds for antimalarial activity.

Meanwhile, research proceeds on two fronts: creating genetic strains of the anopheline mosquito that have plasmodium-inhibiting genes to greatly diminish the potential for spread of the disease and identifying one or more antigens that could be used with powerful new adjuvants in a vaccine to prevent infection.

Cholera

Cholera is a diarrheal disease caused the bacterium *Vibrio cholerae*. Although the infection can often occur without symptoms, the fulminant form seen in epidemics can lead rapidly to dehydration and death. Cholera pandemics, which swept the cities of Asia, Europe, Africa, and the Americas during the nineteenth century, had a profound impact on the development of public health as a discipline and particularly established the need for rigorous surveillance of infectious disease. Given this legacy, it is therefore ironic that this disease remains stubbornly resistant to elimination as a public health hazard. Though treatment through oral and intravenous rehydration therapy has been highly effective, the rapid spread of the disease and the enormous scale of its impact leads to significant mortality, especially among the poor, who often live in crowded conditions without adequate sanitation.

In the first half of the 1990s, almost two million cases of cholera were reported from 115 countries, and refugee camps in Africa have suffered explosive epidemics with enormous mortality. In the new century, surveillance measures must be improved so as more quickly to detect and address epidemics with rehydration therapy for those afflicted and immediate public health measures to interrupt further spread of the disease.

Dengue

Dengue fever is caused by an arbovirus that is transmitted by mosquito vectors, mainly the species *Aedes aegypti*. The fever occurs in up to eighty million persons per year around the world, and about two-thirds of the world's population lives in areas infested by this mosquito (including the United States).

Dengue fever has worsened in recent years. The need for additional research and vigilance concerning this disease has grown even more urgent because a new and often fatal manifestation, dengue hemorrhagic fever, is occurring with increasing frequency. While research is moving ahead in the development of a live attenuated vaccine, the disease could be reined in if nations increased their efforts to control the mosquito vector. Until a vaccine is widely available—or unless control programs eliminate the breeding sites of this mosquito in water containers around domestic settings—this ubiquitous virus will continue to cause high morbidity and mortality.

An outbreak of West Nile virus, formerly unknown in North America, in New York at the end of 1999 demonstrates the ability of "tropical" mosquito-borne viruses like dengue to invade the industrialized world.

CONCLUSION

Overall, the prospects for the control of several tropical diseases in the twenty-first century are indeed positive. Although it is unlikely that the causes of these diseases—be they worms, bacteria, or viruses—will be completely eradicated, we can expect to eliminate the burden of some diseases within the first two decades of the century. At the same time, these potential successes should not engender complacency in the areas of research and surveillance. We may know much about the basic biology and control methods of these tropical diseases, but we should continue to invest in finding even more effective methods of control. In these modern times, tropical disease as a discipline means watching over health concerns in the developing world, and in that respect, the discipline will continue to have great significance in the new century. The concepts of globalization and of "one world" have never been more real than in the present day, and we must address these public health problems as forthrightly as possible—if not out of a humanitarian impulse, then out of our own self-interest.

CHAPTER SEVENTEEN

The Outlook for Eradicating AIDS

Seth F. Berkley

Seth F. Berkley, MD, *is President of the International AIDS Vaccine Initiative, which he founded. He is a specialist in international health and infectious disease epidemiology and has extensive overseas experience, having worked or consulted in more than thirty countries.*

AIDS is the first widespread newly emergent infection of our globally interconnected era. This uniformly fatal viral disease, caused by the human immunodeficiency virus (HIV), was initially identified in homosexual males—a group sometimes stigmatized and marginalized by society. In 1984, when HIV was discovered, there was little precedent for the treatment of viral infections. Rather, developing a preventive vaccine seemed to be the most likely solution. To ensure maximum scientific progress and to focus attention on treatment for those already infected as well as prevention strategies, the gay community initiated a new form of scientific activism. This movement was extremely effective, leading directly to the most intense biomedical scientific research effort ever conducted on an infectious agent, resulting in extraordinary advances in the understanding of pathogenesis, the workings of the immune system, and the development of viral therapeutics. Unfortunately, without advocates, HIV vaccine development was relegated to a low priority.

Less than two decades later, AIDS in the industrialized world is under moderate control. In the developing world, however, the situation remains out of control. Fully 90 to 95 percent of all HIV infections now occur in developing countries. In fact, from a global point of view, it is unlikely that the efforts to control transmission have had a significant impact on the natural spread of the virus. In 1999, there were close to six million new infections. Although recognition of the severity of AIDS has inspired the creation of a new UN body, the United Nations Programme on AIDS, the global effort remains underfunded, and known effective interventions are not widely implemented. Relatively little research has gone into improving preventive technologies or into providing less costly therapeutics for people living with HIV in developing countries.

Only an effective, safe, and globally accessible HIV vaccine has the potential to end the HIV epidemic. Yet until recently, HIV vaccines—particularly for developing countries—were the poor stepchild of AIDS research, commanding less than 10 percent of the research effort and less than 1 percent of global funds spent on HIV. Vaccine development must be accelerated and the resultant vaccine distributed and used throughout the world. A new paradigm of public-private, North-South, industrial-academe partnership is necessary to solve these problems. Such a mechanism will have relevance for other emerging infectious threats around the world.

THE FUTURE OF HIV DISEASE IN INDUSTRIALIZED COUNTRIES

At the turn of the twenty-first century, despite seventy-five thousand new HIV infections per year in industrialized countries, there is a growing sense of complacency about AIDS. With the licensing of eleven antiretroviral drugs (and others available on an experimental basis), AIDS is incorrectly viewed as a chronic and easily treatable condition. Unfortunately, treatment is complicated and expensive, and many patients are unable to tolerate the toxic effects. Because death rates are declining from these improved regimens, the number of persons living with HIV infection is rising. Although treatment can reduce circulating virus to undetectable levels, it does not eradicate it, and patients undergoing therapy can still transmit the virus sexually (Zhang and others, 1998). More persons living with HIV means more potential transmitters. Unfortunately, not only is HIV resistance to these drugs increasing, but transmission of multidrug-resistant strains is also occurring (Hecht and others, 1998). As more patients become careless and compliance declines (in a recent study, only 60 percent of patients took more than 80 percent of the prescribed antiretroviral agents over a seven-day period; Eldred, Wu, Chaisson, and Moore, 1998), we will see an increasing burden of multiply resistant organisms. Finally, more infections are occurring among minority groups, often in poor communities ill equipped to mobilize intensive efforts.

We can be optimistic for continued therapeutic progress. Advances in therapeutics, drug combinations, and immune reconstitution are all progressing, and the private sector is vigorously engaged in drug development (the current market is over $3 billion annually). But it is unlikely that drugs will end the epidemic or become universally available.

THE FUTURE OF HIV DISEASE IN DEVELOPING COUNTRIES

In developing countries, we see a different reality. The epidemic is accelerating. In most of these countries, prevention efforts are inadequate, and antiviral treatment is not available due to high cost, difficulties in use, and severe side effects. In fact, in many impoverished countries, even basic palliative care is not widely available. For the poorest developing countries, therefore, HIV remains a uniformly fatal and untreatable condition.

The effects of this will be seen most clearly in the coming years. Initially, it was easy to deny the seriousness of the epidemic. Although the infection spread rapidly, there is a long disease-free interval during which the many infected persons display no visible symptoms. In countries like South Africa, Cambodia, and India, cases of AIDS are only now presenting, yet the virus has spread widely in their populations.

As the epidemic matures, HIV is beginning to skew all demographic indicators. In countries affected severely and early, death rates are higher, recent improvements in infant and child mortality have been reversed, and population growth has slowed. The largest demographic impacts will be on life expectancies. Recent projections from the U.S. Bureau of the Census (1999) are striking: in six African countries, life expectancies are already down more than twenty years, and the situation is projected to be even worse in 2010 (see Figure 17.1). No other newly emerged infectious disease has come close to having

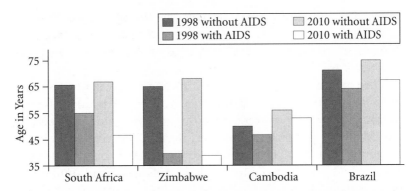

Figure 17.1.   Life Expectancies in Selected Countries, 1998 and 2010.
Source: U.S. Bureau of the Census, 1999, Table 2, p. 57.

such an impact. This magnitude of disease will devastate health care delivery systems, availability of trained workers, family coping-mechanisms, and indices of economic development.

IS GLOBAL ERADICATION OF HIV POSSIBLE?

In the strictest sense, global eradication of the infectious agent, HIV is unlikely, if not impossible. HIV infections can remain asymptomatic for a very long period—often a decade or longer. It is likely that less than 10 percent of the people in the world who are infected are aware of their HIV status. Even with better, less expensive, more rapid testing mechanisms, the vast majority of those infected will not be identified in a timely fashion. This makes targeted interventions for prevention or even early treatment difficult.

On the other hand, with appropriate interventions, HIV could be brought down to a manageable endemic level. It may even be possible to eradicate HIV from selected individuals. The availability of highly active antiretroviral therapy (HAART) agents led prominent scientists in the mid-1990s to believe that aggressive treatment for a number of years might be enough to eradicate HIV infection in a patient. Yet ongoing studies in persons undergoing HAART therapies demonstrate that HIV, even when barely measurable in the blood, continues to infect cells, albeit at a reduced rate. Furthermore, there are resting CD4+ cells in the blood that are latently infected with HIV and decline only slightly despite adequate therapy. Based on these small and limited studies, researchers predict that it might take sixty years or more for the patient to get rid of this reservoir of HIV-infected cells (Finzi and others, 1999).

The combination of HAART treatment and vaccination is more likely as an effective mechanism to cure an individual of HIV. Although there is no precedent for this approach, it is theoretically possible that a person with an early infection and a relatively intact immune system could be put on aggressive HAART. Once viral reproduction had been reduced to very low levels, a series of immunizations, perhaps along with a range of immunomodulators, could lead to a potent immune response that would then keep the infection in check. Recent experiments with immune reconstitution might also yield ways to rebuild a damaged immune system.

WHAT HAS BEEN LEARNED, AND WHAT CAN BE DONE?

Behavior change can work in highly motivated and educated populations as evidenced by the dramatic successes among the gay population in Australia and intravenous drug users in the Netherlands. Yet sustaining change is a challenge. Recidivism, particularly among young persons, is occurring. Intensive behavior change interventions in less well educated or less well motivated populations can also have a dramatic effect; however, widespread implementation among the general population has been difficult. An example of a successful but highly targeted effort is Thailand, where a combination of early HIV surveillance, multisectoral governmental commitment, and targeted interventions in commercial sex establishments led to a measurable slowdown in the spread of the virus. Long-term durability of this success is not clear, as HIV transmission does continue. Uganda has also seen a reduction of HIV incidence in the urban areas, but only after peaking at alarmingly high levels (almost a third of low-risk antenatal women were infected in the capital city, Kampala). In other regions of the country (including many rural areas, where 80 percent of the population lives), HIV continues to spread.

So despite some localized successes, globally we are losing the war against HIV. Political irresponsibility is exemplified by continued denial of the severity of the HIV problem in many countries, when HIV has already infected—and will ultimately kill—more people than all the wars of the twentieth century.

The world also needs improved prevention technologies that work in countries where the epidemic is spreading fastest. Improved barrier methods (such as condoms that are more user-friendly), female-controlled methods of protection (like microbicides), and improved diagnostics and treatment strategies for amplifying cofactors such as sexually transmitted diseases (STDs) will help. Simplified and inexpensive treatment regimens, prophylactic treatment, and immune-supportive regimens to prevent opportunistic infections are also required, as well as assistance in coping with the personal and social consequences of these infections. Vaccines, however, have traditionally been the way to control viral infectious diseases. An affordable, safe, and effective HIV preventive vaccine is the world's best hope for stopping the epidemic.

A POLICY FRAMEWORK FOR THE TWENTY-FIRST CENTURY

A crucial task for the new century is to create the necessary policy and biomedical tools to stop epidemics of emerging infections such as HIV, as well as to assure maximum use of existing technologies.

Information

Global reporting mechanisms are indispensable for identifying new infectious threats, monitoring their spread, and dealing with changes in their epidemiology and susceptibility. Despite almost twenty years of HIV infections, some countries still deny the magnitude of domestic HIV infection, and data are scarce from many areas. Global monitoring of epidemics should become the norm; removed from the realm of politics. Given the rapid globalization that is under way, accurate and timely information about epidemic infectious diseases is an international public good. For HIV, data on incidence, prevalence, change of subtypes, and spread of antiviral resistance should be obtained in a standardized fashion and disseminated globally. (Ironically, the data for HIV are better than for most diseases; however, it is not adequate to monitor and target interventions based solely on real-time information.) The availability of global communication systems and instant computerized analysis could enable the creation of a real-time global system. I can foresee, early in the century, disease maps based on continuously updated real surveillance data, much like TV news programs' weather maps based on continuous satellite surveillance.

Information must be provided to *all* individuals at risk. Adolescents must be educated about the risks of sexual activity and how to have safe sexual encounters. This is true regardless of the status of our HIV interventions, as there are many other risks associated with unsafe sex practices (STDs, unwanted pregnancy and possible unsafe therapeutic abortion, cervical cancer, and sexually transmitted hepatitis B, to name just a few). A recent review demonstrated that in females aged fifteen to forty-four years, up to 12 percent of the deaths and 15 percent of the global burden of disease—the majority of which was due to non-HIV causes—is associated with unsafe sexual activities (Berkley, 1998).

Political Commitment

AIDS has shown us how an epidemic can spread around the world virtually unchecked despite the claims from many politicians that "we do not have 'those' behaviors here." The public must regard this type of political denial as unacceptable. Politicians must be held accountable for dealing with epidemic infectious disease as they are for many other issues of political importance. This includes awareness and openness about the problem as well as providing adequate resources at an early stage when they can be most effective. Responses must be broad and must make use of all available expertise, including all relevant governmental departments and the nongovernmental and private sectors.

Politicians must also do the unthinkable—create programs whose results will not be achieved during their political term. Given the seriousness of the epidemic, politicians as well as policymakers have been forced to deal with the emergency at hand. This is the demand of their constituencies and the source of immediate political benefit. What is required for the future is a focus on the longer-term issues of preventive technology development while continuing to cope with the current epidemic.

Better Use of Existing Technologies

The correct use of male condoms as well as (probably) female condoms dramatically reduces HIV transmission. Treating sexually transmitted infections reduces the risk of transmission of HIV. Providing clean needles for injections reduces bloodborne spread of HIV. Access to counseling and testing reduces risky behavior. Treating HIV-infected pregnant women with AZT and Neverapine reduces perinatal transmission. Each of these technologies is proven—but none is universally used. Widespread use of these interventions now would both slow the existing epidemic and reduce future transmission of the virus.

New Technologies

A modeling study done a few years ago by the World Health Organization (World Bank, 1993) showed that even a tenfold increase in spending on existent interventions would not stop the epidemic. New, more effective prevention technologies are necessary. Although academe and public sector research institutions are excellent at creating new knowledge and discovering scientific breakthroughs, increasingly the expertise to develop products such as vaccines exists only in the private sector. However, HIV vaccine development is expensive, the science is challenging and there is no certainty of success with any one approach. No for-profit company can justify to its shareholders the substantial investment in a full range of potential HIV vaccine technologies, given the cost and risk this would entail. Add to this the inadequate market incentives for companies to invest in product development even for one product and the lack of a global mechanism to create incentives or to finance the development of technologies directly. For national problems, a governmental effort may solve this market failure—however, who should take responsibility for international public goods? It could be argued that multinational agencies should lead, but often these agencies do not have the flexibility, rapid decision pathways, or risk-taking ability to manage complicated product development initiatives.

Decades ago, such a problem at a national level would be tackled by the launching of specialized research efforts (an example is the Los Alamos U.S. nuclear program). Today, however, when industry is competing so intensely for talent, it is not realistic to assume that the public sector can attract and retain the best expertise for vaccine development. In addition, this expertise is not concentrated in any one laboratory, company, or even country. The situation calls for the creation of a "virtual company," one that transcends disciplinary and geographical boundaries. This entity should be global and centrally directed. Although peer-reviewed, researcher-originated research is the best mechanism to pursue new ideas, it is not effective for developing products. Product development requires a linear approach to problem solving and is best milestone- and target-driven. Such an initiative would require a small secretariat to provide the finance and contracts, choose approaches, create talent pools, and ensure that deadlines are met and focus the effort on the critical pathways of product development.

The International AIDS Vaccine Initiative (IAVI) established in 1996, is an example of such a global initiative. It pursues three strategies: (1) creating demand for a vaccine through aggressive communication, education, and advocacy; (2) accelerating scientific progress through a directed product development effort; and (3) creating incentives for industrial involvement in HIV vaccine development. To ensure accessibility, IAVI operates as "social venture capitalists," wherein companies agree to preferential pricing for the public sector of developing countries in return for the financing they receive. They also retain the intellectual property rights for the vaccine for the private sector and for the public sector of industrialized countries but agree that if vaccines are not made available in developing countries in a timely and cost-effective fashion, IAVI can transfer the technology and know-how to another manufacturer. To ensure accessibility and to create a market in developing countries, IAVI is working with the World Bank to investigate mechanisms (using contingent loans, promissory notes, and lines of credit) to create a guaranteed market for a future successful AIDS vaccine.

CONCLUSION

HIV is a global threat of enormous magnitude to which the world has not responded adequately. With appropriate action, including an aggressive effort to use the existing tools and a worldwide effort to create the necessary new tools, HIV could become a minor endemic infectious disease. We cannot guarantee success. It is clear, however, that without an appropriate effort to develop a safe, effective, accessible preventive HIV vaccine, HIV will continue its destructive swath across the developing world. We owe our children, and all of those living in the new century, the best shot science can make to end this epidemic. New and unprecedented mechanisms need to be put in place to ensure simultaneous availability and use of the vaccine in both developed and developing countries. If we cannot do it for HIV, how can we have any hope to succeed with the next emerging epidemic?

References

Berkley, S. F. "Unsafe Sex as a Risk Factor." In C.J.L. Murray and A. D. Lopez. (eds.), *Health Dimensions of Sex and Reproduction.* Cambridge, Mass.: Harvard University Press, 1998.

Eldred, L. J., Wu, A. W., Chaisson, R. E., and Moore, R. D. "Adherence to Antiretroviral and Pneumocystis Prophylaxis in HIV Disease." *Journal of Acquired Immune Deficiency Syndrome and Human Retrovirology,* 1998, *18,* 117–125.

Finzi, D., and others. "Latent Infection of CD4+ T-Cells Provides a Mechanism for Lifelong Persistence of HIV-1 Even in Patients on Effective Combination Therapy." *Nature Medicine,* 1999, *5,* 512–517.

Hecht, F. M., and others. "Sexual Transmission of an HIV-1 Variant Resistant to Multiple Reverse-Transcriptase and Protease Inhibitors." *New England Journal of Medicine,* 1998, *339,* 307–311.

U.S. Bureau of the Census. *World Population Profile, 1998.* Washington, D.C.: U.S. Government Printing Office, 1999.

World Bank. *World Development Report: Investing in Health.* New York: Oxford University Press, 1993.

Zhang, H., and others. "Human Immunodeficiency Virus Type 1 in the Semen of Men Receiving Highly Active Antiretroviral Therapy." *New England Journal of Medicine,* 1998, *339,* 1803–1809.

CHAPTER EIGHTEEN

Future Worldwide Health Effects of Current Smoking Patterns

Richard Peto, Alan D. Lopez

Richard Peto, *is a professor of medical statistics and epidemiology at the University of Oxford and Codirector of the Clinical Trial Service Unit (CTSU). He is involved with large collaborative studies of the hazards of tobacco in many different populations.*

Alan D. Lopez, PhD, *is an epidemiologist at the World Health Organization, where he has worked on both tobacco control and global mortality statistics. He is coauthor of the recent Global Burden of Disease (GBD) study. For a decade, Peto and Lopez have quantified the growing hazards of tobacco, first in developed and then in developing countries.*

Worldwide, the only two major causes of death whose effects are now increasing rapidly are HIV (see Chapter Seventeen) and tobacco. If current smoking patterns persist, there will be about one billion deaths from tobacco during the twenty-first

This research involved collaboration with Jillian Boreham, Zhengming Chen, Roy Collins, Richard Doll, C. K. Gajalakshmi, P. C. Gupta, B.-Q. Liu, and G. Mead and support from the U.K. Medical Research Council, the Imperial Cancer Research Fund, and the British Heart Foundation. Permission is hereby granted to reproduce any part of this chapter.

century, compared to "only" about 0.1 billion (one hundred million) during the whole of the twentieth century. About half of these deaths will be in middle age (thirty-five to sixty-nine years) rather than old age, and those killed by tobacco in middle age lose, on average, more than twenty years of nonsmoker life expectancy (see Exhibit 18.1).

There are two main reasons for this large increase in tobacco deaths. First, the world population in middle and old age will continue to increase. Second, the proportion of the deaths caused by tobacco will increase substantially over the next few decades due to the delayed effects of the large increase in cigarette smoking among young adults over the past few decades (Peto and others, 1994; Doll and others, 1994; World Health Organization, 1997; Ad Hoc Committee, 1996; Murray and Lopez, 1996; Peto, Chen, and Boreham, 1999). Among cigarette smokers, the risk of death from tobacco in middle or old age is really substantial (about one in two) only for those who start smoking in early adult life (Peto and others, 1994; Doll and others, 1994; Peto, 1986; Doll and Peto, 1981). Consequently, when there is a large upsurge in cigarette smoking among the young adults in a particular country, this will produce a large upsurge in tobacco deaths half a century later. Thus the number of deaths from tobacco around the year

---

- ■ **Half are killed by tobacco.** Among persistent cigarette smokers who start early in life and do not quit, about 50 percent will eventually be killed by tobacco.

- ■ **Half of those killed by tobacco die in middle age.** About half of all victims of tobacco die between the ages of thirty-five and sixty nine, with those killed in middle age losing, on average, approximately twenty to twenty-five years of life.

- ■ **Stopping smoking works.** Even in middle age, smokers who quit before they have developed a serious disease avoid *most* of the subsequent risk of death from tobacco. Smokers who quite before middle age avoid *almost all* the risk.

Exhibit 18.1.   Hazards for the Persistent Cigarette Smoker.
Sources: Peto and others, 1994; Doll and others, 1994; based on U.S. and U.K. data.

2000 is strongly influenced by the number of young adults who took up smoking around 1950, and the number of young adults who are taking up smoking around the year 2000 will strongly influence the number of deaths from tobacco around the year 2050 (and beyond).

The main increase in cigarette use by young adults took place during the first half of the twentieth century for men in developed countries but during the second half of the century for women in developed countries and for men in developing countries (Peto and others, 1994; Doll and others, 1994; World Health Organization, 1997). (So far, relatively few women in developing countries have begun to smoke.)

For men in developed countries, the epidemic of tobacco deaths may already be about as large as it will ever be, with tobacco now responsible for about one-third of all male deaths in middle age (Peto and others, 1994). (Continuing increases in male tobacco deaths in countries such as Greece and Portugal are offset by recent decreases elsewhere—for example, in the United Kingdom.) For women in most developed countries, however, the epidemic still has far to go—indeed, in many European countries such as France and Spain, the main increase in tobacco deaths among women is only just beginning. In the United States, however, the proportion of deaths in middle age that is due to tobacco is now almost as great in women as in men (Peto and others, 1994).

Taking both sexes together, U.S. cigarette consumption per adult was one per day in 1910, four per day in 1930, and ten per day in 1950, after which it remained relatively constant for several decades (Peto, Chen, and Boreham, 1999; Peto, 1986; Doll and Peto, 1981). As a delayed result of this pre-1950 increase in cigarette consumption, the proportion of all U.S. deaths at ages thirty-five to sixty-nine years attributed to tobacco rose from 12 percent in 1950 to 33 percent in 1990 (Peto and others, 1994).

In China, which is the largest and best studied of the developing countries, the increase in male cigarette consumption and in tobacco deaths both lag almost exactly forty years behind the United States. (Peto and others, 1999; Liu and others, 1998; Niu and others, 1998) (At present, few young women in China become smokers; Liu and others, 1998.) Chinese male cigarette consumption averaged one per day in 1952, four per day in 1972, and ten per day in 1992, with no further increase during the past few years, and the proportion of Chinese male deaths at ages thirty-five to sixty-nine years attributed to tobacco was 12 percent in 1990 and is projected to be about 33 percent in 2030 (Liu and others, 1998; Niu and others, 1998). Two-thirds of the young men become persistent smokers, and about half of those who do so will eventually be killed by the habit—so about one-third of all the young men in China will eventually be killed by tobacco, if current smoking patterns persist.

China, with 20 percent of the world's population, produces and consumes about 30 percent of the world's cigarettes, and a large nationwide study has now shown that China already suffers almost a million deaths a year from tobacco, a figure that is likely to at least double by 2025. The Chinese study consisted of two parts, one retrospective (Liu and others, 1998), ascertaining the smoking habits of adults who had recently died, and one prospective (Niu and others, 1998), which will continue for decades, monitoring the long-term growth of the epidemic. In recent years, large retrospective and prospective studies have been or are being established in China, India, Latin America, and elsewhere to monitor the current and future hazards not only in developed but also in various developing populations. Results from China (Liu and others, 1998; Niu and others, 1998) and preliminary results from India (Gajalakshmi, 1999; Gupta and Mehta, 2000) show that the hazards are already substantial.

Worldwide, there are now about four million deaths a year caused by tobacco, about evenly split between developed and developing countries. But these numbers reflect smoking patterns several decades ago, and worldwide cigarette consumption has increased substantially over the past half century (World Health Organization, 1997). Currently, about 30 percent of young adults become persistent smokers, and relatively few quit (except in selected populations, such as educated adults in parts of Western Europe and North America). The main diseases by which smoking kills people are substantially different in America, where vascular disease and lung cancer predominate (Peto and others, 1994); in China, where chronic obstructive pulmonary disease causes even more tobacco deaths than lung cancer (Liu and others, 1998; Niu and others, 1998); and in India, where almost half the world's tuberculosis deaths take place and the ability of smoking to increase the risk of death from TB may well be of particular importance (Gajalakshmi, 1999; Gupta and Mehta, 2000). But there is no good reason to expect the overall 50 percent risk of death from persistent cigarette smoking to vary much from one population to another.

There are already a billion smokers, and by 2030 about another billion young adults will have started to smoke. If current smoking patterns persist, worldwide mortality from tobacco is likely to rise from about four million deaths a year currently to about ten million a year around 2030 (increasing by one hundred million per decade) and will rise somewhat further in later decades. This means that tobacco will cause about 150 million deaths in the first quarter of the century and 300 million in the second quarter. Predictions beyond that are inevitably somewhat speculative, but if over the next few decades about a quarter to a third of the young adults become persistent smokers and about half are eventually killed by their habit, about 15 percent of adult mortality in the second half of the century will be due to tobacco, implying some six hundred million to nine hundred million tobacco deaths in 2050–2099.

The number of tobacco deaths before 2050 cannot be greatly reduced unless a substantial proportion of the adults who have already been smoking for some time give up the habit. One reason is that a decrease over the next decade or two in the proportion of children who become smokers will not have its main effects on mortality until the third quarter of the century (see Exhibit 18.2).

The calculations in Exhibit 18.2 show that quitting by adult smokers offers the only realistic way in which widespread changes in smoking status can prevent large numbers of tobacco deaths over the next half century. Widely practicable ways of helping large numbers of young people not to become smokers could avoid hundreds of millions of tobacco deaths in the second half of the century, but not before, whereas widely practicable ways of helping large numbers of adult smokers quit (preferably before middle age) might well avoid one to two hundred million tobacco deaths in the first half of the century. The strategies that are relevant to young people may well be of little relevance to adults, and vice versa, so overemphasis on either at the expense of the other would be inappropriate. In particular, it is often wrongly supposed that it is impossible to get large numbers of adult smokers to quit, but the experience of several countries over the past few decades shows that decreases can occur both in the proportion who start and in the proportion who continue to smoke.

Britain, which is now experiencing the most rapid decrease in the world in premature deaths from tobacco, shows that quite large improvements are possible (Peto and others, 1994). Between 1965 and

1995, annual U.K. cigarette sales fell from 150 billion to 80 billion, and there was a threefold reduction in the machine-measured tar delivery per cigarette (and hence a moderate reduction in the hazard per smoker; Peto, 1986; Doll and Peto, 1981). Over the same period, annual U.K. tobacco deaths in middle age decreased from eighty thousand to forty thousand and are still falling rapidly (Peto and others, 1994). Regarding lung cancer, the U.K. male death rate at ages thirty-five to sixty-nine years has been decreasing at the rate of 40 percent per decade over the past few years. Moreover, as those now in middle age progress into old age over the next decade or two, U.K. mortality in old age from tobacco should also decrease substantially.

Unfortunately, however, although there have been substantial decreases in the prevalence of smoking in some developed populations,

---

- **Effects of adult smokers' quitting on tobacco deaths in the** *first* **half of the twenty-first century:** If many of the adults who now smoke were to quit over the next decade or two, halving global cigarette consumption per adult by the year 2020, this would prevent about one-third of the tobacco deaths in 2020 and would almost halve tobacco deaths in the second quarter of the century. Such changes would avoid 20 to 30 million tobacco deaths in 2000–2025 and 150 million in 2025–2050.

- **Effects of young people's not starting to smoke on tobacco deaths in the** *second* **half of the twenty-first century:** If the proportion of young adults who become smokers were to be progressively reduced by half in the next twenty years, this would avoid hundreds of millions of deaths from tobacco after 2050. However, it would have little effect on the 150 million deaths from tobacco in the first quarter of the century and avoid only 10 or 20 million of the 300 million deaths from tobacco in the second quarter of the century.

Exhibit 18.2.   Effects of Adult Smokers' Quitting on Tobacco Deaths Before 2050, and of Young People's Not Starting on Tobacco Deaths After 2050.

Sources: Peto and others, 1994; Doll and others, 1994.

there have been large increases elsewhere, particularly in Chinese males, over the past decade or two (Peto, Chen, and Boreham, 1999; Liu and others, 1998), and it is difficult to see how worldwide cigarette consumption can be halved over the next couple of decades. Hence the hundred million tobacco deaths in the twentieth century are likely to be followed in the twenty-first by several hundred million—and if present smoking patterns persist, there will be about one billion people killed by tobacco in the next hundred years.

References

Ad Hoc Committee on Health Research. *Investing in Health Research and Development.* Geneva: World Health Organization, 1996.

Doll, R., and others. "Mortality in Relation to Smoking: 40 Years' Observations on Male British Doctors." *British Medical Journal,* 1994, *309,* 901–911.

Doll, R., and Peto, R. "The Causes of Cancer: Quantitative Estimates of Avoidable Risks of Cancer in the United States Today." *Journal of the National Cancer Institute,* 1981, *66,* 1193–1308. (Republished by Oxford University Press as a monograph in 1983.)

Gupta, P. C., and Mehta, H. C. "A Cohort Study of All-Cause Mortality Among Tobacco Users in Bombay, India." *International Journal of Public Health,* 2000, *(forthcoming).*

Liu, B.-Q., Peto, R., and Chen, Z.-M. "Emerging Tobacco Hazards in China: 1. Retrospective Proportional Mortality Study of One Million Deaths." *British Medical Journal,* 1998, *317,* 1411–1422.

Murray, C.J.L., and Lopez, A. D. *The Global Burden of Disease: A Comprehensive Assessment of Mortality and Disability from Diseases, Injuries, and Risk Factors in 1990 and Projected to 2020.* Cambridge, Mass.: Harvard University Press, 1996.

Niu, S. R., Yang, G.-H., and Chen, Z.-M. "Emerging Tobacco Hazards in China: 2. Early Mortality Results from a Prospective Study." *British Medical Journal,* 1998, *317,* 1423–1424.

Peto, R. "Influence of Dose and Duration of Smoking on Lung Cancer Rates." In D. Zaridze and R. Peto (eds.), *Tobacco: A Growing International Health Hazard.* IARC Scientific Publication no. 74. Lyons, France: International Agency for Research on Cancer, 1986.

Peto, R., Chen, Z.-M., and Boreham, J. "Tobacco: The Growing Epidemic." *Nature Medicine,* 1999, *5,* 15–17.

Peto, R., Lopez, A. D., and others. *Mortality from Smoking in Developed Countries, 1950–2000: Indirect Estimates from National Vital Statistics.* Oxford, England: Oxford University Press, 1994.

World Health Organization. *Tobacco or Health: A Global Status Report.* Geneva: World Health Organization, 1997.

CHAPTER NINETEEN

Tobacco Control

Derek Yach

Derek Yach, MBchB, MPH, *is Project Manager for the World Health Organization's Tobacco Free Initiative. From 1995 to 1998, he coordinated WHO's global consultation that led to the adoption by WHO's member states of a new global policy, Health for All in the 21st Century. From 1985 to 1995, he played a leadership role in developing South Africa's epidemiological and community health research and policy capacity. He has published widely on issues related to globalization, tobacco, epidemiology, and health development.*

The twentieth century was characterized by the dramatic increase in an entirely manmade epidemic: that caused by tobacco. Throughout the century, new methods of manufacture, marketing, cigarette design, and distribution were used by the tobacco industry to ensure that tobacco use became ubiquitous. By 2000, almost 1.3 billion adults around the world smoked. On average, children were starting to smoke by their fifteenth birthday; 80 percent of all smokers started by eighteen years of age.

Smoking patterns of the past few decades were causing four million deaths a year by 2000. Current smoking rates will lead to ten million deaths a year by 2030, some 70 percent of them occurring in developing countries. In many countries, although the more affluent are the first to become smokers, this pattern quickly changes, and it is the poor who ultimately suffer the greatest burden of disease from tobacco.

By the late 1950s, tobacco industry scientists privately acknowledged the detrimental impact of tobacco on health. However, it took almost four decades for the major tobacco multinationals to concede this publicly. Since the original epidemiological studies conducted in North America and Europe in the 1950s, there has been a steady stream of studies from countries as diverse as China, India, South Africa, Brazil, and Poland. All clearly show that tobacco is a known or probable cause of more than twenty-five specific diseases. These include ischemic heart disease, chronic respiratory disease, cancers, and stroke. In developing countries, tobacco use exacerbates the impact of underlying additional risks to health resulting from high levels of exposure to tuberculosis, schistosomiasis, and indoor air pollution.

The impact of smoking on the health of the unborn fetus and on nonsmokers is considerable. In recent years, evidence has increasingly shown that in many countries, tobacco results in considerable economic losses and negative environmental consequences. Tobacco is now poised to be the major epidemic of the twenty-first century in developing countries.

In 1998, WHO's Director-General, Dr. Gro Brundtland, established the Tobacco Free Initiative as a special cabinet project. This has led to a substantial increase in effective action against tobacco at the global, regional, and national level. This chapter outlines the future impact of these actions, as well as their likely long-term consequences for the tobacco industry.

BUILDING NATIONAL SUPPORT THROUGH EVIDENCE AND ACTION

National tobacco control is the foundation for public protection against tobacco. While all countries need not repeat studies of the health effects of tobacco, all do need information about the extent of tobacco use domestically in order to assess the potential epidemic they face and to mount effective interventions. These data are also valuable for mobilizing political support for tobacco control no matter what stage of the tobacco epidemic a country is in.

Although surveillance for health effects remains weak in most developing countries, there has been progress in developing a globally standardized approach to measuring tobacco prevalence. The Global Youth Tobacco Survey, which is being implemented in an increasingly large number of countries, will ensure that accurate measures of tobacco use by sex, age, and brand are collected on a regular basis. This basic information will stimulate the development of tobacco control programs and be a means of assessing progress. By 2005, an adult survey that also measures other major risk factors for noncommunicable diseases should be operational in a number of countries.

The majority of countries are concerned about tobacco use among young people and with good intentions have introduced policies and programs that attempt to address this issue. However, these interventions are often less than effective and are not the best use of scarce resources for tobacco control. This concern has led to a review of what really works to reduce youth tobacco use. The findings clearly indicate that policies that work for adults also work for youth. There is clear evidence that among currently known interventions, excise tax increases above inflation have the greatest single impact on youth smoking, particularly because youth are more price sensitive and less addicted then adults. Bans on all forms of promotion, advertising, and marketing benefit both youth and adults.

It is clear that school education programs have limited impact alone. However, they do play a role as part of a comprehensive tobacco control program, including fiscal and legislative policies (incorporating advertising bans and restrictions on smoking in public places), support for cessation programs for both adults and youth, cessation programs, community interventions, and mass media campaigns developed with active input from youth.

Effective implementation of legislation depends on public support. For this reason, media advocacy and communications that frame the tobacco debate in public health terms and encourage vigorous public debate about tobacco control options are essential. There appears to be considerable promise in the twenty-first century for campaigns that highlight how the tobacco industry "dupes" both youth and adults into starting and maintaining tobacco use. National media are likely to become stronger voices for tobacco control over the next decade as their addiction to tobacco advertising revenue is reduced.

For most countries, progress in tobacco control has been slow for three fundamental reasons: lack of funds; weak human and institutional capacity in legislation, economics, and advocacy; and lack of political will. Increasingly, WHO, UNICEF, the World Bank, and a wide range of national and international nongovernmental organizations (NGOs) are working with governments to determine and implement the optimal mix of policies that will work in a particular country. This approach represents a shift from the more "menu-driven" approach to policy development and explicitly builds on national norms, cultural strengths, and political and economic realities.

Dr. Brundtland's global leadership has also encouraged national leaders to be more outspoken about the need for strong action.

REGIONAL SYNERGIES

Simultaneous with national action has been rapid development at regional levels. Regions often share a common language, religion, or political approach. This commonality has already led to innovative approaches in several regions. The best example of this is the European Union (EU). The EU directive on advertising will lead to a progressive ban on all forms of tobacco advertising and promotion with the fifteen current member states by 2006. And with the EU likely to expand over the next decade, this directive could ultimately apply to an additional ten to fifteen countries. The EU program of work in tobacco will expand into other areas over the next few years.

In other regional economic and political blocs, tobacco control is emerging as an issue for attention. Parliamentarians started to join forces across countries in Latin America, French- and Portuguese-speaking African countries, the Persian Gulf states, and the individual nations of Southeast Asia. Regional agreements will expand over the next few years and focus particularly on developing common approaches to reducing smuggling, harmonization of tax systems, mobilization of and by NGOs and health professional bodies, and sharing of research and capacity building.

LETTING TRUTH EMERGE

For decades, the tobacco industry has maintained that tobacco is not a health risk or addictive, that smoking is an adult choice freely made, and that developing countries should focus on priorities other than tobacco, and that successful tobacco control will devastate the economies of many poor countries.

The release since 1998 of internal tobacco industry documents has allowed policymakers to "walk through the minds of the industry." In so doing, they have begun to understand how each of the industry's claims was carefully researched, crafted, and promoted through a network of paid or strongly influenced media supporters, NGOs, front groups, researchers, and policymakers. For decades, tobacco industry-supported scientists in private warned that tobacco was addictive yet denied it in public and even in court testimony. Industry contributions to civil liberties groups, trade unions, and tobacco farmers were earmarked for activities aimed at perpetuating the tobacco industry's arguments.

When WHO announced an inquiry into how the tobacco industry had adversely influenced WHO policy on tobacco over the decades, it joined several other high-level investigations that were announced in 1999. Key among these was the U.S. federal prosecution of the tobacco industry for deception, criminal fraud, and racketeering (under the same law used to indict the Mafia) and the U.K. House of Commons investigations into tobacco industry manipulation of the regulatory environment around tobacco control. These actions all aim to achieve public health goals and do so by countering industry deceptions that have distorted public perceptions of the need for tobacco control.

The reality is that tobacco use begins early in youth: at a time when young people underestimate the health risks and overestimate their potential ability to quit. The World Bank's review of the economics of tobacco use debunked many of the myths about job and revenue losses that effective tobacco control was purported to cause.

The impact of decades of relationship building between tobacco industry representatives and tobacco farmers, retailers, and even finance ministries will take time to alter, but by 2000, the first signs of change were apparent. In the United States, former President Jimmy Carter had taken innovative steps to build a partnership between tobacco farmers and public health officials based on the notion that demand reduction benefits all communities and should be supported as a public good. The special needs of farmers, though, should be acknowledged as requiring attention and support. This dialogue in the United States will in all likelihood globalize.

GLOBAL COMPLEMENTARITY

In this era of globalization, the limits of successful national and regional tobacco control have begun to emerge. The tobacco industry multinationals are structured to take advantage of the global market. Increased consolidation of the industry toward the end of the 1990s left the world with five major tobacco companies: China National Tobacco Corporation (CNTC); Philip Morris, based in the United States; the British-American Tobacco Company (BAT), based in the United Kingdom; Japan Tobacco; and Altadis (resulting from the merger between Seita and Tabacelera) in Spain. Except for CNTC, all other companies embarked on ambitious expansion plans aimed at building up their brands in eastern and central Europe, Asia, and Africa.

In the late 1990s, tobacco control also became more international in scope and started to apply global public goods to its work. The beginning of the development of the Framework Convention on Tobacco Control (FCTC) by WHO's 191 member states in 1999 represented the first time WHO had used the treaty-making right granted in its constitution. This indicates that tobacco is a unique public health problem that demands global legally binding action if success is to be achieved. The FCTC, when it is adopted in the next few years, is likely to focus on controlling the transnational aspects of tobacco use—such things as smuggling, marketing, product regulation, research, and surveillance. The development of the FCTC is in itself leading to enhanced national, NGO, and political commitment to tobacco control worldwide.

In addition, WHO's chair of the United Nations Ad-Hoc Task Force on Tobacco Control is leading to a greater sense of policy coherence among the various sectoral interests that make up the UN. Thus the Food and Agriculture Organization (FAO) is committed to defining where and when demand reduction will harm populations and develop policies to prevent or reduce the impact. The World Bank and International Monetary Fund (IMF) work closely with WHO to implement excise tax policies. UNICEF, UNFPA, UNAIDS, and WHO have started to develop common approaches to working with youth so that the complex mix of risk behaviors is dealt with in a comprehensive manner and that healthy alternatives to tobacco, alcohol, illicit drugs, unsafe sex, and violence are developed. ECOSOC and UNIFEM work with WHO to ensure that women play a stronger leadership role in tobacco control and project their low smoking rate in Asia and Africa as the desirable global norm.

Partnerships with a common sense of purpose are also developing among NGOs and in the private sector. Several hundred NGOs that include health professional bodies, women's groups, cancer and heart associations, environmental groups, and human rights groups as well as tightly focused tobacco control groups have developed strategic alliances at the national and international level. Using the latest information technologies, they are able to mobilize support for the FCTC, for countries under threat from the tobacco industry, and for individuals and communities struggling to introduce local control measures. These local-global linkages are yet another promising force for reversing the tobacco epidemic.

Initially, WHO and NGOs have turned to the pharmaceutical industry for financial and technical support. By 2000, strong working partnerships between public and private groups had led to improved support for the treatment of tobacco dependency, for stronger surveillance systems, and for the use of modern management systems in tobacco control programs. This was just the start. The broader private sector has started to join forces with WHO, the Centers for Disease Control and Prevention (CDC), and other public agencies. Initial reluctance to openly oppose tobacco interests is dissipating, and ethically responsible companies are increasingly distancing themselves from the tobacco industry.

The entertainment industry in Hollywood was recently freed from tobacco product placement by the Master Settlement Agreement, under which tobacco companies agreed to stop all product placement in movies. If tobacco companies are found in violation of the agreement, they are liable for huge fines. The Hollywood entertainment industry and the sports, leisure, and fashion industries are more likely in the future to partner with health organizations rather than the tobacco industry. Investors are also excluding tobacco from highly successful ethical investment funds, due to the questionable nature of the product, coupled with the tobacco industry's uncertain future.

PROSPECTS FOR REAL PROGRESS

All signs point to progress in the twenty-first century. Governments are increasingly moving from general support for tobacco control to implementing measures proven to be effective. NGOs and the private sector are finding that partnerships can improve health. Global actions, such as better surveillance, research, and information sharing, mean that all countries can be equally informed about how best to thwart tobacco industry efforts to prevent policy development. The adoption of the Framework Convention on Tobacco Control and incremental adoption of protocols in the coming decade will make it increasingly difficult for the tobacco industry to seek out new markets.

But there are considerable challenges ahead. The tobacco industry is changing, its products are changing, and its approach to influencing the policy environment is changing. Increased consolidation of the industry means there will be fewer companies, leaner and meaner. New products that could include tobacco with low or no nicotine and nitrosamines will challenge scientists and regulators with claims of safety. New pharmaceutical products that target nicotine-dependent populations may well be introduced not only by the pharmaceutical industry but also by tobacco companies. Constant vigilance will be needed to ensure that new products do lead to public health gains.

By 2000, major tobacco companies like Philip Morris, as part of a new attempt to gain public acceptability and protect itself from future legal actions, had accepted the evidence that tobacco kills and is addictive and had started to invest millions of dollars in programs worldwide to stop children from smoking. Early evaluations of these programs showed that they were ineffective. The public health community will need to carefully analyze and adapt to what the tobacco industry is trying to present as its new "spirit of cooperation."

Finally, as more countries adopt effective policies and the FCTC is increasingly implemented, dramatic reductions in tobacco use should become the norm, with early "achiever" countries acting as a spur to others. With sustained political will, adequate resources, and strong institutions, the twenty-first century could see the end of this entirely manmade epidemic.

Additional Reading

Ciresi, M. V., Walburn, R. B., and Sutton, T. D. *Decades of Deceit: Document Discovery in the Minnesota Tobacco Litigation.*

The World Bank. *Curbing the Epidemic–Governments and the Economics of Tobacco Control.* Washington, D.C., 1999.

Yach, D., and Bettcher, D. "The Globalization of Public Health: I. Threats and Opportunities; II. The Convergence of Self-interest and Altruism." *American Journal of Public Health*, 1998, *88*(5), 735–738; 738–741.

CHAPTER TWENTY

Environmental and Occupational Health

Bernard D. Goldstein

Bernard D. Goldstein, MD, *is Director of the Environmental and Occupational Health Sciences Institute, a joint program of the University of Medicine and Dentistry of New Jersey (UMDNJ) and Rutgers, The State University of New Jersey. He is also Chair of the Department of Environmental and Community Medicine, UMDNJ–Robert Wood Johnson Medical School. Dr. Goldstein served as Assistant Administrator for Research and Development for the U.S. Environmental Protection Agency from 1983 to 1985.*

I n the twentieth century, explosive growth in both basic scientific knowledge and social concern has spurred our understanding of environmental and occupational health threats. I will attempt to anticipate where the science will take us in the twenty-first century and will also touch on emerging social issues that are likely to influence environmental health science. There is much overlap between environmental and occupational health issues, and in some definitions, occupational health is subsumed under the broader term *environmental health*. My focus in this chapter will be on these areas of overlap as they affect human health—but we cannot meet the challenge of protecting human environmental health in the twenty-first century without recognizing that human and ecosystem health are one and the same thing.

ENVIRONMENTAL AND OCCUPATIONAL HEALTH SCIENCE

Environmental health science is in many ways a development of the late twentieth century. Exciting advances in more traditional disciplines—chemistry, biology, physical and earth sciences, ecology, and medicine—have provided new tools. Growing social concern has provided the motivation to apply those tools to the study of environmental health. This concern has also prompted increased investment of research funds, making possible rapid advances in environmental health science that have been the foundation for environmental protection.

Occupational health science traditionally dates itself to Ramazzini, a late-seventeenth-century Italian physician whose insights into the role of work in causing disease established the field of occupational medicine.

The two central scientific disciplines of human environmental health have been toxicology and epidemiology—with exposure assessment now emerging as a discipline in its own right. Toxicology is at the interface of chemistry and biology. It will be challenged in the twenty-first century by the reductionism that has brought biological sciences deeper into molecular structure but farther away from the intact organism. Toxicologists must be able to integrate exciting advances in molecular biology on the cellular, organ, and organism levels. New paradigms are also needed to replace unidirectional models of toxicity so as better to understand the effects of individual agents and mixtures on systems, such as the immune and endocrine, in which modulation in any direction may be of importance.

Epidemiology is now characterized by advances in the ability to tease out confounding factors that previously made it difficult to ascribe cause-and-effect relationships to observed associations. Environmental health epidemiologists face two major challenges. The first is to develop a methodology that will use our improved understanding of the human genome as a basis for unraveling gene-environment interactions. Perhaps the oldest question about disease is, "Why me?" Molecular biology will provide an understanding of the genetic polymorphisms underlying susceptibility to disease. This will greatly increase the power of epidemiological studies to identify the environmental and occupational factors that place people at risk. The second challenge is to determine more precisely the environmental health impacts of changes due to industrial growth and regulatory interventions. This will require building on advances in assessing the value of clinical therapeutic interventions.

The field of exposure assessment, including many aspects of industrial hygiene, has provided new groundwork for understanding and preventing environmental health problems. Simplistic approaches to pollutant control have equated hazard with risk. Yet hazard is an intrinsic property of all chemicals—it is the dose that makes the poison. Without exposure, there is no risk, and it is the province of the field of exposure assessment to estimate exposure to different populations and to provide the basis for prevention through exposure avoidance.

The disciplinary gaps among toxicology, epidemiology, and exposure assessment are being bridged by the hybrid field of molecular epidemiology. This uses the tools of molecular biology to develop biological markers of exposure, effect, and susceptibility that increase the power of epidemiological studies. Molecular epidemiology has been particularly applicable to studies of workers. Surrogates of dose, such as job description or standard industrial hygiene measurements, are being replaced by personal monitoring technologies and by biological markers of exposure.

In the past two decades, risk assessment has become a particularly useful paradigm for approaching environmental problems. However, risk assessment is essentially a tool of secondary prevention (addressing existing exposures) rather than primary prevention (preventing adverse exposures from occurring). This is because it is far more difficult to quantify something that has not occurred. Yet prevention is far more crucial for protecting environmental health (Goldstein, 1996).

The major social value of environmental health science has been the provision of predictive tools—for example, laboratory tests that help avert the development of new chemicals that cause mutations or persist in the environment. Although risk assessment will continue to be important, for the twenty-first century we need additional predictive tools that will allow us to do primary prevention more effectively. We also need to characterize and communicate risks more effectively. This depends on our going beyond poorly understood probabilistic statements (such as a cancer risk of one in a million due to lifetime exposure to a specific pollutant level) to specify characteristics such as duration of exposure and particular populations at risk (Goldstein, 1995). Identifying susceptible individuals will permit targeted approaches to workers' health but will also raise very important ethical issues that society is now only beginning to tackle.

Environmental health science of the twentieth century started with a particular chemical effluent and worked toward understanding its effect. The twenty-first century will be characterized by having the scientific ability to start with the adverse impact on human health and the environment and then working backward to its cause. This attribution of disease to cause will require an understanding of gene-environment interactions.

As we unfold the human genome, we will learn the genetic basis that is necessary, but not sufficient, for many common human diseases. Sufficiency will depend on our environment, in the broadest sense. Lifestyle factors, including what we eat and drink, as well as exposure to chemical and physical agents, will be the determinants of whether and at what age our individual genetic tendencies will lead to disease and death.

Another environmental health trend in the twenty-first century will be a greater focus on noncancer afflictions, particularly those that affect children. Asthma is a major concern. If the increase in incidence observed worldwide continues unabated, it will be a major scourge of the twenty-first century.

For occupational health, the challenge of musculoskeletal problems, including back injury and repetitive motion trauma, will remain highly significant sources of pain and disability for the foreseeable future until understanding of the basics of biostructure and biomechanics approaches our depth of knowledge of biochemistry and physiology.

One of the scientific failures of the twentieth century has been our inability to understand the full implications of the fact that exposure is usually to *mixtures* of pollutants. Central to the issue of environmental justice is understanding the implications of multiple sources of exposure within and across media in poorer and disadvantaged communities, which tend to have larger numbers of polluting sources (Institute of Medicine, 1999). Understanding the interaction of mixtures of both short-acting and persistent hormonal modulators is also important to assess the potential risks of endocrine disruptors. Yet another example is how the current effort to learn the cause of adverse effects epidemiologically associated with airborne particulates is complicated by air pollution being not a single chemical entity but a gas-aerosol complex of multiple chemical and physical species. Imposition of costly environmental control measures requires correctly identifying the cause of these adverse effects and their sources.

Another failure has been our inability to understand the relationship between a variety of nonspecific symptoms and their alleged environmental and workplace causes. Many individuals with complaints that they relate to environmental exposures are grouped under such rubrics as multiple chemical sensitivities or the Gulf War syndrome. Although we cannot reliably demonstrate that the exposures caused disease, these individuals are clearly suffering physically and mentally.

The significant environmental health problems of the twenty-first century will not be solvable by any one discipline working alone (National Research Council, 1996). Multidisciplinary approaches will be crucial. Incorporating the power of social sciences is particularly necessary. For example, land use planning is of central importance to environmental control, whether related to the urbanization of developing countries or the landscape-devouring urban sprawl of the developed world. Yet land use planning rarely connects with environmental health in either academia or decision making (Greenberg, Popper, West, and Krueckenberg, 1994).

SOCIAL ISSUES LIKELY TO AFFECT ENVIRONMENTAL HEALTH SCIENCE

Demands for a clean environment in the twenty-first century will require better measures of human and planetary environmental health. Twentieth-century environmental regulation focused primarily on controlling emissions. But despite significant improvement in emissions reduction, the environment still remains blighted and at further risk of degradation. Control of emissions has hardly kept pace with the expanding industrial base. For example, even in countries with rigorous control of automotive emissions, the decrease in emissions per mile is in a losing race with the rapid increase in number of miles driven, an increase that will continue as poorer countries develop and as urban sprawl envelops the land of developed countries. In addition, for many air and water problems, nonpoint source emissions are of signal importance—an example is the damage done to water bodies by runoff from agricultural activities. Indicators of actual environmental effects that can be directly attributed to sources will be far more effective than judging environmental health solely on the basis of effluent control and ambient levels of pollutants (Moldan and Billharz, 1997).

One healthy trend we are seeing is the greater involvement of stakeholders in environmental health science and of science in society. Scientists are recognizing the value of involvement of communities and of workers in their research activities, and communities are demanding more openness in the development of the environmental health science agenda and in performance and communication in the field (Commission on Risk Assessment and Risk Management, 1998). Access through the Internet to information about local sources of pollution will be a further spur to community involvement. A related recent trend is known as postmodern science. To the extent that it reflects the need for scientists to be responsive to public concerns rather than aloof and to involve communities and workers in their research, including the setting of the research agenda, it will be of great help. But to the extent this represents the nihilism espoused in such fashionable academic movements as deconstructionism, it will only hinder the ability of environmental and occupational health scientists to provide the understanding needed to protect public health and the environment.

Even the definition of *community* will change. The World Wide Web will result in a horizontal world in which geographical proximity will be less important than a community of interests and in which the usual hierarchical national organization will be challenged by groups of like-minded individuals linked by a communication system that knows no boundaries. In such a world, the level of scientific literacy is likely to be the greatest determinant of environmental and occupational health.

As we enter the twenty-first century, two unifying themes are much discussed as guidance for the future survival of our planet: sustainable development and the precautionary principle. Sustainable development is the advancement of the economic and social well-being of the planet's inhabitants in a manner that does not detract from our limited local or global resources. Human health is inextricably part of sustainable development—for example, it is inconceivable that the continent of Africa could develop sustainably without finding a way to prevent malaria and other widespread and debilitating diseases.

Tensions are already apparent in defining sustainability in relation to economic growth and to trade (Costanza and others, 1995), as well as to worker and environmental health issues. Sustainable development will continue to depend on technological progress, which, as in the past, will pose a threat to workers and to the environment. New fibers and structural elements, new energy sources and communications technologies—all will challenge our ability to prevent adverse consequences to worker and environmental health.

The precautionary principle is a classic formulation of basic public health concepts that is now being used to justify acting on environmental problems despite uncertainties. One definition of the principle is expressed as follows: "Where there are threats of serious or irreversible damage, lack of full scientific certainty shall not be used as a reason for postponing cost-effective measures to prevent environmental degradation."

Thus by definition, the level of scientific information on which the precautionary principle is invoked includes some significant extent of uncertainty; otherwise there would be no need to invoke it. There must also be substantial social or economic costs involved, or else, again, the action would be taken without deference to the principle. Accordingly, invoking the precautionary principle carries some finite likelihood that the action will be both mistaken and costly—in fact, the more precautionary we are as a society, the more likely we are to make costly mistakes in the name of precaution. In the twenty-first century, it will be imperative that we both act in a precautionary manner and that we devise means to test whether our actions have been effective. Unfortunately, so far, regulators have shown themselves unwilling to invest the resources in the scientific studies needed to determine whether regulatory actions have in fact been beneficial.

How society will view science and progress in the twenty-first century will be critical to meeting planetary health threats. In our current era, it is easy to forget that technological progress is not inevitable. The worldview during the Middle Ages in Europe was inimical to science and technology—in fact, that era witnessed a retrogression from the level of technological achievement of the Roman Empire. The Industrial Revolution was greeted with opposition that ranged from a romantic yearning for primitive societies to violent Luddite attacks on textile mills. Similar opposition to modern technology may conceivably grow stronger in the coming decades.

The romantic stream of opposition to science and technology today often takes the form of the New Age cult of Gaia, the Earth Goddess, who must be propitiated by restoring the earth to a pristine state. The Luddite strain is also evident in ecoterrorists who justify risking the life of a logger rather than allowing a tree to be cut. They often ally themselves with animal rights activists who are against the testing of chemicals on animals, and some have no compunction against sabotaging research or killing researchers in order to protect animal life. It is not certain whether these groups will gather sufficient strength to slow significantly the development of environmental health knowledge, but the general unwillingness of scientists to take the objections seriously contributes to the problem.

Environmentalism is also increasingly converging with forces that oppose new technology. This is most evident in Europe, where it has focused on biotechnology, although it is difficult at times to distinguish between a genuine response by an environmentally concerned electorate and an attempt at trade protectionism in an area where the United States has technical leadership. The latter is well exemplified by the opposition to the importation of meat obtained from animals treated with bovine growth hormone, despite repeated formal findings by European and international scientific bodies supporting the lack of risk from such treatment. The United States position on global warming is another example of economic well-being given primacy over environmental concerns. This increasing tendency to use the environment for nationalistic purposes related to competitiveness between developed countries or between developing and developed countries is likely to be a major obstacle in dealing with global environmental problems (Johnson, 1995; Porter, 1999).

Society is being challenged by the need to identify and respond to potentially catastrophic changes that come upon us insidiously but irreversibly, as with climate modifications. Catastrophic environmental problems in the twenty-first century may result from destruction by human activities of the various feedback loops that relate our biosphere to the earth's geophysical characteristics. Human activities have decreased the inherent buffering capacity in these loops, and just as an aging human is more vulnerable to relatively minor perturbations in one organ system, so is the biosphere of our planet seemingly more at risk to catastrophic changes that could result from human activities, such as fossil fuel energy use, deforestation, erosion, and desertification, whose indirect planetary impacts have previously been well buffered.

War is unfortunately the most likely cause of environmental degradation resulting directly and indirectly in adverse effects on human health. It is possible that environmental degradation will itself lead to mass movement of populations or to military action (Percival and Homer-Dixon, 1996).

Many environmental threats in the twenty-first century will coincide with the dying out of the post–World War II baby boomers. Future historians may call them the fortunate generation. Their fortune was to have been born after the discovery of penicillin, to have lived in an age of selfish overconsumption of resources, and to have died before the oil ran out. There are also major threats to global freshwater resources, with timelines that appear to coincide with the shift to major new energy sources (Postel, Daily, and Ehrlich, 1996). Desalination and other approaches to obtaining fresh water for the twenty-first century also have significant energy implications.

Each of the many scenarios as to what will replace petroleum as our major energy source has its own environmental and occupational health implications that need to be thoroughly explored before adoption. Unfortunately, if we follow the same scenario as occurred with the recent switch to oxygenated gasoline, to which one hundred million Americans in the general population and the petrochemical workforce were exposed without adequate advance testing, there could be major environmental health problems caused by new engines or fuels.

Rapid homogenization of our globe has characterized this fortunate generation, as reflected in the advent of telecommunication and an increase in the speed of travel. This homogenization also extends to infectious diseases. Just as a monoculture of corn increases the likelihood of significant damage due to a single new vector, so does the homogenization of the human environment have a potentially significant impact on our resistance to new vectors. New organisms, or antibiotic-resistant agents, can be spread at dramatic speed in our new world of frequent international travel.

CONCLUSION: TWO MAJOR CROSSCUTTING ISSUES

I have divided this chapter rather arbitrarily, separating the environmental and occupational health issues that will be driven primarily by changes in our scientific knowledge from those in which the science will be driven by social issues. I conclude that there are similarly two central driving forces. The first is population growth. In the twenty-first century, either we will find a means of stabilizing human population levels or we will conduct the ultimate Malthusian experiment.

Second, we must remember that there is only one sure prediction for the twenty-first century: there will be major environmental and occupational health problems that no one today envisions. The implication is that we need a scientific community capable of responding rapidly and flexibly to the unpredictable.

References

Communicating Risk in a Changing World. Washington, D.C.: The Presidential/Congressional Commision on Risk Assessment and Risk Management, 1998, 5–9.

Costanza, R., and others. "Sustainable Trade: A New Paradigm for World Welfare." *Environment,* 1995, *37,* 16–20, 39–43.

Goldstein, B. D. "The Who, What, When, Where, and Why of Risk Characterization." *Policy Studies Journal,* 1995, *23,* 70–75.

Goldstein, B. D. "Risk Assessment as a Governmental Indicator." *Technology,* 1996, *333A,* 59–62.

Greenberg, M., Popper, F., West, B., and Krueckenberg, D. "Linking City Planning and Public Health in the United States." *Journal of Planning Literature,* 1994, *8,* 235–239.

Committee on Environmental Justice, Institute of Medicine. *Toward Environmental Justice: Research, Education, and Health Policy Needs.* Washington, D.C.: National Academy of Sciences, National Academy Press, 1999.

Johnson, P. "Observations: Arguing for Free Trade." *Commentary,* August 1995, *100,* 50–51.

Moldan, B., and Billharz, S.(eds.). "Sustainability Indicators." *SCOPE,* 1997, *58,* 6.

National Research Council. National Forum on Science and Technology Goals. *Linking Science and Technology to Society's Environmental Goals,* 1996, 5.

Percival, V., and Homer-Dixon, T. "Environmental Scarcity and Violent Conflict: The Case of Rwanda." *Journal of Environment and Development,* 5, 1996, 270–291.

Porter, G. "Trade Competition and Pollution Standards: 'Race to the Bottom' or 'Stuck at the Bottom'?" *Journal of Environment and Development,* 8, 1999, 133–151.

Postel, S. L., Daily, G. C., and Ehrlich, P. R. "Human Appropriation of Renewable Fresh Water." *Science, 271,* 1996, 785–788.

CHAPTER TWENTY-ONE

Environmental Health

Anthony J. McMichael, Alistair Woodward

Anthony J. McMichael, MBBS, PhD, *is Professor of Epidemiology at the London School of Hygiene and Tropical Medicine. His research interests for more than twenty-five years have encompassed the causes of occupational diseases, dietary causes of cancer, and environmental risks to health. He has a major interest in the health risks of global environmental change and chairs the health impact assessment panel of the United Nations' intergovernmental Panel on Climate Change.*

Alistair Woodward, MBBS, PhD, *is a public health physician and epidemiologist who is currently Professor of Public Health at the Wellington School of Medicine, New Zealand. A graduate in medicine from the University of Adelaide, he undertook his teaching in public health in Australia and the United Kingdom. His interests in research and teaching include environmental health, the social determinants of health, and tobacco control.*

Population health indices have broadly improved in the past half century. Infant mortality rates have generally fallen; life expectancy has risen. This improvement resulted from gains in material living conditions, the retreat of infectious diseases, reduced exposures to occupational and ambient environmental hazards, changes in personal and community behavior, advances in medical and public health technology, and better health care. However, the gains have been unevenly shared around the world and may be readily undone—as shown, for example, by the plunging life expectancy of men in the former Soviet Union in the early 1990s and in several severely AIDS-afflicted sub-Saharan African countries over the past decade.

With a mixture of good management and luck, we can extend and consolidate improvements in human health during the twenty-first century. Challenges to be faced include continuing changes in infectious disease patterns as human ecology, mobility, and environmental encroachment evolve; conflicts that may occur in response to dwindling natural resources; and unprecedented changes in the type and scale of environmental hazards to human health.

At the 1972 United Nations Conference on the Environment in Stockholm, concerns focused on the increasing release of chemical contaminants into local environments, the prospects of depletion of certain strategic materials, and the environmental consequences of urbanization. The industrial intensification in Western countries that accompanied the economic growth in the two decades after World War II was compounded by rapid programmed industrialization in Soviet bloc countries and new, often poorly controlled, and increasingly debt-driven industrial and agricultural growth in newly independent Third World countries. The world experienced various serious episodes of air pollution (as in London in 1952), organic mercury poisoning (in Minamata, Japan, in 1956), heavy metals accumulations (especially lead and cadmium), pesticide toxicity, and scares from environmental ionizing radiation exposures.

Three decades later, as we enter the twenty-first century, those same toxicological environmental problems persist widely around the world. Since 1972, we have had Bhopal, Seveso, Chernobyl, and other dramatic local disasters. Air pollution is an increasing problem in many large cities in the developing world. Meanwhile, against the global backdrop, a new and unfamiliar set of environmental problems is emerging. These problems were, apparently, beyond the perceptual horizon at the Stockholm Conference. However, by the 1992 UN Conference on Environment and Development, in Rio de Janeiro, they were beginning to command attention. Indeed, one of them, global climate change, was addressed directly by the adoption of the UN Framework Convention on Climate Change.

THE MAIN TYPES OF GLOBAL ENVIRONMENTAL CHANGE

Global climate change, occurring because of human augmentation of the greenhouse effect in the lower atmosphere, is now a potent symbol of emerging and unprecedented large-scale environmental changes. These changes pose a hazard to human health during the twenty-first century. Average world temperatures increased during the last quarter of the twentieth century, and the pace of increase actually quickened as the 1990s ended. Weather patterns in many regions displayed increasing instability in the 1990s. Scientists, the public, and policymakers have become increasingly aware of these human-induced climatic changes, and questions about future health consequences are now clearly on the environmental health agenda. Meanwhile, higher in the atmosphere, depletion of stratospheric ozone by human-made gases such as chlorofluorocarbons (CFCs) has been documented over several decades. Ambient terrestrial levels of ultraviolet irradiation are estimated to have increased by around 10 percent at mid-to-high latitudes since 1980. This exposure is projected to peak within the first two decades of the twenty-first century.

The great significance of these changes in the lower and middle atmospheres is that they provide a clear signal, perhaps the most unambiguous yet, of planetary overload. The size and intensity of the total human enterprise has now become so great that several of the earth's biophysical systems are being stressed beyond limits. This enormous aggregate impact of humankind is a function of our still-increasing numbers, our levels of consumption of energy and materials, and our high level of waste generation. We have manifestly exceeded the capacity of the troposphere and stratosphere to act as "sinks" for our industrial and agricultural gaseous wastes. Likewise, as the human demand for space, materials, and food increases, so populations and species of plants and animals around the world are being extinguished at an accelerating rate—apparently faster than the great natural extinctions that have occurred in eons past. Alongside that loss of biodiversity, there is increasing translocation of "invasive" species into nonnatural environments via intensified food production, trade, and mobility.

Since the 1940s, there has been a marked upturn in the human "fixation" of nitrogen, converted from the inert form to biologically active nitrate and ammonium ions. Most of the sixfold increase has been due to the use of nitrogenous fertilizers. Likewise, we have markedly altered the geochemical cycling of sulfur in the biosphere. These two chemical changes are affecting the acidity and nutrient balances of the world's soils and waterways. Meanwhile, the ever-increasing demands of agricultural and livestock production are adding further stresses to the world's arable lands and pastures. We enter the twenty-first century with an estimated one-third of the world's previously productive land seriously damaged by erosion, compaction, salination, waterlogging, and chemicalized destruction of organic content. Similar pressures on the world's ocean fisheries have left most of them severely depleted or seriously stressed. These changes to the integrity of soils and waterways and to the productivity of fisheries are compromising the capacity of the world to continue sustainably to provide sufficient food for its people.

Three other worldwide environmental changes portend risks to future human health. First, freshwater aquifers are being depleted of their "fossil water" on all continents. Agricultural and industrial demand now often greatly exceeds the rate of natural recharge. Second, many long-lived and biologically active chemicals have become widely distributed across the globe. Lead and other heavy metals are present at increasing concentrations in remote environments such as the polar ice caps. As semivolatile organic chemical pollutants (such as polychlorinated biphenyls, or PCBs) are disseminated toward the poles via a sequential "distillation" process *across* the cells of the lower atmosphere, their concentrations are increasing in polar mammals and fish and in the human groups that eat these animals. Chemical pollutants are thus no longer just an issue of local toxicity.

Third, urbanization is occurring in all countries. By 2050, the great majority of humans will live in medium-to-large cities. There are various environmental benefits of compact city living. However, urban populations have a large and mostly displaced environmental impact, best described as an "ecological footprint." Modern Western cities typically require an area of the earth's surface around 150 times greater than that of the city, to supply needs and absorb wastes. Some of the health risks consequent on urban living are thus displaced to populations remote in space and time. Urbanization also tends to concentrate certain environmental health problems—including air pollution, traffic hazards, noise, industrial exposures, and microbiological and chemical contamination along extended food chains. Rapid urbanization amplifies the role of cities as gateways for new and disseminated infections. Population movement from rural areas into cities and variously intensified urban-rural, interurban, and intraurban contacts create new opportunities for otherwise marginal microbes—as happened in the launching of the poorly transmissible HIV/AIDS virus in the 1980s. Likewise, the modern advance of dengue fever in tropical and subtropical zones has been aided by the urban expansion of breeding sites for the mosquito vector.

The reported rates of food poisoning have increased in Western countries during the past two decades—and nearly doubled in the United Kingdom between the mid-1980s and the mid-1990s. The reasons for this increase are not clear. They are likely to include changes in dietary habits (for example, more frequent consumption of reheated and precooked foods), increased long-distance trade in perishables (the spread of the potentially lethal *E. coli 0157* in North America and Europe in the mid-1990s, for example, was aided by distribution of bacterially contaminated beef from South America), and factors in the local environment. In New Zealand, the typical summer peaks in foodborne infections have recently extended further into the autumn months, in association with rising temperatures over the past decade.

What is driving these environmental changes? The impact of human activity worldwide is a function of levels of consumption, modes of consumption and waste generation (dependent on prevailing technologies), and the number of people. The reasons for increasing consumption of physical and biological resources include increasing affluence of large populations in developing countries, the rise of a culture that measures social worth in terms of what is owned and used, and aggressive international marketing by powerful corporations. In some respects, new technologies are "environment friendly" (for example, energy-efficient heating and lighting, biodegradable detergents), but in some, new modes of consumption are more destructive than the old (examples include intensive fishing practices and the increasing use of coal-fired power stations in some countries). The determinants of population growth are complex and vary between countries and over time. But there is a strong link in less developed countries with poverty and lack of social services, particularly education.

OTHER ANTICIPATED HEALTH IMPACTS OF GLOBAL CHANGE

One of the most striking trends in the global economic environment over the past fifty years has been the rapid growth in international trade—in goods, services, and human resources. Where trade leads to both economic *and* social development, one expects to see health gains. However, if one of the parties is impoverished by the exchange or there is widely unequal distribution of the benefits of the trade, the health of the disadvantaged population is likely to suffer. International trade may also act as an accidental carrier of health threats. An example is the spread of disease vectors such as mosquitoes, which have been carried by plane and ship to relatively isolated parts of the globe (such as New Zealand) where human populations are highly susceptible to infectious diseases such as dengue and Ross River fever.

The genetic engineering of food species (which often entails the insertion of genes from unrelated species into crop plants) may help increase world food production—and may do so in ways that lessen pressures on the environment (as by reducing insecticide use). However, there are unresolved concerns about how genetically modified (GM) crops might pose risks to human health. Some preliminary but inconclusive evidence indicates that potential toxins could result from the product of the "transgenic" gene itself, from other changes in plant chemistry induced by the rest of the transgenic "construct" (gene promoters and the like), or from the altered functioning of host organism genes. Various scenarios of altered balance between species have been posited by scientists, entailing the unplanned spread of either transgenic plants or their inserted genes into wider nature. By analogy, there have been various examples in recent years of how human disturbances of agroecosystems and adjoining natural ecosystems have resulted in the unexpected introduction or increase of infectious diseases—Junin virus in Argentina, Machupo virus in Bolivia, Lyme disease in the northeastern United States, hantavirus pulmonary syndrome in the U.S. Southwest, and so on. Similar chains of ecological consequence could follow the inadvertent spread of transgenic organisms or hybrids into natural ecosystems. Although this may be unlikely, other experiences in recent decades underscore the need for heightened precaution in our increasingly intrusive interventions in the natural world. Our capacity to modulate the molecular basis of life itself holds great promise, but necessitates a precautionary approach lest human health and other living organisms and systems be endangered.

UNDERSTANDING THE SCIENTIFIC CAVEATS AND UNCERTAINTIES

It is important to understand the unusual and difficult challenges that these global environmental changes present to population health scientists. Traditional environmental health research proceeds locally and empirically, observing exposures (chemical, physical, or microbiological) and associated health outcomes, and assessing and quantifying the causal relationships. The new and unfamiliar challenge that is posed by the prospect of worsening trends in these large-scale environmental changes is to reasonably foresee and estimate the health consequences in future decades. This requires working from projected scenarios of future environmental conditions—for example, climatic conditions as modeled by climatologists for the years 2020 and 2050—and applying existing knowledge or theory about how climatic variation affects a particular health outcome. If we know how death rates in urban populations in southern Canada are affected by heat waves in today's world, can we model how they would respond to a summer season in a future warmer world in which the frequency of heat waves is, say, tripled?

A more complicated example refers to estimating the ways in which changes in world climatic conditions would affect the potential geographical range of transmission of mosquito-borne infectious diseases such as malaria and dengue fever. Considerable developmental research has recently been done on such tasks, building and testing mathematical models that give indications of the direction, timing, and extent of change. For example, from multiple simulations by computer, conducted by various research groups, it seems likely that malaria will significantly extend its geographical range of potential transmission during the twenty-first century as average temperatures rise by several degrees Celsius. Similar types of modeling, allowing also for future trends in trade and economic development, have estimated the impacts of climate change on world yields of cereal grains. A slight downturn appears likely overall, greatest in regions where supplies are already marginal (such as in food-insecure South Asia, parts of western Asia and northern Africa, and Central America). This would result in a climate-induced increment in the number of malnourished people during the coming century.

The impact of global environmental change will, more generally, differ between populations. Other causes of heightened vulnerability to disease and injury due to climate change include environmental impoverishment (such as the clearing of indigenous forests that serve valuable flood control and water purification functions), population growth (leading, for example, to settlement in cyclone-prone coastal areas), and reduction in basic public health services (such as disease surveillance and vector control). The impacts will also vary across sectors. For example, in resource-rich countries, the agribusiness industry may be able to adapt to a changing environment if the rate of change fits the time frame for investment in new technology (and provided there are no unexpected frame-jumping changes, such as the emergence of new pests). However, in the same countries, certain ecosystems that are central to human health may be less resilient, unable to cope with environmental change that is unprecedentedly rapid, and not susceptible to technological rescue.

CONCLUSION

Forecasting the health impacts of global environmental changes is an inexact science. Future scenarios of environmental change contain many approximations. Impacts on complex environmental and ecological systems are uncertain—and may well include intrinsically unforeseeable "surprises" (such as the emergence of new diseases because of altered climatic conditions). Sources of uncertainty include gaps in the data, the inherently variable nature of many of the phenomena being studied, and the subjective judgments required for construction of plausible scenarios. Nevertheless, scientists have no real alternative since (1) today's emerging large-scale environmental trends are likely to evolve during the twenty-first century, (2) many of these environmental changes entail serious risks of irreversibility (the loss of species is certainly irreversible), and (3) governments and public are asking scientists to estimate the likely health consequences.

The fact that the risks to human well-being and health are spatially and temporally distant and uncertain does not justify discounting the hazard. Rather, this is a situation in which care is required. A major challenge in the new century will be to protect and extend the recent gains in human health. To do this, we must understand and sustain the life-supporting functions of our physical and biological environment.

CHAPTER TWENTY-TWO

Family and Reproductive Health

Allan Rosenfield, Elizabeth Tyler Crone

Allan Rosenfield, MD, *is Dean of the Mailman School of Public Health, Columbia University, and De Lamar Professor of Public Health and of Obstetrics and Gynecology. He is the author of more than 110 articles in the fields of population, women's reproductive health, obstetrics and gynecology, human rights, and health policy.*
    Elizabeth Tyler Crone, MPH, *is Program Officer at the Spunk Fund, a small, private foundation with an emphasis on child health and international development.*

The 1994 International Conference on Population and Development (ICPD), held in Cairo (the third such conference, following earlier ones in 1974 and 1984), established a new paradigm for programs in population and reproductive health and set the agenda for the twenty-first century. The overall theme was comprehensive sexual and reproductive health care for women and men of reproductive age. The resulting Programme of Action called for both an expansion of reproductive health services and recognition of the importance of women making free, informed choices to meet their reproductive goals with minimal risk. Still acknowledging population imperatives in parts of the world where rates of growth are the highest, the 1994 ICPD demonstrated a shift from what had been largely a demographic agenda to one that focused on reproductive health more broadly.

Among specific areas to be included in a comprehensive reproductive heath program are the provision of contraceptive services; the prevention, screening, and treatment of sexually transmitted diseases (STDs) and HIV/AIDS; the provision of maternity care to reduce high rates of maternal mortality; the provision of safe abortion where they are legal and the treatment of incomplete abortions where they are illegal; the provision of care to adolescents; the involvement of men; and most broadly, the empowerment of women.

A major challenge for the twenty-first century is to develop the means to implement the goals set in 1994. Unfortunately, insufficient progress has been made in achieving these goals, in part because of several obstacles. Although estimates of the costs to expand contraceptive services were reasonable, the costs of the rest of the reproductive health agenda had been underestimated. Much more information is needed on the costs of STD and HIV prevention screening and treatment, of efforts to decrease maternal mortality, and of additional components of reproductive health beyond family planning. The essential goals of the empowerment of women and pursuit of gender equity are exceptionally difficult to budget. Furthermore, the implementation of comprehensive, integrated services where resources are limited is a serious challenge. We will briefly review the progress made so far and then comment on hopes for the future.

Because the United States had played a positive role at the 1994 ICPD and had committed a substantial increase in funding for the ICPD program, the ensuing 1994 U.S. elections were a major setback, as the new Congress reversed the government's support for the ICPD goals. Because the United States was the largest single bilateral donor, this political reversal had a significant impact. In part due to the U.S. political change, there has been a decrease in international assistance and development aid generally and in support of reproductive health initiatives specifically. Family planning assistance through USAID dropped from $542 million in 1995 to $385 million in 1999. More generally, funding for reproductive health initiatives has not met the goals set by the ICPD. Annual global spending on family planning and the prevention of STDs falls short of the needs projected by the ICPD.

In addition, in many parts of the developing world, the past several years have seen a worsening of the economy. The gap between human needs and available resources has intensified, perhaps best seen in the economic and social toll of both HIV/AIDS and other STDs and the disproportionate burden of maternal mortality in less developed regions. For success to be reached in the achievement of these goals, strong political commitment and the ensuing global partnerships, inter-governmental cooperation, and cross-sectoral alliances must be in place.

Progress since the 1994 ICPD has been disappointing:

- There has been little, if any, evidence of a decrease in the morbidity related to STDs and reproductive tract infections.

- The challenges of HIV/AIDS have increased, with uneven hope for the future in poor countries. One solution, the development of an AIDS vaccine, is unlikely in the foreseeable future.

- The "safe motherhood" agenda has so far had little impact in decreasing the high rates of maternal mortality in poor countries.

- Complications of unsafe illegal abortions continue to cause significant morbidity and mortality in many poor countries.

- Adolescent pregnancy remains a daunting challenge.

FAMILY PLANNING

The first part of the Cairo agenda was in effect introduced in the late 1960s with the development of national voluntary family planning efforts first in Asia, then in Latin America, and thereafter in sub-Saharan Africa. In the intervening years, the development of programs to provide contraceptive services has been one of very few public health success stories of the twentieth century. As of 1998, fully 56 percent of all married women used a modern method of contraception (67 percent in the more developed world and 54 percent in the less developed world, 43 percent excluding China; Population Reference Bureau, 1998). Since the prevalence of contraceptives in the developing world in the 1960s was estimated to be less than 5 percent, the increases over the past thirty years are truly dramatic. Nonetheless, it is estimated that more than 150 million couples in developing countries still have significant unmet needs for contraception.

SEXUALLY TRANSMITTED DISEASES (STDs) AND HIV/AIDS

The true magnitude of STDs is typically underestimated because many are asymptomatic and carry a social stigma. Recent estimates indicate that STDs are among the most common causes of illness around the world: 12 million cases of syphilis, 62 million cases of gonorrhea, 89 million cases of chlamydia, and 170 million cases of trichomoniasis—a cumulative total of over 333 million cases of the four major curable STDs in persons of reproductive age (Gerbase and others, 1998). Approximately one million people are infected with a new STD each day. With effective educational programs, many of these cases could be prevented, and with screening and early intervention, the majority of infections could be cured at early stages of infection, thus preventing long-term complications.

In disability-adjusted life years lost for women of reproductive age, STDs are second only to maternal mortality. STDs and HIV necessitate an increase in the number of female-controlled methods to prevent transmission as well as improved prevention, screening, and treatment efforts. STDs can lead to pelvic inflammatory disease and ultimately infertility. If left untreated in pregnant women, STDs may result in low-birthweight infants as well as eye and lung damage in newborns. STDs are also an important cofactor in the transmission of HIV.

HIV/AIDS is the most serious epidemic of the twentieth century and destined to retain that dubious honor in the twenty-first, taking a horrific toll in Africa, Asia, and Latin America. Despite increased knowledge about the prevention of HIV transmission, sixteen thousand people become newly infected every day. At the end of 1998, 33.4 million people were estimated to be living with HIV. Approximately 13.9 million people have died from AIDS since the beginning of the epidemic. HIV is increasingly affecting women: almost half of the adults around the world living with HIV or AIDS today are female. The impact on those in their reproductive years has been without parallel and has rippled through all segments of society. One in every three children orphaned by HIV/AIDS is less than five years old. Almost all of the nearly six hundred thousand children infected with HIV each year are infected by their mothers before or during birth or through breast-feeding (Joint United Programme, 1998).

Life expectancy in parts of southern Africa is falling, and decades of progress in child health are being negated by this epidemic. What does an epidemic of this proportion and with this devastating a toll on human life necessitate? Governments must provide strong political commitment and significant financial support for a broad and frank preventive educational campaign to bring about behavior change. Advances in drug therapies have postponed disease and lengthened life in some regions of the world. Yet these essential drugs are largely inaccessible in the developing world, where more than 95 percent of HIV-infected persons live and where 95 percent of all deaths from AIDS have occurred. Short regimens of antiretrovirals have greatly reduced maternal-fetal transmission in the developed world, and this therapy is being introduced in some developing countries. Given the depth and complexity of the epidemic and the lack of resources in many of the poorer countries of the world, however, highest priority must be given by the donor community (both public and private) to the development of an effective vaccine. Vaccine development will be the ethical, economic, and scientific challenge of the next twenty years.

ADOLESCENT PREGNANCY

Adolescent pregnancy has been increasingly recognized as an urgent reproductive health problem. Inconsistent data lead to ineffective estimates of the magnitude of the issue. Further, the success of prevention efforts has been uneven at best. In 1995 alone, young women aged fifteen to nineteen gave birth to seventeen million infants (World Health Organization, 1998). Maternal mortality from pregnancy-related complications is one of the major causes of death for girls in this age bracket. The problems are magnified by WHO estimates that the number of young women aged fifteen to nineteen will increase from 251 million in 1995 to 307 million in 2025.

The reproductive health needs of young women are great and necessitate the appropriate provision of services. Young women need access to reproductive health care, including sexuality education, provision of contraceptives, and screening and treatment for STDs. Transition to adulthood has become increasingly fraught with violence and lost opportunities. Therefore, we need to ensure the health of the world's adolescents so that these young people can enjoy life as healthy adults.

MATERNAL MORTALITY

The World Health Organization estimates that 585,000 women die each year of pregnancy-related complications (World Health Organization and UNICEF, 1996). Put more dramatically, more than one woman dies every minute from a complication of pregnancy. Well over 95 percent of these deaths take place in poor countries in Asia, Africa, and Latin America. For example, a woman's lifetime risk of maternal mortality in northern Europe is 1 in 4,000, while the risk in West Africa is 1 in 12.5. As serious a tragedy as these numbers represent, in all likelihood these are underestimates of the problem. After a dozen years of what has been called the Safe Motherhood initiative, there has been little visible impact on this tragic problem.

There is increasing agreement that all women must have access to emergency obstetrical services to manage the most serious complications that lead to death, namely obstructed labor and ruptured uterus, postpartum hemorrhage, eclampsia, postpartum infection, and complications of unsafe abortion. With such services readily available, this problem can be dramatically reduced, as it was in the Western world a century ago.

ABORTION

One consequence of the global unmet need for contraception is the global abortion rate. The abortion rate approximated thirty-five per thousand women aged fifteen to forty-four in 1995 (Henshaw, Singh, and Haas, 1999). Twenty-six percent of all pregnancies, excluding miscarriages and stillbirths, were terminated in 1995. Unsafe abortion remains a fundamental threat to public health and a dire consequence of both unmet need for contraception and inconsistent access to safe abortion services around the world. Of the approximately forty-six million abortions performed globally in 1995, an estimated twenty million were illegal. Women who have unwanted pregnancies should have access to reliable information, to safe abortion services where abortion is legal, and to effective postabortion care where abortion is illegal. The human toll of unsafe abortion is far too great: between sixty thousand and one hundred thousand women die each year from abortion-related complications.

EMPOWERMENT OF WOMEN

Fundamental to all of these goals is the empowerment of women. The recognition of women's rights as basic human rights and the advancement of women's status are crucial elements in the ICPD action program. While reproductive health advocates and providers must provide leadership on the issue of gender equality, the empowerment of women is one area of reproductive health that cannot be accomplished without the explicit commitment of a broad range of policymakers in both the public and the private sector.

CONCLUSION

Although the ICPD set the agenda for the twenty-first century, the action program contained no true blueprint for the implementation of reproductive health initiatives. The challenge is to develop and disseminate the tools with which to implement this agenda. Issues of prioritization, financing, and implementation must be reviewed and resolved. With competition for scarce resources and the inherently political nature of the reproductive health agenda, implementing the goals set in 1994 will require broad global cooperation and intersectoral alliances.

Despite the monetary price of such comprehensive programs, the cost of ignoring reproductive health needs, as evidenced in the social, economic, and health burden of maternal mortality, STDs, and HIV/AIDS, is tremendous. A high level of commitment at both the national and international level and the mobilization of necessary resources will be fundamental to the successful implementation of the reproductive health agenda for the twenty-first century.

References

Gerbase, A. C., and others. "Global Prevalence and Incidence Estimates of Selected Curable STDs." *Sexually Transmitted Infections,* 1998, *74* (suppl. 1), S12–S16.

Henshaw, S. K., Singh, S., and Haas, T. "The Incidence of Abortion World-wide." *International Family Planning Perspectives,* 1999, *25* (suppl.), S30–S38.

Joint United Programme on HIV/AIDS and World Health Organization. *Report on the Global HIV/AIDS Epidemic.* Geneva: Joint United Programme on HIV/AIDS and World Health Organization, 1998.

Population Reference Bureau. *World Population Data Sheet, 1998.* Washington, D.C.: Population Reference Bureau, 1998.

World Health Organization. *World Health Report, 1998.* Geneva: World Health Organization, 1998.

World Health Organization and UNICEF. *Revised 1990 Estimates of Maternal Mortality.* Geneva: World Health Organization and UNICEF, 1996.

CHAPTER TWENTY-THREE

Maternal and Child Health

Pierre Buekens, J. T. Boerma

Pierre Buekens, MD, PhD, Chair, and **J. T. Boerma, MD, PhD, Research Associate Professor,** *are both with the Department of Maternal and Child Health of the School of Public Health at the University of North Carolina at Chapel Hill. Dr. Buekens is an obstetrician-gynecologist and a perinatal epidemiologist and is President of the Association of Teachers in Maternal and Child Health. Dr. Boerma is a demographer who has worked in HIV prevention programs in developing countries since the mid-1980s.*

Great progress was made during the twentieth century in the field of maternal and child health (MCH), although inequalities persist and in several instances have increased. In the twenty-first century, we will have to address this unfinished agenda and face new challenges for an unprecedented number of children and women in the world.

MORE WOMEN AND CHILDREN

The number of women of childbearing age in less developed regions will increase from about 500 million in 1965 to 1.6 billion in 2015. Even though fertility (the number of children per woman) in 2015 is likely to be much lower than fifty years earlier, this tripling of the number of women implies that many more births will occur in each year of the twenty-first century than the 123 million births in the less developed regions in 1998. The number of children in the century before us will also exceed those in the last part of the century just ended, especially in the less developed regions of the world. In 1965, there were about 385 million children under the age of five years and 592 million aged five to fourteen years in the less developed regions. Fifty years later, in 2015, there will be 623 million children under five and 1.2 billion aged five to fourteen (Heligman, Chen, and Babakol, 1993). About one in three of these children will be living in India or China. The proportion of children living in urban areas will have increased from 21 percent in 1965 and 33 percent in 1990 to 51 percent in 2015. Maternal education levels, one of the most important determinants of child survival and development, are likely to increase. Urbanization and higher levels of education will lead to a higher demand for and use of health services. At the same time, inequalities in access to health services will probably continue to increase.

The increase in absolute numbers of women of reproductive age and of children do not automatically imply that MCH will be a priority on the national and international health agenda, as was the case in the last decades of the twentieth century. First, mainly due to a decline in fertility, the relative proportion of the populations in less developed regions who are children under fifteen will decrease, from 42 percent in 1965 to 29 percent in 2015. Second, significant progress has been made in the control of most communicable childhood diseases, which has led to a changing disease profile in the population dominated by noncommunicable conditions of adults and the elderly. However, one consequence of the changing disease profile will be the increased importance of perinatal and fetal health, which are less influenced by communicable diseases than later ages but are major determinants of later life. In other words, the early and late phases of the life cycle will be of increased priority. More attention will also have to be paid to women's health, including maternal health.

UNFINISHED AGENDA AND NEW CHALLENGES

MCH programs in the twenty-first century will have to address an unfinished agenda and emerging problems (Mosley, Bobadilla, and Jamison, 1993). The unfinished agenda includes efforts to decrease maternal mortality and morbidity, which cannot be achieved by preventive measures only. In the 1990s, the estimated number of maternal deaths was 585,000 per year (Maine and Rosenfield, 1999). The main causes of death are hemorrhages, infections, hypertensive disorders, obstructed labor, and complications of abortion. Only access to emergency obstetrical care and postabortion care could significantly decrease the mortality linked to these complications. In the absence of such programs, the number of maternal deaths will probably increase, as will the number of cases of maternal morbidity.

The challenge for the twenty-first century will be to increase access to emergency obstetrical care without increasing the number of unnecessary interventions. The frequency of cesarean sections is high in many countries of the world, especially in Latin America. For example, the cesarean section rate was 30 percent in southern Brazil in 1993 (Barros, Victora, and Morris, 1996). Other obstetrical interventions, such as oxytocics, are also often overused (Dujardin and others, 1995).

The rates of low-birthweight babies (under 2.5 kg) remained high during the twentieth century, especially in South Asia. Low-birthweight rates are high when babies are suffering from intrauterine growth retardation or when they are born preterm (less than thirty-seven weeks). Intrauterine growth retardation is the main challenge for developing countries, where it is estimated that 11 percent of the infants born at term are low-birthweight (de Onis, Blossner, and Villar, 1998). This is six times more frequently than in industrialized countries, where the corresponding rate is approximately 2 percent.

In industrialized countries, the main challenge is the increasing number of preterm births. In the United States, for example, preterm births rose slightly but steadily between 1981 and 1997 (see Figure 23.1). Part of the increase is due to a higher incidence of multiple births owing to fertility-enhancing therapies (fertility drugs and techniques such as in vitro fertilization; Ventura, Martin, Curtin, and Mathews, 1999a, 1999b). The increase in preterm births might also partly be due to other medical interventions, including preterm inductions and cesarean sections (Kramer, 1998). The short-term objective for the first decade of the twenty-first century should be to limit the increase of preterm births. The long-term objective should be to prevent preterm births, but unfortunately, most interventions designed to prevent them do not work (Goldenberg and Rouse, 1998). Even though the frequency of preterm babies is increasing, their survival is improving. In many countries, the increased survival of very preterm babies is a success but also a cause for concern. The number of survivors with moderate or severe morbidity is increasing. Improving the survival outcome of very low birthweight infants is thus a challenge.

Only recently has the full importance of micronutrient deficiencies for MCH become clear. Deficiency of folic acid at the time of conception is strongly associated with neural tube defects. Deficiencies of iron, iodine, vitamin A, and zinc each contribute to children's disease incidence and case fatality and also affect their ability to learn. Most micronutients can easily be added to food (in sugar or salt) or given in an oral tablet or capsule. In the twenty-first century, food fortification programs may become the main intervention against the micronutrient deficiencies. Progress in the battle against protein-energy malnutrition among young children has been slow, and much more needs to be done in the new century to redress this global inequality. Continuing to promote breastfeeding will also be a challenge as more women seek paid employment, perhaps in difficult working conditions.

Another piece of unfinished business is the eradication, elimination, or control of vaccine-preventable diseases of childhood, such as measles, poliomyelitis and tetanus. During the last decades of the twentieth century, great progress was made. The eradication of polio in the Americas through high levels of routine immunization coverage, active surveillance, national immunization days, and mopping-up campaigns needs to be replicated in other continents and for other diseases.

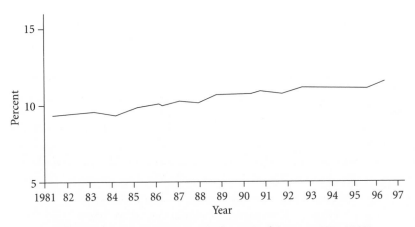

Figure 23.1.   Preterm Births in the United States, 1981–1997.

Sources: Ventura, Martin, Curtin, and Mathews, 1999a, 1999b.

Tropical diseases may receive more attention in the new century, particularly if global warming continues and climates change to favor the spread of vectors of tropical diseases to more temperate zones. Malaria will continue to be a major public health problem in Africa and Asia. A prolonged effort to strengthen curative health care for malaria patients and to enhance strategic vector control measures is required. The ubiquitous helminthic infections have a significant impact on child development and learning abilities, so control of such infections needs to be a priority intervention as well.

The AIDS pandemic also presents an unprecedented challenge to the health of mothers and children. This is most evident in sub-Saharan Africa, where the epidemic is most severe and older than other parts of the world. In several countries with generalized epidemics, a reversal of the infant and child mortality decline is likely to occur; it has already been observed in Kenya, for example (see Figure 23.2). This change in mortality trend may partly be due to the AIDS epidemic, although decline in MCH services in the context of poor economic growth is also likely to be a contributing factor.

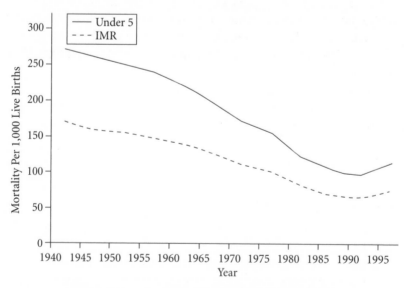

Figure 23.2.   Trends in Infant Mortality Rates and
Under-Five Mortality Rates in Kenya, 1940–1995.

Sources: Estimates from census and survey data.

NEW INTERVENTIONS

A range of new vaccines has been developed or is under development to reduce mortality and morbidity in childhood. These include vaccines against various pathogens causing pneumonia and diarrheal diseases, the two main killers in childhood. A major challenge is to deliver these vaccines to the children who need them most.

New drug treatments are being developed, against communicable and perhaps also noncommunicable diseases. A recent example is the antiretroviral treatment for HIV infection or prevention of HIV transmission from mother to child. The costs of the new treatments, however, are very high. Few countries in the least developed regions of the world, where the AIDS epidemic is worst, will be able to pay for the antiretroviral treatment, even if drug prices come down. Increasing resistance against antimicrobial drugs is another problem that will be more prominent in the new century and may enhance inequity. Unregulated use and other factors have contributed to the development of drug resistance for many diseases. Newly developed, more potent antimicrobial drugs are available throughout the world, but in developing countries their use is confined to patients who are wealthy enough to afford the treatment (Hart and Kariuki, 1998).

CONCLUSION

Maternal and child health programs will contend with unprecedented numbers of women and children in the twenty-first century. Inequities between regions of the world and between and within countries are likely to become larger if no concerted efforts are made to redress the imbalance.

References

Barros, F. C., Victora, C. G., and Morris, S. S. "Caesarean Sections in Brazil." *Lancet,* 1996, *347,* 839.

de Onis, M., Blossner, M., and Villar, J. "Levels and Patterns of Intrauterine Growth Retardation in Developing Countries." *European Journal of Clinical Nutrition,* 1998, *2* (suppl 1), S5–S15.

Dujardin, B., and others. "Oxytocics in Developing Countries." *International Journal of Gynecology and Obstetrics,* 1995, *50,* 243–251.

Goldenberg, R., and Rouse, D. "Prevention of Premature Birth." *New England Journal of Medicine,* 1998, *339,* 313–320.

Hart, C. A., and Kariuki, S. "Antimicrobial Resistance in Developing Countries." *Lancet,* 1998, *317,* 647–650.

Heligman, L., Chen, N., and Babakol, O. "Shifts in the Structure of Population and Death in Less Developed Regions." In: J. N. Gribble and S. H. Preston (eds.), *The Epidemiological Transition: Policy and Planning Implications for Developing Countries.* Washington, D.C.: National Academy Press, 1993.

Kramer, M. "Preventing Preterm Births: Are We Making Progress?" *Prenatal and Neonatal Medicine,* 1998, *3,* 10–12.

Maine, D., and Rosenfield, A. "The Safe Motherhood Initiative: Why Has It Stalled?" *American Journal of Public Health,* 1999, *89,* 480–482.

Mosley, W. H., Bobadilla, J. L., and Jamison, D. T. "The Health Transition: Implications for Health Policy in Developing Countries." In D. T. Jamison, W. H. Mosley, A. R. Measham, and J. L. Bobadilla (eds.), *Disease Control Priorities in the Developing Countries.* Oxford, England: Oxford University Press, 1993.

Ventura, S., Martin, J., Curtin, S., and Mathews, T. "Births: Final Data for 1997." *National Vital Statistics Reports,* 1999a, *47* (18), 13–14.

Ventura, S., Martin, J., Curtin, S., and Mathews, T. "Report of Final Statistics, 1997." *Monthly Vital Statistics Reports,* 1999b, *46* (11 suppl.), 80.

CHAPTER TWENTY-FOUR

Midwifery

Judith P. Rooks, Ruth Watson Lubic

Judith P. Rooks, CNM, MPH, MS, is a nurse-midwife and epidemiologist with a long career as a researcher, writer, teacher, and consultant in maternal health and family planning in the United States and developing countries. She is the author of more than sixty scientific and professional papers, as well as the comprehensive book Midwifery and Childbirth in America. *She is an Associate of the Pacific Institute for Women's Health in Los Angeles and a consultant to the Maternity Center Association in New York City.*

Ruth Watson Lubic, CNM, EdD, is a nurse-midwife and anthropologist known for her work in developing the freestanding birth center model. She has received many honors, including honorary degrees and special recognition from eight universities, a MacArthur Fellowship, and membership in the National Academy of Sciences Institute of Medicine. She is President and CEO of the District of Columbia Developing Families Center.

Nearly half of all births in developing countries occur without the assistance of a trained health care provider (World Health Organization, 1993; Peters, 1999). Many mothers and babies die or are harmed as a result. Each year, more than half a million women die because of pregnancy; 99 percent of those deaths occur in less developed countries. Maternal mortality is the health indicator for which the differential between developing and industrialized countries is greatest. Approximately one of every twelve women in West Africa will die as a result of pregnancy, compared to only one of every four thousand women in northern Europe (Maine and Rosenfield, 1999). Most women who die because of pregnancy and childbirth are poor and live in remote rural areas or urban slums (Kwast, 1991).

At the same time, the wealthiest countries are moving toward a highly medicalized form of childbirth. Technical, often invasive procedures developed for use during high-risk pregnancies are being applied to an ever-expanding proportion of births, increasing costs and resulting in high cesarean section rates. This continues despite conclusive evidence that frequent or routine use of these methods is either unlikely to be beneficial or results in trade-offs between beneficial and adverse effects (Enkin, Keirse, Renfrew, and Neilson, 1995). Electronic fetal monitoring and intravenous infusions are used routinely in the United States, and oxytocin augmentation of labor is increasing. More than 18 percent of all labors were induced in 1997—more than twice the proportion in 1989 (Curtin, 1999). Epidural analgesia is the first response to labor pain in many American hospitals. Cesarean section on demand among trendsetting elites and a series of *British Medical Journal* articles discussing elective cesarean sections as an ideal method of birth "for modern mothers" portend more to come. But low birthweight and inadequate parenting are the greatest threats to the lives and health of infants in most wealthy countries. Indiscriminate use of high-tech childbirth makes no contribution to better pregnancy outcomes and draws attention and resources from other important aspects of maternity care.

Medical practices in the United States and other Western countries exert an influence in the poorer, less developed countries. Overuse of oxytocin during labor is a problem in many developing countries, and cesarean section rates are high and increasing in major hospitals in some large Latin American and Asian cities. Cesareans accounted for nearly a third of all births in Brazil in 1986 (Notzon, 1990) and an even higher percentage of births in Chile from 1986 to 1994 (Murray and Pradenas, 1997). Cesarean section rates in these countries, as in the United States, are highest among well-educated, upper-class women who receive their care from private physicians. Thus high-tech obstetric care, including cesarean section, acquires the patina of modernity and "the best care money can buy," creating even more demand for these methods, while many poor women in the same countries lack access to essential preventive and emergency care.

At the beginning of the new century, the human community must make a commitment to protecting the lives and health of all childbearing women and their babies. Health care is an essential component of such protection. It will require provision of maternity care that is geographically and financially accessible and culturally acceptable to every pregnant woman. It should cost no more than necessary and must be based on firm scientific evidence of safety and effectiveness. Although the physical health of the mother and baby are of greatest importance, the care should also address the other needs of a pregnant woman—understanding and support for her personal and social transition into motherhood; encouragement, comfort measures, and direct physical assistance during labor and birth; and information and guidance related to breastfeeding and mothercraft. A strong midwifery profession is essential to providing this kind of care. This chapter explains the inherent strengths of midwifery and problems that limit the effectiveness of the midwifery profession and provides a strategy to give midwives the means to implement their model for the primary care of pregnant women as an essential part of the basis for healthy childbearing in the twenty-first century.

STRENGTHS OF MIDWIFERY AND THE MIDWIFERY MODEL OF CARE

Ideal maternity care combines primary midwifery care with access to medical obstetric care for women with serious complications. Both professions make essential contributions.

Historically, midwifery arose from the domestic and community role of women helping other women. The midwifery model of care is based on a caregiving role that builds a partnership between the midwife and the pregnant woman, who is respected as a critical decision maker and actor in promoting her own health and that of her family and her unborn child.

Midwives are also the guardians of normal birth. While constantly looking for signs of abnormality and increased risk, midwives view pregnancy as a fundamentally healthy physiological process and expect labor to proceed normally and successfully, until there is evidence to the contrary. By avoiding unnecessary interventions, midwives support the normal physiology of labor, delivery, and breastfeeding.

Although every obstetrical procedure has important uses and may be lifesaving in some cases, frequent or routine use of those procedures does not produce any benefit (Enkin, Keirse, Renfrew, and Neilson, 1995; World Health Organization, 1996). Comprehensive reviews of the best clinical epidemiological studies of effective care for low-risk pregnant women lead to recommendations for care that are virtually identical to the midwifery model.

Although many midwives work exclusively in hospitals, midwifery has a strong history of being based in communities. Midwives are the furthest extension of the formal health care system in most developing countries. Indonesia is trying to train enough midwives to place one in every village, whereas health centers staffed by doctors and nurses are based in cities and towns. Midwives in Sweden provide prenatal and postpartum care and family planning in "mothercare centers" located in residential communities and provide sex education and counseling in store-front "youth clinics" located in areas accessible to teens. Nurse-midwives in the United States operate birth centers in residential areas and a nationwide *community-based* distance learning program that makes midwifery education available to nurses who live in rural areas and small towns. Midwives often provide a critical link between the medical culture of the hospital and the traditional culture of the community; many work in public health.

Midwifery requires a high level of independent responsibility. It tends to attract intelligent, committed women who are willing and able to act independently.

PROBLEMS THAT LIMIT THE EFFECTIVENESS OF MIDWIFERY

The benefits of midwifery care cannot be realized if there are too few midwives or they are not well educated or lack control of their practice and thus cannot implement the midwifery model of care. At least one of these problems decreases the effectiveness of midwives in almost every country.

Midwifery in most developing countries is severely limited by both quantitatively and qualitatively inadequate initial education of midwives, poor supervisory and material support for midwives deployed to rural areas, lack of continuing education, and unreliable access to the transportation and communication necessary to transfer a critically ill woman to a hospital. Although planners try to provide one midwife for every two hundred yearly births (Kwast and Bentley, 1991),the actual number of midwives in most developing countries is only one-sixth to one-sixtieth of the number needed. A 1990 meeting of a World Health Organization task force on human resources for maternal health and safe motherhood noted enormous problems, including "a worldwide decline, and in some countries a disappearance, of the intermediate level provider of maternal care, usually the midwife or nurse-midwife, with no provision for her replacement" and "in many countries . . . a failure to identify and train a category of personnel at the first referral level to perform essential obstetric functions" (World Health Organization, 1990, p. 3). In addition, inadequacies in both the scientific base and clinical experience components of initial midwifery education compromise the effectiveness of midwives in many developing countries. Lack of access to clinical experience under the preceptorship of experienced, practicing midwives is a critical problem. As a result, many midwives working in rural areas are unable to provide lifesaving care during an obstetric emergency.

Most of these conditions flow from the wider fabric of poverty, weak infrastructure, and the problems of large, underfinanced ministry of health bureaucracies overwhelmed by unmet needs. Superimposed on these generic limitations are additional problems related to gender and role discrimination, which affects midwives as well as the women they serve. This problem is augmented by a lack of university degrees, which are available to a few nurses in most countries but rarely to midwives who are not also nurses; weak or nonexistent midwifery organizations; and a lack of opportunities for midwives to develop as leaders. Midwives are usually not present when decisions are being made about "safe motherhood" programs and other aspects of maternal and infant health care. Thus their insights and perspective are missing. These limitations flow in part from ignorance and confusion about the appropriate role of midwifery and how it relates to both medicine and nursing. Midwifery schools are often headed by physicians, who may not understand either the midwifery model of care or the educational needs of midwifery students. Where only nurses have degrees, midwives may be "supervised" by nurses who have higher status but no midwifery training and experience. In some countries, midwifery is losing its attraction to the brightest young women, who want to move into the modernizing sectors of their societies and see midwifery as a traditional female role.

The problems of midwifery in the industrialized countries are of a lower order but important given the impact—and creeping influence—of hypermedicalized pregnancy care throughout most of the Western world. Midwifery education is of high quality in most Western countries and attracts intelligent, highly motivated women, who compete for entrance into midwifery schools. Midwifery organizations are strong, and midwives have been supported by women's groups and consumer organizations that are dissatisfied with current maternity care and promote midwifery as the solution. New laws and policies supporting—in some cases mandating—greater reliance on midwives have been passed in Australia, New Zealand, the United Kingdom, Canada, and many U.S. states. Spanish obstetricians tried but failed to convince their government to close midwifery schools, and the German Obstetrical Society was unable to convince the German government to revoke a law that requires a midwife at every birth (Rooks, 1997). But the medicalization of childbirth is marching forward nonetheless, driven by the authority of medicine and a general Western cultural belief in the benefits of technology. Midwives practicing under policies written by obstetricians are also increasing their use of obstetric interventions.

During the twentieth century, childbirth moved into hospitals in most Western countries and thus entered a domain dominated by medicine and its focus on pathology. The invention and development of anesthesia and antisepsis, allowing relatively safe cesarean deliveries, and of antibiotics, blood transfusions, drugs to treat pregnancy-induced hypertension, and methods to dull the pain of labor demonstrated the power of medicine and further eclipsed the authority of midwives. Poor understanding of midwifery flows in part from the close association between midwifery and nursing in many countries, and the necessary, universal, close association between midwifery and medicine. Nursing education is required for entrance into midwifery education in some countries. Training the same person in both professions is an advantage where midwives must assume a large responsibility for primary health care; this explains why three of every four midwives in developing countries are also nurses (Peters, 1995). But midwifery is not part of nursing, just as it is not part of medicine. Although midwives must collaborate with physicians, midwifery and medical obstetrics are separate but *complementary* professions—with different philosophies and overlapping but distinct purposes and bodies of knowledge.

STRATEGIES TO IMPROVE MATERNITY CARE THROUGH MIDWIFERY

Solving the problems of maternity care and midwifery in developing countries will require substantial sustained investments to expand and improve the basic education of midwives. The International Confederation of Midwives has developed a document that defines the global "essential competencies for midwifery." These competencies should be incorporated into the blueprint for midwifery education in every country, which must teach the midwifery model of care and give every midwife the knowledge and skills needed to save life during an obstetric emergency. Midwifery educators in developing countries should adapt some of the methods used to increase access to appropriate clinical experience for midwifery students in Western countries, such as the large distance learning program that places students under the tutelage of experienced nurse-midwives in active practices throughout the United States. This program uses modern communications technology to bind geographically disparate academic faculty, clinical preceptors, and students into a cohesive learning community. Increasing access, decreasing costs, and greater ease of communicating through the Internet, facsimile transmission of documents, audiotapes, and videocassettes should make it possible to use a similar approach to expand clinical training opportunities for midwifery students in even the poorest countries.

In addition, midwifery should be recognized and supported as a separate discipline and profession. Such recognition would strengthen the midwifery profession throughout the world, but especially in the poorest countries, which need effective midwifery leaders and organizations to improve midwifery education and services and provide a voice for the experience and perspective of midwives in creating maternal health care policies. Midwives are the backbone of the maternal health care system, the problems of which cannot be solved without strengthening midwifery. And the profession cannot be strengthened sufficiently without leadership and authority from within the profession. Further strengthening of midwifery will also make it easier for midwives to develop truly collaborative, collegial relationships with physicians.

Recognition of midwifery as an autonomous discipline and profession is also needed in Europe, North America, and the former Soviet republics—to empower midwives to control their own education and practice and to further develop the scientific base for the care unique to midwifery. Research is needed to objectively assess the effectiveness of specific elements of midwifery practice and to examine the influence of women's care and other experiences during pregnancy and birth on maternal-infant bonding and the woman's assimilation of her role as mother.

TRENDS

Although most midwives are employed by the government health service of their country, some midwives throughout the world are starting small private practices and birth centers in order to implement the midwifery model of care, meet needs that are not being met by government services, and control the quality of the care they provide. Individual midwives operating small private clinics and birth centers can provide low-cost, culturally acceptable care in communities where women live. This is part of a worldwide trend toward an increasing role for private sector health care. Midwives are also collaborating with women's organizations and making other efforts to listen to women, trying to address their criticisms and focusing on client satisfaction as an important, measurable outcome of maternity care. The demands of private practice and the expressed concerns of women have led to an increased focus on providing continuity of care—with one or a small group of midwives accepting responsibility for all phases of the primary care of a caseload of pregnant women. All of these trends bring midwives back to their roots in the community and the origins of the word *midwife,* which literally means "with woman."

Other trends that will affect midwifery in the twenty-first century include pressure to provide cost-effective, "evidence-based" health care; a developing consensus that client satisfaction is necessary for effective reproductive health care for women; and the threat of antibiotic-resistant nosocomial infections, which could increase support for birth centers that are near but physically separate from hospitals. All of these trends support midwifery.

References

Curtin S. "Recent Changes in Birth Attendant, Place of Delivery, and the Use of Obstetric Interventions, United States, 1989–97." *Journal of Nurse-Midwifery,* 1999, *44,* 349–354.

Enkin, M., Keirse, M.J.N.C., Renfrew, M. J., and Neilson, J. P. *A Guide to Effective Care in Pregnancy and Childbirth.* (2nd ed.). New York: Oxford University Press, 1995.

Kwast, B. E. "Safe Motherhood: A Challenge to Midwifery Practice." *World Health Forum*, 1991, *12*, 1–24.

Kwast, B. E., and Bentley, J. "Introducing Confident Midwives: Midwifery Education—Action for Safe Motherhood." *Midwifery*, 1991, *7*, 8–19.

Maine, D., and Rosenfield, A. "The Safe Motherhood Initiative: Why Has It Stalled?" *American Journal of Public Health*, 1999, *89*, 480–482.

Murray, S. F., and Pradenas, S. F. "Cesarean Birth Trends in Chile, 1986 to 1994." *Birth*, 1997, *24*, 258–263.

Notzon, F. C. "International Differences in the Use of Obstetric Interventions." *Journal of the American Medical Association*, 1990, *263*, 3286–3291.

Peters, M. H. "Midwives and the Achievement of Safer Motherhood." *International Journal of Gynecology and Obstetrics*, 1995, *50* (suppl. 2), S89–S92.

Peters, M. H. "Safe Motherhood: A Journey." *Journal of Nurse-Midwifery*, 1999, *44*, 145–150.

Rooks, J. *Midwifery and Childbirth in America*. Philadelphia: Temple University Press, 1997.

World Health Organization. *Human Resource Development for Maternal Health and Safe Motherhood: Report of a Task Force Meeting, Geneva, 2–4 April 1990*. Geneva: World Health Organization, Maternal and Child Health and Family Planning, Division of Family Health, 1990.

World Health Organization. *Coverage of Maternity Care. A Tabulation of Available Information*. Geneva: World Health Organization, Division of Family Health, 1993.

World Health Organization. *Care in Normal Birth: A Practical Guide*. Geneva: World Health Organization, 1996.

CHAPTER TWENTY-FIVE

Building the Capacity of Schools to Improve Health

Lloyd J. Kolbe, Jack T. Jones,
Isolde Birdthistle, and Cheryl Vince Whitman

Lloyd J. Kolbe, PhD, *is Founding Director of the Division of Adolescent and School Health, National Center for Chronic Disease Prevention and Health Promotion, U.S. Centers for Disease Control and Prevention (CDC), Atlanta. He is a member of the U.S. Senior Biomedical Research Service and serves as Director of the World Health Organization's Collaborating Center on Health Education and Promotion for School-Age Children and Youth.*

Jack T. Jones, MPH, *is School Health Team Leader for the World Health Organization in Geneva. He has been assigned by the CDC to WHO's Department of Health Promotion since 1992. He serves as leader for the WHO School Health Team and is responsible for organizing the affairs of WHO's Global School Health Initiative.*

Isolde Birdthistle, MS, *is Senior Research and Development Associate at Education Development Center, Inc. (EDC), in Newton, Massachusetts. She has been assigned by EDC to WHO's Department of Health Promotion to further the work of the Global School Health Initiative, particularly in the areas of violence and injury prevention, adolescent reproductive health, and rapid assessment of school health programs.*

*Cheryl Vince Whitman, EdM, is Senior Vice President of
the Education Development Center, Inc. She also serves as EDC's
Director of Health and Human Development Programs and as
Director of the World Health Organization's Collaborating Center
to Promote Health Through Schools and Communities.*

Among the world's nearly six billion people, more than two billion are younger than twenty years old, and one billion are enrolled in schools. Eighty percent of the developing world's children now enroll in school, and 60 percent complete at least four years. The formal education system thus provides the world's most powerful means to dispense vital information and skills for its citizens.

In developing regions, where four-fifths of the world's people live, noncommunicable diseases such as heart disease and depression are rapidly replacing infectious diseases and malnutrition as the leading causes of disability and premature death. By 2020, tobacco is expected to kill more people than any single disease; injuries, both unintentional (such as traffic accidents) and intentional (suicide, violence, war), could rival infectious diseases as a source of ill health; and reproductive health conditions resulting from HIV infection, other sexually transmitted diseases (STDs), and unintended pregnancy may cause 10 percent of the world's burden of illness.

The leading causes of premature death and disability in the twenty-first century could be markedly reduced by enabling schools to educate young people about how to avoid these causes and by enabling schools to provide simple health services for young people. For example, the World Bank (1993) has suggested that one of the most cost-effective ways to improve health in most regions of the world is to implement an "essential public health package" that includes (1) an expanded program on immunization, including micronutrient supplementation; (2) school health programs to treat worm infections and micronutrient deficiencies and to provide health education; (3) programs to increase public knowledge about family planning and nutrition, about self-cure or indications for seeking care, and about vector control and disease surveillance activities; (4) programs to reduce consumption of tobacco, alcohol, and other drugs; and

(5) AIDS prevention programs with a strong STD component. Modern school health programs could provide one of the most efficient means available for most nations to continuously provide all five elements of such "essential packages" for young people.

NATURE AND EFFECTIVENESS OF MODERN SCHOOL HEALTH PROGRAMS

The modern school health program can include eight interactive components: (1) a healthy biophysical and psychosocial school environment; (2) health education; (3) health services; (4) psychological, counseling, and social services; (5) food services; (6) physical education and physical activities; (7) health programs for faculty and staff; and (8) integrated efforts of schools and communities to improve the health of young people (Marx, Wooley, and Northrop, 1998). School administrators, teachers, and other school staff, health officials, colleges, families, and the community can work as a team to implement such programs.

Obviously, not all health programs implemented by schools are effective in achieving their objectives. However, research has shown that carefully designed school health programs can improve health and education outcomes among large populations of young people. For example, carefully designed school programs in the United States have reduced tobacco use, improved eating and physical activity behaviors, reduced obesity among girls, increased standardized test scores and math grades while reducing absences, and increased school commitment and attachment while decreasing heavy drinking, sexual intercourse, multiple sexual partners, and pregnancy.

REASONS FOR NATIONS TO IMPLEMENT SCHOOL HEALTH PROGRAMS

Students who suffer health problems—who are hungry or depressed, ill or injured, abusing drugs or pregnant—do not learn as well as children who are healthy. Furthermore, parents who attain more education have healthier children than parents who attain less education; and children of parents who attain more education are also less likely to engage in various health risk behaviors. Effective school health education can enable young people to protect their own health, the health of families for which they will become responsible, and the health of communities in which they will reside. In the United States, the state directors of health and the state directors of education jointly concluded that "healthy kids make better students, and better students make healthy communities" (Council of Chief State School Officers and Association of State and Territorial Health Officials, 1999). Recent national surveys in the United States have shown that the public, school administrators, and students believe that education about health is at least as important as education about mathematics, science, and language. In 1998, Education International (which represents teachers' unions in virtually every nation in the world) proclaimed that schools are the irreplaceable and most useful place in a country to improve both health and education and called on all governments to strengthen policies and resources for school health programs (Education International, 1998).

COMMON BARRIERS TO
IMPLEMENTING PROGRAMS

The World Health Organization has suggested that school health programs are inadequately developed in every nation because of: inadequate understanding and acceptance of school health programs; inadequate vision and strategic planning; inadequate collaboration and coordination among responsible parties; the lack of a sense of ownership and responsibility; and the lack of resources (financial, human, materials, and organizational infrastructure). To address these barriers, WHO developed ten recommendations that would enable the world's schools to develop more fully the potential of future generations and called on all member states of the United Nations, relevant international organizations, relevant nongovernmental organizations, and schools around the world to implement these recommendations (World Health Organization, 1997). We will next summarize the various national and international efforts to implement these recommendations (World Health Organization, 2000).

STRATEGIES IMPLEMENTED
BY THE LARGEST NATIONS

As part of WHO's Global School Health Initiative, ten nations that contain at least one hundred million people are working independently and together to improve school health programs. These ten nations comprise about half of the world's population.

Bangladesh implemented a five-year plan to improve school health education, school health services (including deworming and vitamin A supplementation), and school water and sanitation facilities. Many nongovernmental organizations that provide education for young people are involved; and committees at the national, district, and school levels monitor activities.

Brazil used its new national school curriculum guidelines, called "Parameters for the National Curriculum," as a bridge to integrate education about health, the environment, multiculturalism, and ethics with education about more traditional subjects such as science and language. Local health and education agencies are providing leadership for these efforts to improve school health education.

China established regulations for school health programs that provide guidelines for school health program management, health education, school environment and facilities, mental health, nutrition, safety, health inspection, physical examination, health services, and special health services for girls and disabled students.

India set up state health education bureaus in all its states and union territories to implement school health education programs; and each year paramedics administer medical checkups in schools to detect common health problems among one hundred million primary school students.

Indonesia set up a school health coordinating committee to unite the efforts of the Ministries of Health, Education and Culture, Religious Affairs, and Interior. Schools are implementing supplementary feeding programs and antidrug and antitobacco campaigns and are involved in eliminating *Aedes aegypti* breeding places to help control dengue hemorrhagic fever.

Mexico launched its School Health Care Program nationwide in approximately twenty-five thousand preschool centers and thirty thousand primary schools to improve the health of its young people. The program provides health education, detects and addresses health problems, improves preschool and school environments, and encourages social participation.

Nigeria introduced health education into the curriculum of all primary schools as one component of a national strategy for providing primary health care and is monitoring specific indicators to ensure that program implementation is effective.

Pakistan has implemented School Health Program Five-Year Plans. The Seventh Plan recommended that all children have a complete medical checkup when they enter school and a comprehensive quarterly checkup as long as they remain in school. The Eighth Plan recommended that the program be reoriented to help schoolchildren develop healthy lifestyles.

Russian Federation school health activities are organized collaboratively by the Federal Ministries of Health and Education, 89 regional departments of health and education, and 260 Preventive Medicine Centers. Regional programs have clearly defined goals for altering unhealthy behaviors and include efforts to reach not only students but their families and communities as well.

The United States suffers serious health, education, and social problems caused by six types of behavior usually established during youth: behaviors that cause unintentional or intentional injuries, alcohol and drug abuse, sexual risk behaviors, tobacco use, unhealthy diets, and insufficient physical activity. The U.S. Centers for Disease Control and Prevention (CDC) implements four interrelated strategies to prevent many of these behaviors (Kolbe, Collins, and Cortese, 1997). First, CDC monitors the prevalence of these behaviors in each state and large city and the extent to which schools implement effective policies and programs to prevent these behaviors. Second, CDC synthesizes research to identify effective school health policies and programs. Third, CDC enables state and large-city education and health departments and national nongovernmental organizations to collaboratively help schools in their respective jurisdictions implement effective policies and programs. Fourth, CDC evaluates the efforts of state and large-city education and health departments to reduce critical risk behaviors among young people in their respective jurisdictions. (More detailed and up-to-date information about school health programs in the United States can be found on the Education Development Center's Web site at http://www.edc.org/HealthIsAcademic and on CDC's Web site at http://www.cdc.gov/nccdphp/dash.)

STRATEGIES IMPLEMENTED BY INTERNATIONAL AGENCIES

As outlined next, six United Nations agencies and Education International are working independently and together to help schools improve the health of nations.

The *Food and Agriculture Organization (FAO)* of the United Nations uses school-based nutrition education as a means to promote lifelong healthful eating habits. Schoolchildren are a priority target group for FAO because nutrition education at an early age can increase learning potential and healthy development and simultaneously decrease nutritional disorders and diet-related diseases later in life. FAO assists member states through nutrition advocacy and promotion; technical assistance (for example, developing curricula, evaluating pilot projects); development of nutrition education materials, such as the Planning Guide for Ministry Officials; and collaboration with research and training institutions and other organizations.

The *United Nations Educational, Scientific and Cultural Organization (UNESCO)* promotes health mainly through school-based education to prevent disease and other risks to health, helps children acquire sustainable values and life skills, and helps create a culture of peace. UNESCO has links with national education authorities, educational institutions, and community-based organizations and is therefore in a position to help front-line education decision makers and policymakers renew curricula and adopt new teaching techniques. Through its teacher training, community-based activities, networks, and connections with universities, UNESCO influences formal and nonformal teaching and learning strategies.

The *United Nations Population Fund (UNFPA)* supports population education, family life, and sexuality education in schools. UNFPA's strategies include learning what works (using lessons learned and evaluation findings to enhance population education), supporting a comprehensive approach to population education (with participatory teaching methods in seventy developing countries), working through a variety of channels to promote consistent messages (for example, through parents, mass media, churches), and implementing extracurricular activities associated with school programs.

The *United Nations Children's Fund (UNICEF)* strives to meet and protect children's rights to education, hygiene, nutrition, and development through schools. UNICEF helps schools develop a basic school health package that includes policies on gender, HIV/AIDS discrimination, and tobacco, in addition to policies that support health-promoting schools and adolescent- and child-friendly schools; efforts to improve school water and sanitation; skills-based health and hygiene education, including life skills; and specific health, hygiene, and nutrition interventions.

The *World Bank* coordinates information about school health and nutrition approaches through its International School Health Initiative. World Bank strategies include providing access to expert advice; providing a clearinghouse of good practice examples; developing practical tool kits for implementation; making information available through the Internet and the World Bank Advisory Services; building partnerships with governments, international agencies, and national nongovernmental organizations; and assisting task teams to prepare school health components for World Bank projects. (More detailed and up-to-date information about World Bank efforts to improve school health programs can be found on the Internet at http://www.worldbank.org/html/schools.)

The *World Health Organization's Global School Health Initiative* includes four strategies:

Research: WHO consolidates research and expert opinion to describe the nature and effectiveness of school health programs.

Building Capacity to Advocate: WHO publishes research findings jointly with other UN agencies and partners to help people advocate for improved school health programs.

Strengthening National Capacities: WHO helps countries develop national strategies to improve school health programs and fosters collaboration between health and education agencies.

Creating Networks and Alliances: WHO helps establish Networks for the Development of Health Promoting Schools and helps form global alliances, such as the alliance among Education International, WHO, UNAIDS, and UNESCO, that enable teachers' organizations worldwide to improve health through schools.

(More detailed and up-to-date information about WHO efforts to improve school health programs can be found on the Internet at http://www.who.int/hpr.)

Education International (EI) brings together 294 national organizations representing 23 million education workers in 152 countries and territories. At the Second World Congress of Education International, members passed a resolution to support the development of school health programs. EI encourages the development of comprehensive school health programs and helps its affiliates implement school health-related policies, curricula, and training.

CONCLUSION

Modern school health programs could become one of the most efficient means nations might employ to improve the health, education, quality of life, and productivity of their people in the twenty-first century. But to implement such programs, international, national, provincial, and local agencies, education and health professionals, parents, and communities will need to learn how schools can improve health, they will need to make a commitment to implement effective programs, and they will need to work *together* in new ways on behalf of young people.

References

Council of Chief State School Officials and Association of State and Territorial Health Officials. *Why Support a Coordinated Approach to School Health? School Health Starter Kit.* Wsahington, D.C.: Council of Chief State School Officers, 1999.

Education International. *Highlights from the Second World Congress of Education International.* Brussels: Education International, 1998.

Kolbe, L. J., Collins, J., and Cortese, P. "Building the Capacity of Schools to Improve the Health of the Nation: A Call for Assistance from Psychologists." *American Psychologist,* 1997, *52,* 256–265.

Marx, E., Wooley, S., and Northrop, D. (eds.). *Health Is Academic: A Guide to Coordinated School Health Programs.* New York: Teachers College Press, 1998.

World Bank. *World Development Report 1993: Investing in Health—World Development Indicators.* New York: Oxford University Press, 1993.

World Health Organization. *Promoting Health Through Schools: Report of a WHO Expert Committee on Comprehensive School Health Education and Promotion.* Geneva: World Health Organization, 1997.

World Health Organization. *Improving Health Through Schools: National and International Strategies.* Geneva: World Health Organization, 2000.

CHAPTER TWENTY-SIX

Women's Health

Adrienne Germain

Adrienne Germain *is President of the International Women's Health Coalition, a nongovernmental organization that promotes women's sexual and reproductive rights and health worldwide. Trained in sociology and demography, she has written articles and edited books on women's health, rights, and development. She was a U.S. delegate to the United Nations' world conferences on population, development, and women in the 1990s and an architect of the 1994 shift in population policy from demographic targets to individual health, rights, and well being.*

As we enter the twenty-first century, girls' and women's health is in grave danger from threats of human origin. Discrimination, sexism, gender inequality, and inequity are the root causes of much of girls' and women's ill health and death. If policymakers, communities, and families choose to end these threats right now, the prognosis for women's health in the new century will be quite favorable. If not, we can expect increasing suffering and misery, not only for women, but also for their families.

Although new technologies and intensified research are needed, the need is even greater for strengthening basic health systems, creating the political will for women's equality, and respecting women's rights. Maternal mortality and morbidity are a central case in point. Despite our having the necessary technologies and knowledge, every minute of every day, at least one woman dies somewhere in the world because there is no one to help her through childbirth or to provide a safe abortion (WHO, 1999).

Who was the woman who died in the minute just past, and why did she die? It could have been Hanatu, a girl of twelve in northern Nigeria, the second wife of a much older and very conservative man who denied her permission to go to a health center. It could have been Salma, a twenty-eight-year-old rural Bangladeshi woman in her fourth pregnancy who did not have the bus fare to get to a nearby clinic. It could have been Betania, a middle-class teenager in Recife, Brazil, pregnant by rape, refused an abortion by the municipal hospital. She died terrified and alone after a desperate attempt to abort herself.

In addition to the nearly six hundred thousand women who die every year in these sorts of circumstances (WHO, 1996), some fifteen million are left disabled or chronically ill (WHO, 1995). Worldwide, maternal mortality represents the largest gap in human well-being between poor and rich countries (WHO, 1999): women in Africa and South Asia are up to two hundred times more likely than women in the United States to die from causes related to pregnancy (WHO, 1996). The sexism, gender inequality, and inequity that are responsible for poor maternal health policy and inadequate resource allocation manifest themselves in a number of ways that must be changed in the twenty-first century.

First, we must make maternal health a political and budgetary priority. For $2 to $3 per person per year, in most poor countries with *existing* technologies, we could significantly reduce maternal death and illness (World Bank, 1999). Why have we so far failed to do this? One reason is that the deaths are largely invisible and undervalued, even in the United States. They attract no headlines, and the women die one by one, many at home or on the journey to a distant or poorly equipped health facility. Most of the women who die are poor and young, with no political power or representation. Legislators and policymakers often think their deaths are a low priority, given the nearly twelve million deaths of children under age five every year (UNICEF, 1998). In fact, these deaths of women and children are intimately linked. For example, we cannot reduce the eight million stillbirths and newborn deaths and the twenty million low-birthweight babies born annually (UNICEF, 1998) without taking better care of women before, during, and after they give birth. A mother's death also dramatically affects the health and survival of her living children: in Bangladesh, for example, children up to age ten whose mothers die are three to ten times more likely to die within two years than those with both parents living (Chen and others, 1974).

Second, we must get policy right. International agencies and public health specialists, in the poorest countries where maternal mortality is highest, have provided primarily inexpensive "technical fixes" and have avoided dealing with health system and socioeconomic factors. As we know from Western history, women like Hanatu and Salma must have ready access to skilled and equipped health care providers at delivery and after giving birth (61 percent of maternal deaths in developing countries occur after delivery)(Starrs, 1999). We must not only make essential obstetric care available to all women but also engage both families and communities in ensuring that women can access that care.

Third, we must ensure access to safe abortion. Many international agencies and national governments, cowed by anti-abortion politics and archaic laws, refuse to provide easily accessible, safe abortion, one of the simplest, lowest-cost lifesaving interventions. As a result, twenty million unsafe abortions occur each year (WHO, 1998). These cause 13 to 15 percent of all maternal deaths overall; in some countries, they account for 35 to 50 percent (WHO, 1998). We could save the lives of at least seventy-five thousand women every year (WHO, 1998) and spare millions untold suffering with a very modest investment in training and equipment. But we are not doing it.

Fourth, we must allocate sufficient resources to contraceptive services. Worldwide, an estimated one hundred fifty million *married* couples who want to regulate their fertility lack access to a method of contraception that is safe and acceptable to them (UNFPA, 1997). But the actual number without access is even larger. Young, unmarried people are generally not included in estimates of the unmet need for contraceptives. They are commonly excluded from services, leaving them at high risk of sexually transmitted diseases (STDs), unwanted pregnancies, and botched abortions.

Fifth, we must ensure equal access to services. Even in the United States, the world's richest country, women's lifetime risk of maternal death has not budged in fifteen years (UNFPA, 1997), primarily because poor women of color do not have adequate pregnancy care.

Maternal deaths and ill health are only one of the many ways that sexism, power imbalances, and gender inequality and inequity—in families, communities, the health professions, governments, and the courts—kill and maim women.[1] Women are subject to violence and unable to protect themselves from other risks associated with sexuality from a very young age. Sexual abuse of girls is rampant; rape and domestic violence in developed and developing countries account for one out of five healthy days of life lost to women aged fifteen to forty-nine (World Bank, 1993). Such violence, and fear of it, is in part responsible for the higher prevalence of depression among women than among men worldwide (Astbury, 1999). And the majority of women beaten by their men have no forum for redress, support services, or place of refuge (Heise, 1999).

Sexism also manifests itself in gross violations of women's human rights—in the name of religion, morality, or "culture." For example, a dozen Latin American countries exonerate rapists if they marry their victims, and several Arab countries condone the murder of women to protect family honor. Female genital mutilation, suffered by two million girls and young women each year, is usually described as a "cultural" practice and justified in the name of Islam. But such violation of the fundamental right to security of the person is in no way justifiable. Right-wing groups in the United States campaign not only against abortion but also against modern contraception and would have women stay at home, subordinate to husband, father, or brother.

Other dangers stemming from the power imbalance between women and men have just as much or more potential to injure and kill. The World Health Organization estimates that 330 million new STD infections occur annually, at least half among young people (WHO, February 5, 1999). Women are more vulnerable than men due not only to biological differences but also to social factors. When men who have sex with multiple partners refuse to use condoms, the women in their lives often end up with STDs, including HIV/AIDS. Further, it has become common for older men to seek younger and younger women with whom to have "safe" sex—in villages in Uganda, in the cities of India, and in sections of Washington, D.C. (WHO, 2000; UNAIDS, 1999; Penos Institute, 1996). Across the world, male privilege is also variously reflected in giving sons preferential access to health care, sex-selective abortion, female infanticide, or trafficking in women.

Death in childbirth, botched abortions, sexually transmitted diseases and HIV/AIDS, violence, coercion, poverty, discrimination, sexism, oppression—as long as these are allowed to happen to one woman anywhere, no woman is safe.

In the twenty-first century, we must give higher priority to making the world a healthful place for girls and women. In 1994, at the International Conference on Population and Development held in Cairo, and again in 1995, at the Fourth World Conference on Women held in Beijing, the world's governments agreed on sweeping twenty-year agendas to address these injustices. In the years since these agreements were made, examples of progress are many. In the countries where we described women dying due to lack of health care in pregnancy, new programs and policies are emerging.

In 1998, after three years of intensive work, Bangladesh completed its first comprehensive national health and population sector program, based on the definition of reproductive health used in the Cairo conference agreement. Recognizing that maternal mortality in Bangladesh is as high today as it was twenty-five years ago, the government, civil society, international agencies, and donors worked together to design ways to broaden the existing national family planning program to encompass more comprehensive reproductive health care, including essential obstetric services, continued access to menstrual regulation (early abortion), improvements in the quality of contraceptive services, and programs for young people.

Brazilian law allows abortion only in the case of rape or incest or to save the life of the woman. The national women's health movement and health professionals have blocked attempts to outlaw abortion altogether. Just as remarkable, they have endeavored to ensure that women who are allowed by law to have an abortion can receive safe services in public hospitals by persuading at least thirteen hospitals in seven cities to train and equip staff.

In 1995, Action Health Incorporated (AHI), one of Nigeria's most effective nongovernmental organizations working for sexual and reproductive health and rights, opened a reproductive health clinic for young people—a radical act in most countries. Responding to adolescents' needs, including alarming rates of HIV infection—62 percent of AIDS cases from 1986 to 1995 were among young women aged fifteen to twenty-nine (Federal Government of Nigeria, 1996)—the clinic provides counseling, testing, treatment, and referral for contraception, pregnancy, STDs including HIV/AIDS, and sexual violence. AHI and several other Nigerian organizations also provide programs to build girls' self-esteem and work with boys and girls to teach them how to build respectful, responsible relationships. As a result, the government recently agreed to create a national adolescent health policy and to develop sexuality education curricula for schools.

In addition to these country-specific examples, two other general areas of progress are technology development and increases in women's capacity to mobilize. Considerable progress has been made on the development of microbicides, substances that women can use intravaginally to protect themselves against STDs. More governments are subsidizing access to female condoms in Africa and Latin America. The U.S. Food and Drug Administration has approved emergency contraception to prevent pregnancy after unprotected intercourse, which means that it can be made more easily available worldwide. Work is also progressing to develop less expensive means to diagnose and treat STDs.

Twenty years ago, women's organizations in Africa, Asia, and Latin America were relatively few and scattered. They had not coalesced into movements with social and political force, nationally or internationally; they were largely absent from the health and family planning arenas. After years of organizing at the grassroots level, women all over the globe are now playing vital roles in the policies and programs that determine their health and well-being. We shaped the agendas set in Cairo and Beijing, and we are changing national programs and policies as well. We are joined every day by more and more men who realize that they and their communities will benefit.

As encouraging as these examples are, an enormous amount remains to be done. The women's health agenda for the twenty-first century must therefore include all of the following:

- A "rights-based" approach to sexual and reproductive health care that both ensures girls' and women's access to services and respects their autonomy
- Appropriate policies and sufficient budgetary allocations by governments and donors for sexual and reproductive health, particularly in order to reduce maternal death and injury to a minimum and to curtail the STD and HIV epidemics
- Access to female condoms, development and distribution of microbicides, and simple, inexpensive STD diagnostics and treatments
- Access to safe abortion for all who need it
- Sexual health information and services for young people that include emphasis on gender equality and equity
- Zero tolerance of harmful practices, violence against women, and sex discrimination

Achieving this ambitious agenda is within our reach. Governments and international institutions, with support from health professionals and advocates, can reorder financial and political priorities away from the military, corruption, and special interests toward equity and the well-being of people—what Amartya Sen, 1998 Nobel laureate in economics, has described as "a better deal for the basic requirements of good living, rather than efficient killing" (WHO, May 18, 1999) Ultimately, however, the health of women in the twenty-first century will not be determined by money, improved policies, and new technology alone. There will have to be social justice for women.

We must counter the forces, including political and ideological fanatics, that oppress and discriminate against women around the globe, that render women voiceless, and that deny them rights essential to their health. This will require sustained and increased investment in the international health and rights movements, public education, and advocacy to, in the words of Nobel laureate in literature Wole Soyinka, bring down the "blood-soaked banner of fanaticism billowing across the skies of [the second] millennium" (Soyinka, 1999). Much of that blood has been women's. We must not let that be the case in the new century.

Note

1. Our focus is girls and women through childbearing age and health problems specific to women. Communicable and noncommunicable diseases and other health risks that affect men are also serious problems for women, and health issues faced by older women will become more prevalent in the twenty-first century as populations age. These issues are covered in other chapters in this book.

References

Astbury, J. "Promoting Women's Mental Health," Geneva: World Health Organization, 1999. 29 pp. (in press) In Heise, L., Ellsberg, M., and Gottemoeller, M. *Population Reports: Ending Violence Against Women,* Series L, *11,* 1999.

Centers for Disease Control and Prevention. "Maternal Morbidity–United States, 1982–1996." *Morbidity and Mortality Weekly Report,* 1998, *47,* 705–707.

Chen, L. C., Gesche, M. C., Ahmed, S., Chowdhury, A. I., and Mosley, W. H. "Maternal Mortality in Rural Bangladesh." *Studies in Family Planning,* 1974, *5,* 334–341.

Federal Government of Nigeria, National AIDS and STD Program. 1996. AIDS Cases Reporting Profile: A Decade of the Nigerian Experience, 1986–1995 in Action Health Incorporated. "Fact Sheet," Lagos.

Heise, L., Ellsberg, M., and Gottemoeller, M. *Population Reports: Ending Violence Against Women,* Series L, *11,* 1999.

Panos Institute. *AIDS and Young People: A Generation at Risk?* Panos AIDS Briefing No. 4, London, July 1996.

Soyinka, Wole. "Every Dictator's Nightmare," *New York Times Magazine,* April 18, 1999, 90–92.

Starrs, A. *Safe Motherhood Action Agenda: Priorities for the Next Decade.* New York: Family Care International in Collaboration with the Interagency Group for Safe Motherhood, 1999.

UNAIDS. *Gender and HIV/AIDS: Taking Stock of Research and Programs.* Geneva: UNAIDS, 1999.

UNICEF. *The State of the World's Children 1998.* New York: UNICEF, 1998.

United Nations Population Fund (UNFPA). *The State of the World Population 1997.* New York: UNFPA, 1997.

Vaughn, J. P., and AbouZahr, C. "Reproductive Health: Widening Horizons." *International Journal of Public Health; Bulletin 2000.* 2000, *78,* 569.

World Bank. *Safe Motherhood and the World Bank: Lessons from 10 Years of Experience.* Washington, D.C.: World Bank, 1999.

World Bank. *World Development Report 1993: Investing in Health.* Oxford, England and New York: Oxford University Press, 1993.

World Health Organization. "Women and HIV/AIDS," Fact Sheet No 242, Geneva: World Health Organization, 2000.

World Health Organization. *UN Agencies Joint Statement for Reducing Maternal Mortality.* Geneva: World Health Organization, 1999.

World Health Organization press release, Feb. 5, 1999.

World Health Organization press release, May 18, 1999.

World Health Organization. *Global and Regional Estimates of Incidence of and Mortality Due to Unsafe Abortion with a Listing of Available Country Data.* Geneva: World Health Organization, 1998.

World Health Organization. *Revised 1990 Estimates of Maternal Mortality: A New Approach by WHO and UNICEF.* Geneva: World Health Organization, 1996.

World Health Organization. *The Mothercare Project.* Geneva: World Health Organization, 1995.

CHAPTER TWENTY-SEVEN

Undernutrition

Barbara A. Underwood

Barbara A. Underwood, PhD, *is President of the International Union of Nutritional Sciences and Scholar in Residence on the Food and Nutrition Board of the National Academy of Sciences' Institute of Medicine. She served as focal leader for micronutrients at the World Health Organization in Geneva and Director for International Programs at the National Institutes of Health's National Eye Institute. She has also held faculty positions at the Massachusetts Institute of Technology, Pennsylvania State University, Columbia University, and the University of Maryland. She has participated in international programs and research for more than three decades and is the author of more than 150 research articles, reviews, and book chapters on nutrition.*

Five decades ago, international agencies and public health officials began to recognize severe protein and energy malnutrition (PEM) and classic signs of vitamin and mineral deficiencies as problems worthy of attention and expenditure of resources. Global programs to combat severe PEM were slow to start, however, and several early attempts were aborted. Nonetheless, momentum toward the elimination of severe deficiencies identified as public health problems accelerated on a global scale in parallel with progress in medical treatment and control measures that accompanied economic progress and social development. In most countries today, mortality rates among infants and young children are at historic lows, and life expectancy is at historic highs. Severe forms of PEM still occur but are associated most commonly with devastating natural disasters and civil unrest that have led to displacement of persons, prolonged crop failures, or lasting economic crises. Yet even when such emergency circumstances prevail, the relief community is better prepared than ever before to respond rapidly and to minimize the disastrous effects of severe malnutrition and disease. The prevalence of classic clinically evident vitamin and mineral deficiencies has also declined in nearly all countries.

In the face of these advances, a shift in concern occurred about 1990 from overt clinical nutritional deficiencies to "hidden hunger" and the consequences for human health and world development of populations subjected to persistent undernutrition. This veiled problem still persists on an unacceptable global scale, especially among underprivileged people residing in countries with slowly advancing economies. Even the most optimistic estimates indicate that this situation will continue in most of these countries well into the new century unless there is a significant shift in the way the problem is confronted. Vertical national programs that distribute food packages or micronutrient supplements, subsidized largely through external agency funds, have successfully muted the problem in some of the countries most affected but are unlikely to provide sustainable control when these countries must assume the full burden of implementation in the future.

Indeed, selective micronutrient undernutrition may also be a problem in some middle-income countries. Lessons learned from experience beginning in the 1930s and 1940s in the United States and several European countries indicate that at the middle-income level of economic and technical advancement, selective fortification of the food supply is a sustainable option for prevention of micronutrient deficiencies when central quality control can be maintained and distribution channels permeate the country.

MEASURING PROGRESS

Achieved stature (height for age), a product of the dynamic interaction among genetics, environment, and diet during growth, is the index of choice for monitoring the prevalence of persistent undernutrition.

Post–World War II secular trends among the Japanese, including those who migrated to developed Western countries, reveal how population-based improvements in reaching genetic potential in height have paralleled improved household dietary diversification and environmental sanitation. Similar secular trends are occurring worldwide (except in sub-Saharan Africa) as progress is made in interrupting the malnutrition-infection cycle, which is devastating to health and well-being, and improving household food security. In its *Third Report on the World Nutrition Situation,* the UN Subcommittee on Nutrition tracked regional progress from 1980 through 1995 (United Nations, 1997). It indicates that the situation in sub-Saharan African countries has been static or deteriorating, whereas rates of improvement have been greatest in Southeast Asia, South Asia, and Latin America. However, data from the World Health Organization global database on child growth and malnutrition (de Onis and Blossner, 1997) reveal that rates of improved stature are quite variable across countries in a given region so that such regional gains must be interpreted with caution.

Progress in the control of severe vitamin and mineral malnutrition over the past decade has also been quite remarkable. Political will and the commitment of resources to implement known effective interventions intensified following the 1990 UNICEF-sponsored World Summit for Children; the 1991 multiple-agency-sponsored Conference on Ending Hidden Hunger; and the 1992 International Conference on Nutrition sponsored by WHO and the Food and Agriculture Organization (FAO). In these very visible forums, representatives at the highest political levels from most countries around the world made commitments to achieving specific health and nutritional improvement goals by the start of the new century, especially for children and pregnant mothers. The implementation of country-level nutrition planning and prevention programs was stimulated as a result, financed largely by international funding of focused interventions.

For example, iodized salt is now available in most countries, distributed even in the remote areas that had been previously plagued by the health consequences of inadequate iodine intakes (goiter and cretinism). Similarly, in the short run, repetitive periodic distribution of high-dose vitamin A supplements has contributed to a reduction in impaired ocular health and blinding malnutrition, and in areas where clinical deficiency was formerly rampant, is believed to be contributing to a decline in young child mortality. On the other hand, anemia from iron deficiency, the most globally common of the micronutrient deficiencies, has been less amenable to improvement. This may be because the internationally generated political commitments were initially less forceful and comprehensive in this area than in others. As a result, global determination to address this problem may not have been sufficient to stimulate remedial activity by local health workers and politicians.

ADULT UNDERNUTRITION: A CHALLENGE FOR THE FUTURE

Adult PEM is now appearing on nutritional radar screens. Political awareness is growing regarding the significance of the problem for national and global economic and social development, as well as for individual quality of life. Adult PEM is manifested as slimness or low body mass index (BMI). Slenderness may be fashionable, but not when it occurs among the impoverished and is associated with reduced physical capacity, higher rates of illness, and premature mortality. Although limited data are available to document the prevalence of low BMI, some estimates indicate that 30 to 50 percent of adults in South Asia and 15 to 30 percent in Africa are underweight. Data are also accumulating on the importance of adequate intake of micronutrients (vitamin A, iron, iodine, and folic acid, to name but a few) in the preconception and gestational periods of a woman's life cycle to lessen risk of defects in fetal development, reduce infant mortality and morbidity, and improve maternal survival and health.

Seasonal variations in food availability and energy expenditure contribute to adult undernutrition, with potentially adverse effects on rural women in particular. In many countries, these women constitute one-third of the total workforce and often three-quarters of the informal work sector and provide over half of the country's food supply. These working fertile women and their progeny are particularly vulnerable during pregnancy, when field and household work demands do not diminish and food consumption does not increase. Recent data support the hypothesis that lasting risks for the development of diet-related diseases in later life, including hypertension, diabetes, obesity, and heart disease, are associated with fetal and infant undernutrition. The global implications for future adult health of not aggressively combating gestational and infant undernutrition among the poor now are obvious. Clearly, health and development planners need to take a life-cycle perspective in preventive nutrition planning.

MALNUTRITION IN TRANSITION

The demographic transition involving longer life spans and increasing urban populations that took place during the past century in the developed world is now occurring on a global scale. Emerging at the same time are the nutrition-related chronic diseases that are already the major killers among relatively sedentary populations who overindulge in Westernized diets high in cholesterol, saturated fats, and calories and low in fiber, vegetables, and fruits. Before the 1980s, the least developed countries had limited affluent populations with the capacity to mimic Western lifestyles and eating habits, but this situation is rapidly changing with no evidence that the trend is slowing. Relatively inexpensive, convenient fast-food restaurants have penetrated ever deeper into traditional and emerging markets, and rural migrant families moving to urban centers have relinquished traditional dietary patterns for convenient food. Urban jobs and household work are often less demanding of energy than rural activities. There may be more free time, but there are also more limited opportunities for inexpensive entertainment, while low-cost urban housing deprives inhabitants of traditional relaxation. Consequently, obesity is emerging as a global malnutrition problem, a problem that is not restricted to the affluent even in developing countries that are also faced with continuing undernutrition. The dilemma for nutrition and health leaders in such settings is how to communicate consistent and relevant nutrition and health messages to address the range of problems observed with changing social, economic, and ecological conditions. It is likely that these conditions will continue to change and even accelerate in the new century.

SHIFTING ECONOMIC WINDS AND SUBSIDIES

Whereas progress in combating undernutrition has occurred in recent years on many fronts, these accomplishments have been made largely through subsidies to local health budgets with international funding of public health programs specifically targeting nutritional improvement. Indeed, over the past two decades, many countries have been plagued by an economic crisis resulting in greater unemployment or underemployment, as well as stagnant or declining government budgets available for health expenditures. This situation has particularly affected low- and middle-income countries that have made important development progress. Although global population growth rates have slowed, the total world population continues to grow; according to projections, the world's population will increase from about six billion today to nearly eight billion in 2020, with most of this growth occurring in the less developed world. Furthermore, the global population is aging, and individuals over age forty-five years are expected to number two billion by 2020, doubling their population in a mere twenty-five years (UN World Population Prospects, 1996). Again, this will occur increasingly in developing nations.

The growing and graying world population is shifting the balance of health concerns between communicable and noncommunicable diseases, even in the less developed countries. National health budgets are increasingly being stretched to combat both infectious diseases still afflicting younger populations and chronic diseases of growing numbers of the elderly. Urbanization has also been accelerating in the developing world, with over 60 percent of the world's population expected to inhabit cities by the year 2020 (UN World Population Prospects, 1995). Much of this internal migration results from young people leaving rural areas in search of increased urban opportunities, which have diminished in several countries as a result of the growing economic crisis.

NUTRITION AT THE START OF THE NEW CENTURY

The well-publicized year 2000 nutritional goals articulated at the international conferences mentioned earlier have not been achieved. Undernutrition will continue to impede national and world development well into the twenty-first century. The problem will continue to take a toll on child health in subtle forms that impair physical growth and intellectual achievement and on adult health in ways that reduce work productivity and earning capacity and increase the risk of premature death and chronic health problems. The affluent countries of the world and international funding groups must recognize their continued responsibility in the twenty-first century to assist the less affluent in achieving their national and local development goals, but they must do it in ways identified as appropriate by local authorities. National political and decision-empowered authorities must also recognize that it is in their best interest to invest in improved health for their entire population, but with sustainable disparity-reducing programs especially targeted to the poor.

Difficult decisions lie ahead. Accelerated economic growth in the less developed countries could contribute to addressing the problem of undernutrition if increased revenues were applied to human development rather than military budgets and if political stability were maintained. Thailand provides a notable example: severe and moderate underweight was almost eliminated in less than ten years, and mild underweight was reduced to about 10 percent prevalence, based on Thai growth standards, in fifteen years. These achievements were made possible by developing a coherent national policy articulated through explicit actions with government support for community-based improvements. Programs addressed not only nutrition but also a range of social, educational, health, and agricultural issues that were identified—through community participation, village by village—as constraints amenable to progress. A committed stable government, an improving economy, and purposeful strategic planning with clear goals were crucial factors in transforming the Thai nation's health in such a short period (Winichagon, Kachondham, Attig, and Tontisirin, 1992). The recent economic crisis in Thailand may have slowed economic growth temporarily, but gains in the control of undernutrition are apparently being sustained, most probably as a result of the capacity and commitment engendered by the process of community participation.

There are examples in other countries of health benefits accruing even in the absence of improved per capita income and with a virtually stagnant national economy. Examples include Costa Rica, China, and the state of Kerala in southwestern India. Costa Rica abolished its armed forces in 1949, redirected resources to social welfare and development, and focused the health system on preventive medicine equitably dispersed and involving community participation. Where vitamin A deficiency had previously been evident, it became possible to discontinue the national vitamin A fortification of sugar because adequate vitamin A status had been achieved through other means. In China, the blinding vitamin A deficiency, widespread before the 1949 revolution, subsequently declined following the institution of policies favoring greater evenhandedness in the distribution of food and health services. In Kerala, a reduction in the gender disparity in social services that had been in effect for many years, including education of women, has played a key role in the low occurrence of vitamin A deficiency. This contrasts with widespread clinical vitamin A deficiency reported in several other Indian states where gender disparities and limited access to social services still persist.

NUTRITION PARADIGMS FOR THE TWENTY-FIRST CENTURY

As with most issues impeding individual and national development, the causes of undernutrition are dynamic, complex, and context dependent. Sustained progress in overcoming undernutrition depends on establishing principles based on an amalgam of scientific findings with efficient operating practices. However, the local context must be the determinant in the flexible and appropriate application of those principles and practices, thus empowering communities to make optimal use of their human, natural, and economic resources. Sustained resolution of undernutrition is unlikely through narrowly focused national nutrient-specific public health policies and activities, an approach that characterized past donor-driven programs. Moreover, policies that lack some degree of individual and community participation are also unlikely to lead to sustainable changes in behavior. Apparently simple, age-specific, immediate solutions will need to be recast in the larger context of an entire life cycle, and closer links between knowledge and its implementation will have to be forged.

CRUCIAL ELEMENTS OF A FUTURE ACTION PARADIGM

The tenet of human rights advocates that adequate food and nutrition is a basic right has increasingly been receiving lip service recognition by political leaders. The future of the world's health, however, will depend in part on replacing moving lips with moving, flexible hands and minds, focused on empowering people to achieve their own food and nutrition security. The paternalistic, vertical charity paradigm traditionally followed by food, nutrition, and health institutions must give way to holistic, flexible approaches that include community capacity building, direct involvement, and responsibility. Poor communities must be mobilized to participate and commit to self-improvement. Gender and economic disparities must be reduced, and women must be elevated and empowered through literacy and other status-enhancing programs and economic opportunities. Nutrition and health education and communication must become proactive in creating demand for services, and they must focus on eliminating constraints that can potentially be addressed using available resources, augmented as necessary by external aid. Changed behaviors will not be achieved through programs imposed by central governments but through decentralized policies that empower local residents to engage in decision making and foster their capacity to manage, evaluate, and adjust as progress occurs incrementally and local conditions improve. This paradigm is focused on building self-esteem and confidence, crucial elements in sustaining healthy environments and encouraging wise choices that yield personal benefits while contributing to improved community, national, and global well-being. As incremental change occurs community by community, the future of the world's health will improve. Providers of external aid can accelerate this process by freeing those funds for integration with local resources in ways that are synergistic with, rather than a replacement for, local capacity building.

References

United Nations. *Third Report on the World Nutrition Situation.* Geneva: United Nations, Administrative Committee on Coordination, Subcommittee on Nutrition, 1997.

United Nations. *Ending Malnutrition by 2020: An Agenda for Change in the Millennium.* Geneva: United Nations, Administrative Committee on Coordination, Subcommittee on Nutrition, Commission on the Nutrition Challenges of the 21st Century, 1999.

United Nations Population Division. *World Population Prospects: The 1994 Revision.* New York: United Nations, 1995.

United Nations Population Division. *World Population Prospects: The 1995 Revision.* New York: United Nations, 1996.

Winichagon, P., Kachondham, Y., Attig, B. A., and Tontisirin, K. (eds.). *Integrating Food and Nutrition into Development: Thailand's Experiences and Future Visions.* Bangkok, Thailand: UNICEF, 1992.

WHO Programme of Nutrition. de Onis, M., and Blossner, M. (eds.). *WHO Global Database on Child Growth and Malnutrition.* Geneva: World Health Organization, 1997.

Additional Reading

Muñoz, C. & Scrimshaw, N. S. *The National and Health Transition of Democratic Costa Rica.* Boston, Mass.: International Foundation for Developing Countries, 1995.

CHAPTER TWENTY-EIGHT

The Nutritional Crisis to Come

W.P.T. James

W.P.T. James *is Chairman of the special UN Millennium Commission on Global Issues Relating to Nutrition up to 2020 and one of eight scientists elected by the European Commission to deal with public health policies in Europe. He is also responsible for the funding and organization of global initiatives relating to food and health, with particular emphasis on the pandemic of obesity and the implementation of preventive and management strategies. For seventeen years, he was the Director of the Rowett Research Institute in Scotland.*

I have been privileged to chair a commission on the future of global health in relation to food and nutrition for an inter-UN group reporting to the Secretary General's main administrative coordinating committee. We were challenged to explain why, despite relatively sustained economic growth, there had been such a minimal reduction in the prevalence of childhood malnutrition. Major progress had been made in dealing with the multiple disorders induced by iodine deficiency. Vitamin A deficiency was also being combated, but the preschool childhood problem of early stunting was unremitting. Our analyses suggested that a billion more children would grow up stunted, suffering the associated mental impairment, before the year 2020. The problem, especially acute in the Indian subcontinent, persisted because of the lack of public health strategies focused on the welfare of girls and women. They therefore grow up short, thin, malnourished, and anemic; they then go on in pregnancy to produce small, vulnerable babies of low birthweight who would have to experience an unusual major growth spurt to catch up with the international standards for appropriate child growth. Catch-up growth is almost impossible in an environment where exclusive breast-feeding also entails the consumption of water, teas, and herbal drinks using an almost universally contaminated water supply with rudimentary sanitation affecting at least 1.5 billion people in the Indian subcontinent alone. Attempts to combat low birthweights are handicapped by the frequency of infections and the low energy and animal protein intake of societies geared to vegetarian diets. Grains, vegetables, and fruits are cooked to the point where many vitamins are destroyed; such culinary patterns were developed to limit the endemic enteric diseases, but in practice they result in multiple vitamin deficiencies. Folate deficiency, a particularly large problem, exacerbates anemia, limits fetal growth when mothers become deficient during pregnancy, and amplifies the risk of cardiovascular disease in adults (James, 1997). Our renewed emphasis on the care and well-being of young girls and mothers has now led to a major shift in UNICEF policies in Asia.

These classic nutritional problems have been expanded by recent confirmations of widespread adult malnutrition and obesity in the developing world (see Exhibit 28.1). The focus on childhood problems had led to the neglect of adult malnutrition, which we classified first into three (James, Ferro-Luzzi, and Waterlow, 1988) and then into five grades (Ferro-Luzzi and James, 1996) of chronic energy deficiency (CED) based on the degree of low adult weight for height. Weights are expressed as calculated by the body mass index (BMI), where weight in kilograms is divided by the square of the height in meters (see Table 28.1). Whereas a BMI below 18.5 (a Grade I CED) handicaps adults' physical capacity to work, a BMI below 17.0 (Grade II) for men and women is linked to intercurrent infections, with time spent in bed rather than working. This level of CED was evident in adult men and women in Latin America, Africa, and Asia (Shetty and James, 1994), with 10 to 15 percent of adults affected in Latin America, 15 to 40 percent, depending on famine and war, affected in Africa, and fully 50 to 70 percent of Indian adults in rural societies affected. Malnourished adult women are handicapping their children's future not just during pregnancy but subsequently during childhood when frequent feeding and mental stimulation are so crucial to brain development (Grantham-McGregor, Fernald, and Sethuraman, 1999). Thus we are witnessing an intergenerational life cycle of handicap with maternal as well as child care now the priority.

OBESITY AND CHRONIC DISEASES IN THE DEVELOPING WORLD

In 1995, as my colleagues and I assessed the degree of adult malnutrition in different countries, we saw a shift in the distribution of adult weights; as the average weight of a population increased, particularly with mechanization, the right-hand tail of the distribution was being accentuated. Thus our original classification of adult weights (see Table 28.1), now accepted by WHO (Ferro-Luzzi and James, 1996), identified adults as "overweight" with a BMI of 25.0 or more and "obese" with a BMI of 30.0 or higher. Now, throughout the developing world, we are beginning to see a surprisingly high proportion of overweight adults. Obesity is also affecting an astonishing proportion

Grades	BMI	Grades	BMI
Overweight		Underweight	
Extreme obesity	40.0+	Chronic energy	17.0–18.4
Severe obesity	35.0–39.9	Deficiency (I)	
Obesity	30.0–34.9	Moderate (II)	16.0–16.9
Pre-obese/overweight	25.0–29.9	Severe (III)	13.0–15.9
Normal weight	18.5–24.9	Extreme (IV)	10.0–12.9
		Terminal (V)	< 10.0

Table 28.1.   Adult Malnutrition and Obesity, Classified on the Basis of the Body Mass Index (BMI) Weight.

Note: WHO classifies a "normal" weight range with 3 degrees of underweight and 4 of overweight, but terminologies differ slightly. New Asian guidelines suggest that a BMI of 23–24 is an at-risk category because of emerging evidence of susceptibility in that range to diabetes, hypertension, and abnormal plasma lipid levels linked to coronary heart disease.

- Each year, thirty million infants in the developing world are born with intrauterine growth retardation. This represents about 24 percent of the births in these countries. Interventions on a population basis are urgently needed to prevent fetal growth retardation.

- More than 150 million preschool children worldwide are still underweight and more than 200 million children remain stunted. Underweight and stunting, however, are only the tip of the iceberg —suboptimal growth affects many more. Stunting is linked to mental impairment. At current rates of improvement, about one billion children will be growing up by 2020 with impaired mental development.

- In Africa and Asia, high proportions of women are undernourished. This is made worse by seasonal food shortages. Around 243 million adults in developing countries are undernourished (Body Mass Index of less than 17 mg/m^2); their work capacity and resistance to infection are lowered as a result.

- Maternal undernutrition exacerbates infantile anemia, which impairs brain development. Anemia is also highly prevalent in schoolchildren and adolescents. Maternal anemia is pandemic, over 80 percent in some countries, and is associated with very high rates of maternal mortality.

- Evidence from both developing and industrialized countries links maternal and early childhood undernutrition to increased susceptibility in adult life to noncommunicable diseases such as diabetes, heart disease, and hypertension.

- Overweight and obesity are rapidly growing in all regions, affecting children and adults alike. These problems have replaced more traditional public health concerns in many developing countries.

- A fundamental link is emerging between maternal and childhood malnutrition and the child's subsequent marked sensitivity to abdominal obesity, diabetes, high blood pressure, and coronary heart disease. These changes are exacerbated by the switch to high-fat, energy-dense diets and physical inactivity around the globe.

Exhibit 28.1. A Summary of Global Nutritional Challenges.

of deprived adults in central and eastern Europe. We were already aware that obesity was reaching epidemic proportions in western Europe, North America, and the Pacific Islands, but its rapid emergence in Asia, Latin America, and Africa was surprising (see Table 28.2).

Simultaneously, WHO, in its collation of adult chronic diseases, was finding that the health burden of hypertension, coronary artery disease, diabetes, and cancers was dominated by the burden in the developing rather than the developed world (see Exhibit 28.1), so suddenly the diseases formerly described as those of affluence were placing a double burden—of diseases related to malnutrition and at the same time of diseases of purported nutritional excess—on many very poor countries with limited resources and poor health service structures.

THE DIETARY BASIS OF THE GLOBAL BURDEN OF DISEASE

Figure 28.1 shows the fundamental links between diet, physical inactivity, and the major adult diseases traditionally associated with the Western world. It is clear that excess weight gain is very closely linked to diabetes; it also readily induces hypertension and amplifies abnormal changes in circulating lipid levels, particularly by inducing a rise in plasma triglycerides and a fall in high-density lipoprotein cholesterol. A multiplicity of risk factors have additional effects on the likelihood of developing coronary heart disease (CHD). Thus the U.S. diet is so energy dense that it readily induces obesity, but the remarkable drops in saturated fatty acid intake have led to a fall in CHD despite the escalating roles of obesity. Our global analysis of diet and cancer (World Cancer Research Fund, 1997) also shows that obesity and physical inactivity are particularly conducive to the development of colon cancer and postmenopausal breast and endometrial cancers. Other nutritional factors, including salted fish, overcooked red meat, and particularly a lack of vegetables and fruit, have an impact on the development of cancer. Rapid childhood growth rates, together with the early onset of puberty in response to high protein and energy feeding, also enhance the risk of later breast cancer.

Given this perspective and the five- to tenfold range in rates of obe-

Region	Country	Year	Age Range	Men	Women
Europe	Czech Republic	1995	20–65	22.6	25.6
	Former East Germany	1992	25–69	21.0	27.0
	Former West West Germany	1990	25–69	17.0	19.0
	Finland	1991–93	20–75	14.0	11.0
	Netherlands	1995	20–59	8.4	8.3
	Sweden	1988–89	16–84	5.3	9.1
	UK England	1997	16–64	17.0	20.0
	Scotland	1995	16–64	16.0	17.0
	Russia	1996	18–59	10.8	27.9
	Malta	1984	25–64	22.0	35.0
North America	Canada	1991	18–74	15.0	15.0
	USA	1988–94	20–74	19.9	24.9
Central and South America	Mexico (urban)	1995	Adults	11.0	23.0
	Brazil	1989	25–64	5.9	13.3
	Curaçao	1993–94	18+	19.0	36.0
Middle East	Iran, Islamic Republic of	1993–94	20–74	2.5	7.7
	(south) Cyprus	1989–90	35–64	19.0	24.0
	Kuwait	1994	18+	32.0	44.0
	Jordan (urban)	1994–96	25+	32.7	59.8
	Morocco	1984–85	20+	2.3	14.6
	Bahrain (urban)	1991–92	20–65	9.5	30.3
	Saudi Arabia	1990–93	15+	16.0	24.0
Australia and Oceania	Australia	1995	25–64	18.0	18.0
	Nauru	1994	25–69	80.0	79.0
	New Zealand	1989	18–64	10.0	13.0
	Samoa (urban)	1991	25–69	58.0	77.0
	Papua New Guinea (urban)	1991	25–69	36.6	54.3
South and East Asia	Japan	1990–94	15–84	1.8	2.6
	India (urban Delhi middle-class)	1997	Adults	2.31	9.84
	China	1992	20–45	1.2	1.64
	Kyrgyzstan	1993	18–59	4.2	10.7
	Malaysia	—	18–60	5.0	8.0
	Singapore	1992	adults	4.0	6.0
Africa	Mauritius	1992	25–74	5.3	15.2
	Tanzania	1986–89	35–64	0.6	3.6
	Rodrigues (Creoles)	1992	25–69	10.0	31.0
	South Africa (blacks)	1990	15–64	7.9	44.4

Table 28.2.   Obesity Around the World.

Source: Obesity Task Force.

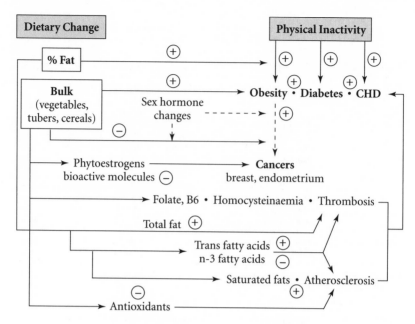

Figure 28.1.   The Interactions of Diet and Physical Inactivity in Adult Chronic Diseases.

sity, diabetes, hypertension, coronary heart disease, and cancers around the world, it is becoming increasingly accepted that these chronic conditions reflect the impact of environmental-genetic interactions, with diet, physical inactivity, and smoking being the principal contributors. These may explain 80 percent of the variance, the impact of smoking having been well established (Peto and others, 1992).

ASIAN METABOLIC SYNDROME (SYNDROME X)

The selective deposition of fat in the abdominal area is now recognized as particularly hazardous because of its links with the development of diabetes, abnormal blood lipids, and hypertension; this complex is designated "syndrome X" or the "Asian metabolic syndrome" of obesity. Traditionally, the distribution of fat has been ascribed predominantly to genetic influences, with men being char-

		Waist Circumference (cm)	
		Increased Risk	Substantially Increased Risk
WHO (Caucasians)[a]	Men	94+	102+
	Women	80	88+
Asians[b]	Men	80+	86+
	Women	74+	80+

Table 28.3.   Proposed Cutoff Waist Measurements in Caucasians and Asians, Based on the Risk of Diabetes and Other Complications of Weight Gain.

[a]WHO data on Americans and Europeans.
[b]Data based on Hong Kong Chinese.

acteristically prone to depositing fat intra-abdominally, especially in the omentum. Women tend to deposit fat around the hips and limbs. Now, however, there is increasing evidence that early events, particularly growth in utero, alter the deposition of body fat. Thus Barker (1998) showed a twentyfold increased risk of syndrome X in adults who had been of low birthweight. New analyses also suggest that simple measures of waist circumference are a good general index of both the amount of intra-abdominal fat and the risk of metabolic complications, although some investigators persist in expressing the risk in terms of the ratio of waist to hip circumference. Different cutoff levels of waist circumference or waist-to-hip ratio have been defined for men and women separately (see Table 28.3). New Asian data show that a fifth of adults in Indian cities have excessive waist values even though their BMIs are within the normal limits of 18.5–25.0, and in overweight Indians, nearly two-thirds of the adults have abdominal obesity, far higher rates than those found in the United Kingdom or in other Caucasian populations.

New analyses from Japan and Hong Kong reveal that the risk of developing diabetes, hypertension, and abnormal blood lipids rises very rapidly above a BMI of 20: the risk of diabetes doubles when BMI reaches only 23 or 24 and increases fourfold with a BMI of 26 or 27. Yet until recently, these higher BMIs were classified as normal in the United States. Careful analyses of data on adult Chinese in Hong Kong also show escalating rates of metabolic complications and particularly of diabetes at far lower waist circumference values (see Table 28.3). It is therefore not surprising that WHO predicts a dramatic escalation in the burden of diabetes, particularly in Asia. In China, there are already eighteen million diabetics, projected to rise to thirty-eight million in the next twenty years. In India, however, 12 percent of urban slum dwellers already have undiagnosed diabetes, and a further 18 percent show the prediabetic condition of impaired glucose tolerance.

THE BASIS OF DIABETES SUSCEPTIBILITY IN ASIA

There is increasing evidence from Jamaica, from Poona in India, and from Europe that fetal conditions program the future child's susceptibility to diabetes. Low birthweight and disproportionately sized babies reveal the signs of a diabetic predisposition by four to six years of age. What features of the maternal and infant diet explain this susceptibility is unclear, but folic acid, animal protein, zinc, iron, and n-3 fatty acid deficiencies are all being considered as key candidates. Yajnik from Poona is now finding that Indian mothers seem unable to grow lean protein-rich fetuses, particularly if the mothers are thin, short, and have small head circumferences themselves, their smaller heads being taken as an index of their own childhood and indeed fetal deprivation (Yajnik, 2000). Mothers eating no green leafy vegetables (a rich source of folic acid) are prone to produce small babies with limited muscle and relatively more fat who are then at particular risk of being short and underweight, but with a higher proportion of fat and increased susceptibility to diabetes later in life. The diabetes stems from early impairment of insulin production in the pancreas or the development of insulin resistance at a young age. Increasing evidence is emerging of Indian children and adults having a poor lean tissue mass, meaning that they are relatively much fatter for the same BMI than Caucasians. Malays have a slightly higher lean-to-fat ratio than Indians, and the Chinese have values closer to Western ratios. Only Papua New Guineans and some other Pacific Islanders seem to have higher amounts of lean tissue at body weights equivalent to Caucasians'. These altered ratios of lean to fat tissue do seem to relate to abdominal obesity, with all its associated risks, but we await new analyses on the link between lean tissue growth and insulin sensitivity.

GENETIC OR NUTRITIONAL
SUSCEPTIBILITY TO CHRONIC DISEASE?

Recent advances in molecular biology have now allowed the discovery of new hormones and receptors that enhance the propensity toward many diseases. We have learned that a congenital absence of the newly discovered leptin hormone induces remarkable childhood obesity, but in practically all obese subjects, blood leptin levels increase in proportion to their excess body fat. Attempts to define subtle changes in the control of leptin secretion or in its signaling effectiveness at the brain or other tissue leptin receptor level have not yet allowed a clear definition of subgroups in a society or different ethnic groups with particular propensities toward obesity. Many genes seem to be involved in the complex neurophysiological control of both food intake and the metabolic responses to food. It was recently shown in France that a single gene change in the β_2 adrenergic receptor involved in the stimulation of the sympathetic nervous system increased average BMI in the one-third of French adults who are affected. The risk of obesity was tripled in subjects who were inactive. The challenge is therefore to establish whether there is a "thrifty" genotype in the Asian populations, how this may relate to the remarkable propensity to deposit fat rather than lean tissue, whether additional genes are involved in the selective deposition of abdominal fat, and whether particular genes are involved in the enhanced risk of diabetes. If such genes are found at high frequency in the Asian populations, they may parallel other disparities in genetic clustering, as for lactase and alcohol dehydrogenase deficiencies, which are far more common in Japanese, Chinese, and Indians. The implications for public health will then mean that even greater emphasis has to be given to preventive measures.

A plausible alternative explanation for Asians' sensitivity to adult chronic diseases is based on Björntorp's striking demonstration that in Swedes, abdominal obesity relates strongly to an excess secretion of the stress hormone cortisol and abnormalities in the hypothalamic control of the adrenal's secretion of cortisol (Björntorp and others, 1999). Intriguingly, experimental evidence shows that a poor maternal protein intake reduces the placenta's capacity to degrade the mother's cortisol, so the fetus becomes exposed to higher adrenal hormone levels, which then induce a permanent propensity to high blood pressure in the offspring. If the fetus adapts to recognize the higher fetal cortisol, its own cortisol control system may be reset, leading to sustained high cortisol levels throughout life but particularly when stress occurs. In Cushing's disease, induced by a cortisol-secreting tumor, the body loses protein, gains fat, and redistributes it to the abdominal area. It is therefore tempting to speculate that the thin, short Asian women on a vegetarian diet where rice, with its low protein content, is the staple are particularly prone to producing small babies conditioned to expect high cortisol levels and with a low body protein content. Whether the ethnic genetic differences or the customary Asian diets and infection-induced stress are primarily responsible for the escalating rates of abdominal obesity, diabetes, and cardiovascular disease remains uncertain, but the question is of exceptional public health importance.

WHY THE OBESITY EPIDEMIC?

These propensities toward the Asian metabolic syndrome still leave unexplained the reason for the now almost universal excessive weight gain affecting not only adults in urban areas throughout the world but children too. Two factors are fundamentally involved: physical inactivity and an energy-dense, fat-rich diet. The dramatic fall in physical activity over the past four decades has come with the proliferation of motor vehicles and their enormous impact on urban planning, the mechanization of almost all work, reduced demand for physical work in the household, the revolution in office work brought by computerization, and the escalation of television viewing. All these changes induce the majority of the population to spend practically all their working hours sitting down. Thus the demand for energy may have dropped by 500 to 750 kilocalories per person per day since World War II. This means that humans' appetite control systems are constantly challenged to reduce food intake. A gamut of behavioral changes in meal patterns are evident: the avoidance of breakfast, the elimination of three large meals a day, the neglect of the dessert course at main meals, and (except in the United States) the substantial reduction in portion sizes—all reflect behavioral responses to the need for lower energy and food intake.

At low levels of physical activity, diet composition becomes crucial, and diet density gains in importance. The human brain seems oblivious to the high energy value of dietary fat, which in evolutionary terms was a scarce commodity. High-fat, varied diets are particularly conducive to obesity in every experimental setting for animals and humans when physical activity is restricted. Thus to maintain energy balance under sedentary conditions, a diet containing only 20 percent fat is necessary; people who sustain high levels of physical activity may be able to tolerate a fat intake as high as 40 percent. Once weight gain has occurred, however, both animals and humans seem to induce some neurophysiological adaptive mechanism that "resets" the brain's appreciation of what normal body weight should be. Thus lower-fat diets may not induce substantial weight losses in obese individuals, particularly if, as in the United States, the diet remains very energy dense because of the use of sugars, fructose syrups, and maltodextrins as fat substitutes in low-fat foods. This may explain the American paradox of escalating obesity despite lowered fat intake.

Analyses of activity patterns suggest that preventing obesity requires a rethinking of town planning, with pedestrian precincts, walkways, cycle paths, and new building designs that allow people to remain spontaneously on their feet for longer periods of time. School and community activities and a host of other initiatives also need to be devised that do not rely on the naive assumption that social patterns of behavior can be changed by simply urging people to increase their sports and vigorous leisure activities. Only in Norway does there seem to have been a major cultural shift involving the whole society to increase leisure activity levels. At present, urban development, Western industrial policies, and technological innovation are all geared toward allowing us to engage in as little physical activity as possible.

The food patterns of society are changing rapidly. The spread of fast foods, eating while walking and conversing, and rising reliance on cafés and restaurants make tracking the fat content of the foods one consumes nearly impossible. All these changes favor weight gain. Adopting these behavioral changes, encouraged by intense advertising, is regarded by the Third World as a measure of affluence. The food, catering, and entertainment industries amplify these tendencies in the developing world, with urban slum dwellers readily taking to foods that provide once rare and sought-after fatty, sugary, and salty tastes for which humans have evolved special taste buds. These foods are also less perishable than the traditional foods of rural origin, and their organoleptic and practical advantages make their appeal almost irresistible.

These trends mean that we are likely to see remarkably high rates of diabetes, hypertension, coronary disease, and cancer in the twenty-first century, overwhelming health services in the developing world.

We therefore need to shift the perceptions of governments and society to recognize that much of their health burden is preventable if changes can be induced by a multiplicity of schemes in the lifestyle of the general population.

References

Barker, D.J.P. *Mothers, Babies and Health in Later Life*. (2nd ed.) Edinburgh: Churchill Livingstone, 1998.

Björntorp, P., Holm, G., and Rosmond, R. "Hypothalamic Arousal, Insulin Resistance, and Type 2 Diabetes Mellitus." *Diabetic Medicine*, 1999, *16*, 373–383.

Ferro-Luzzi, A., and James, W.P.T. "Adult Malnutrition: Simple Assessment Techniques for Use in Emergencies." *British Journal of Nutrition*, 1996, *75*, 3–10.

Grantham-McGregor, S. M, Fernald, L. C., and Sethuraman, K. "Effects of Health and Nutrition on Cognitive and Behavioral Development in Children in the First Three Years of Life." *Food and Nutrition Bulletin, 20*, 1999, 53–99.

James, W.P.T. "Long-Term Fetal Programming of Body Composition and Longevity." *Nutrition Reviews*, 1997, *55*, S31–S42.

James, W.P.T., Ferro-Luzzi, A., and Waterlow, J. C. "Definition of Chronic Energy Deficiency in Adults: Report of a Working Party of the International Dietary Energy Consultative Group." *European Journal of Clinical Nutrition*, 1988, *42*, 969–981.

Peto, R., and others. "Mortality from Tobacco in Developed Countries: Indirect Estimation from National Vital Statistics." *Lancet*, 1992, *339*, 1268–1278.

Shetty, P. S., and James, W.P.T. *Body Mass Index. A Measure of Chronic Energy Deficiency in Adults*. FAO Food and Nutrition Paper no. 56. Rome: United Nations Food and Agriculture Organization, 1994.

World Cancer Research Fund. *Food, Nutrition and the Prevention of Cancer: A Global Perspective*. Washington, D.C.: American Institute for Cancer Research, 1997.

Yasnik, C. "Interactions of Perturbations in Intrauterine Growth and Growth During Childhood on the Risk of Adult-Onset Disease." *Proceeding of the Nutrition Society*, 2000, *59*, 1–9.

CHAPTER TWENTY-NINE

Population and Health

Joseph Chamie

Joseph Chamie, PhD, *is Director of the Population Division, Department for Economic and Social Affairs, United Nations Secretariat in New York and served as the Deputy Secretary-General for the 1994 United Nations International Conference for Population and Development. In addition to completing many studies issued under United Nations authorship, he has also published under his own name in such areas as fertility, marriage, population estimates and projections, international migration, and population policy.*

Throughout human history, the size, levels, structure, and distribution of populations have greatly affected the health of societies, and the twenty-first century will be no exception. The significance of the twenty-first century is that it comes after the twentieth century—a period when an unprecedented global demographic revolution took place. As this revolution continues to unfold in the coming decades, the world will move through uncharted demographic territory.

The views expressed in this chapter are those of the author and do not necessarily reflect those of the United Nations. The figures cited are from United Nations World Population Prospects (1999).

The rapid growth of world population is a relatively recent phenomenon. Over most of the distant past, population growth was relatively slow, and the number of people in the world did not increase significantly for long stretches. Periods of growth were followed by periods of decline. Life was harsh, health conditions were poor, and death rates were high. War, pestilence, and famine kept population in check. Infant, child, and adult deaths, especially maternal mortality, were common, and relatively few people reached sixty years of age. Birthrates were also high; contraception was rare, and women had numerous pregnancies. Because both fertility and mortality were high, world population changed little over long periods of time.

Indeed, the population explosion is a modern phenomenon: most of the growth of the world population has occurred in the past two thousand years. It is estimated that two thousand years ago, the world's population was about 300 million people; ten centuries later, it may have reached 310 million people. It rose to 500 million around 1500, and the 1 billion mark was reached around 1800 (see Table 29.1).

As the table shows, in stark contrast to the past, the twentieth century was a century of revolutionary demographic proportions, unparalleled during all preceding centuries. At the beginning of that extraordinary century, the world's population was 1.65 billion; at the end it stood at an estimated at 6.06 billion, yielding an incredible and

Year	Population (Billions)
1	0.30
1000	0.31
1500	0.50
1800	0.98
1900	1.65
1925	1.96
1950	2.52
1975	4.07
2000	6.06
2025	7.82
2050	8.91
2075	9.32
2100	9.46

Table 29.1. World Population Estimates and Projections, Year 1 to 2100 (Medium Variant).

Source: United Nations Population Division, *World Population Prospects: The 1998 Revision* (United Nations, 1999).

unprecedented increase of 4.41 billion people in a period of one hundred years. Moreover, 80 percent of this growth, or 3.54 billion, took place in the second half of the century. In addition, the twentieth century holds the record for both the highest annual rate of population growth for the world, 2.04 percent in the late 1960s, and the largest annual increase in the world's history, 86 million in the late 1980s.

The rapid growth of world population is not over. The population of the world is projected to continue to increase well into the twenty-first century, but at a slower pace than occurred in the demographically historic twentieth century. For example, world population is projected, according to the medium variant, to reach 8.91 billion by 2050 and 9.46 billion by the year 2100 (see Table 29.1).

Behind these global population estimates and projections lie enormous diversity and differences between and within regions. For example, among the more developed regions, little population growth is taking place. In fact, the current population of the more developed regions of 1.19 billion is projected to decline slightly to 1.16 billion by 2050 and 1.04 billion by 2100 (medium variant). In contrast, the current population of the less developed regions of 4.87 billion is expected to increase to 7.75 billion by 2050 and 8.42 billion by 2100 (see Table 29.2).

With respect to the growth and distribution of major geographical regions, enormous diversity exists. As Table 29.2 shows, the most rapidly growing area is Africa. Between 1950 and 2000, the population of Africa more than tripled, increasing from 220 million to 780 million. This trend is expected to continue, with the African continent projected to have 1.8 billion inhabitants by 2050 and 2.2 billion by 2100 (medium variant). Thus in a matter of 150 years, it is expected that Africa will have witnessed a tenfold increase in its population. Asia, which currently accounts for about 60 percent of the world's population, is projected to experience a fourfold increase over this period of 150 years, from 1.4 billion to 5.4 billion. The population of Latin America and the Caribbean will likely see a fivefold increase over this period, from 170 million to 880 million.

In contrast to the less developed regions, the populations of Europe and Japan are now in a period of decline, and these trends are expected to continue well into the future. By 2100, for example, it is projected that the European population will to be nearly 30 percent smaller than it is today, dropping from 730 million to 550 million. However, due to relatively higher fertility and international migration,

Major Area	1900	1950	2000	2050	2100
	Population (Millions)				
World	1,650	¯2,521	6,055	8,909	9,459
More developed	540	813	1,188	1,155	1,041
Less developed	1,110	1,709	4,867	7,754	8,418
Africa	133	221	784	1,766	2,215
Asia	947	1,402	3,683	5,268	5,416
Europe	408	547	729	628	515
Latin America	74	167	519	809	877
Northern America	82	172	310	392	388
Oceania	6	13	30	46	49
	Distribution (%)				
World	100.0	100.0	100.0	100.0	100.0
More developed	32.7	32.2	19.6	13.0	11.0
Less developed	67.3	67.8	80.4	87.0	89.0
Africa	8.1	8.8	12.9	19.8	23.4
Asia	7.4	5.6	60.8	59.1	57.3
Europe	24.7	21.7	12.0	7.0	5.4
Latin America	4.5	6.6	8.6	9.1	9.3
Northern America	5.0	6.8	5.1	4.4	4.1
Oceania	0.4	0.5	0.5	0.5	0.5

Table 29.2. Population for World and Major Areas, 1900-2100 (Medium Variant).

Source: United Nations Population Division, World Population Prospects: The 1998 Revision (United Nations, 1999).

Australia, Canada, New Zealand, and the United States are expected to continue growing.

As a result of differential growth patterns among the regions, the distribution of the world's population is undergoing rapid change. For instance, whereas in 1950 the populations of Europe and Africa accounted for 21.7 and 8.8 percent, respectively, of the world total, now the European and African proportions are roughly equivalent, 12.0 and 12.9 percent, respectively. Moreover, it is projected that by 2050, when Europe's population will be about 7 percent of the world total, the African population will account for 20 percent.

At the national level, the top ten contributors to world population growth today are shown in Table 29.3. Of the net addition of 78 million per year, India's contribution is about 21 percent, or about 16 mil-

		Annual Share of World		
Rank	Country	Annual Addition	Percent	Cumulative Percent
1	India	16.0	20.6	20.6
2	China	11.4	14.7	35.3
3	Pakistan	4.0	5.2	40.5
4	Indonesia	2.9	3.8	44.3
5	Nigeria	2.5	3.2	47.5
6	United States	2.3	2.9	50.4
7	Brazil	2.2	2.8	53.2
8	Bangladesh	2.1	2.7	55.9
9	Mexico	1.5	2.0	57.9
10	Philippines	1.5	2.0	59.9
	Subtotal	46.5	59.9	59.9
	World Total	77.7	100.0	100.0

Table 29.3. Top Ten Contributors to World Population Growth, 1995-2000 (Annual Additions in Millions).

Source: United Nations Population Division, *World Population Prospects: The 1998 Revision* (United Nations, 1999).

lion people. Following India is China, with a 15 percent contribution, or 11.4 million people. As a consequence of a more rapid rate of growth, India's population is projected to match China's in 2045, when both countries will contain around 1.5 billion people, and to surpass it thereafter. Currently, the top five countries—India, China, Pakistan, Indonesia, and Nigeria—account for almost half of world population growth. With the addition of the next five countries—the United States, Brazil, Bangladesh, Mexico, and the Philippines—the percentage reaches 60 percent.

At the other extreme, eighteen countries, all in Europe, have negative rates of natural increase, ranging from −0.52 percent in Latvia to −0.01 percent in Portugal (see Table 29.4). The populations of most of these countries, which are predominantly in eastern Europe, are projected to decline markedly in the coming decades. For example, the population of the Russian Federation is projected to decline from its current level of 147 million to 121 million by 2050.

The cause for the slowdown in population growth rates is smaller family size, which is due to the desire among couples for fewer children. With the increased availability of contraception, especially

Country	Annual Rate of Natural Increase (%)
Latvia	−0.52
Bulgaria	−0.47
Estonia	−0.47
Ukraine	−0.43
Russian Federation	−0.42
Hungary	−0.38
Belarus	−0.34
Romania	−0.23
Czech Republic	−0.22
Lithuania	−0.16
Germany	−0.16
Italy	−0.14
Slovenia	−0.10
Croatia	−0.09
Sweden	−0.09
Greece	−0.03
Spain	−0.02
Portugal	−0.01

Table 29.4. Countries with a Negative Annual Rate of Natural Increase, 1995-2000.

Source: United Nations Population Division, *World Population Prospects: The 1998 Revision* (United Nations, 1999).

modern methods, couples are increasingly able to limit their fertility and can effectively choose both the number and spacing of children they desire. The world average is around 2.7 children per woman, which is about half the level of just a few decades ago. Specific country examples demonstrate the remarkable changes that have taken place over the recent past. Twenty-five years ago, for instance, women in Brazil were having on average about 6 children; now the average is less than half that, at around 2.5. Similarly, in Kenya, the average number of children per woman was about 8.5; now it is around 4.5. And in Viet Nam, the average, once around 6, is now less than 3 children per woman.

Among the developed countries and some developing countries, fertility levels are below replacement, that is, below roughly two children per couple. The combined population of these sixty-one countries (2.6 billion) amounts to about 44 percent of the world total. The populations of thirty countries are projected to decline in the medium term. Austria's population, for example, is projected to decrease from

8.1 million to 7.1 million by 2050. In contrast, the populations of thirty-one countries will continue to increase. The population of China, for example, is expected to increase from 1.3 billion to nearly 1.5 billion by 2050.

An important consequence of declining rates of fertility and mortality, particularly the transition to low levels of fertility, is the aging of populations. Whereas the number of persons aged sixty years and older is estimated to be nearly 600 million today, this number is expected to more than triple—reaching 2 billion—over the next fifty years. Moreover, by 2050, the number of older persons (sixty and older) will for the first time in history exceed the number of children (under fifteen years of age).

The magnitude, tempo, and consequences of global population aging are issues of considerable significance and concern for both developed and developing countries. Many societies, especially in the more developed regions, have already attained age structures older than ever seen in the past. For example, whereas the median age of Europe's population was twenty-nine years in 1950, today it is thirty-seven years, and by 2050 the median age is projected to reach forty-seven years. The proportion of Europe's population that is elderly (60 years and over) has increased from 12 percent in 1950 to 20 percent today; by 2050, it is expected to be 35 percent.

Less developed regions are also experiencing rapid shifts in the relative numbers of children, working-age population, and older persons. For these regions as a whole, the proportion of children (under fifteen years of age) has decreased from about 40 percent in the 1950s and 1960s to about 33 percent today; by 2050, the proportion of children is expected to be approximately 20 percent. In contrast, while the proportion of persons sixty years and older has remained around 6 to 7 percent during this last half century, it is projected to triple by 2050, reaching 22 percent. In addition, the tempo of population aging will be even faster in some developing countries due to relatively rapid declines in their levels of fertility. In China, Cuba, and Thailand, for example, close to a third of the population will be sixty years or older by the middle of the twenty-first century.

Also noteworthy is the fact that the older population is itself aging. More people are reaching old age—eighty, ninety, even one hundred years. This group will be increasing markedly both arithmetically and proportionally. Today, close to 70 million persons are aged eighty years and over; in fifty years' time, this number is expected to reach 370 million. Moreover, it should be noted that the growth of the oldest old (eighty and above) could be even more rapid than expected today. Unforeseen breakthroughs in medical science may extend life expectancy among the elderly well beyond current projections.

Also, at present, the oldest old (eighty and older) account for about one out of every ten older persons (aged sixty and up); by 2050, nearly one out of every five older persons will have celebrated an eightieth birthday. Even more dramatic growth is expected in the population of centenarians (aged one hundred years and older). This exceptional subgroup of the population is projected to increase fifteenfold over the next fifty years, growing from about 145,000 in 2000 to 2.2 million persons by 2050.

Furthermore, because women live longer than men in the vast majority of countries, the feminization of older population groups is a global phenomenon. Among people sixty years and older, 55 percent are women. Among the oldest old (eighty and up), there are nearly two women for every man, and among centenarians, there are about four women for every man.

In addition to fertility and mortality, the other basic component of population change is migration, both internal and international. During the twentieth century, international migration was of minor demographic significance for most nations. However, at the beginning of the century, migration was a major factor of population change in the Western Hemisphere as well as in Australia and New Zealand. In addition, at the end of the century, international migration continued to be an important factor of population growth for Northern America, Australia, and some European nations. The current low levels of fertility for most developed countries imply that even moderate sustained levels of international migration can contribute to increased rates of population growth.

Another major demographic transformation during the twentieth century was increased urbanization and the growth of giant urban centers. Because both fertility and mortality are normally lower in urban areas than in rural areas, the process of urbanization itself leads to lower national fertility and mortality rates. In addition, urbanization affects public and private health needs as well as the means to meet these needs.

Currently, approximately 47 percent of the world's population lives in urban areas, and the urban population is growing at 2.3 percent per year, which is three times faster than its rural counterpart. By 2006, and for the first time in human history, a majority of the world population is expected to be urban; and by 2030, fully 60 percent of all people will be living in urban areas.

The giant urban centers of the world are becoming both larger and more numerous. The largest cities in the world are Tokyo, with a population of 28 million, Mexico City (18 million), and São Paulo (17 million). By 2015, Lagos will be the third largest in the world (25 million), after Tokyo (29 million) and Bombay (26 million). Over the past thirty years, the number of cities with 10 million or more inhabitants grew from three to eighteen. It is projected that by 2015, twenty-six cities will have a population of 10 million or more (four in the more developed regions and twenty-two in the less developed regions).

In sum, the population of the world in the twenty-first century will in all likelihood be significantly larger, older, more urban, and more concentrated in less developed regions. Nevertheless, much of the world's demographic future remains uncertain. For instance, according to the medium variant of the United Nations projections, world population in the year 2050 is expected to be 8.91 billion. However, the high and low variants of these projections, which are also certainly possible, range from 10.67 billion to 7.34 billion for the year 2050. Thus decisions, policies, and actions taken today and tomorrow will greatly affect the well-being, living standards, and health conditions of men, women, and children in the coming decades and beyond.

Reference

United Nations Population Division. *World Population Prospects: The 1998 Revision.* New York: United Nations, 1999.

CHAPTER THIRTY

Interpersonal Violence

Lee Ann Hoff

Lee Ann Hoff, PhD, is a Professor in the College of Health Professions, University of Massachusetts Lowell, and Adjunct Professor in the Faculty of Health Sciences, University of Ottawa, Canada. Known for her work on international violence issues, she is the author of People in Crisis: Understanding and Helping *and coauthor (with Kazimiera Adamowski) of* Creating Excellence in Crisis Care: A Guide to Effective Training and Program Design.

Afrer centuries of being considered a private matter, interpersonal violence has taken center stage as a human rights violation and a public health problem. In virtually every country, women and children are the major victims of male aggression and homicide, both inside and outside the home (U.S. Department of State, 1998). Survivors of trauma from abuse, along with their advocates, have been the major players in bringing this issue to international attention. In dozens of speakouts and workshops at the 1995 UN Conference on Women, in Beijing, and the 1985 World Conference of th UN Decade for Women, in Nairobi, women outlined the

---

The author wishes to thank David Keepnews and Cynthia Medich for their suggestions on this chapter.

devastating effects of violence in their lives (United Nations, 1996a).[1] These declarations consistently acknowledge the importance of competent, compassionate health care in the arduous healing process, which for some people lasts a lifetime. Despite their pivotal role, health professionals have only recently acted on their enormous potential for alleviating pain and suffering from violence.

This chapter addresses (1) the unique position of health and social service professionals in preventing violence and providing comprehensive health care to survivors, (2) some commonalities and differences across cultures in addressing violence, and (3) progress, gaps, and international approaches to strengthening health professionals' knowledge and skills on behalf of individuals at risk or already traumatized by abuse.

POTENTIAL FOR PREVENTING AND ALLEVIATING EFFECTS OF VIOLENCE

Epidemiological, clinical, and social studies overwhelmingly document the negative sequelae of violence on the health status of individual survivors, their assailants, the entire family, and all of society (Stark and Flitcraft, 1996).[2] Although official data worldwide are limited, the United Nations (1996b) reports that up to 38 percent of the world's women have histories of assault by an intimate partner, with estimates as high as 60 percent in some countries. In the United States, women are more likely to be assaulted, raped, or killed by a current or former male partner than by all other assailants combined (American Medical Association, 1992). The human and economic toll exacted is incalculable. Recently, even the corporate sector has recognized the cost of this epidemic in lowered performance, spillover of violence from home to workplace, and absenteeism of victims and their assailants.

Although most violence among intimates and against family members occurs "behind closed doors," survivors of traumatic abuse— whether attacked in public or in private—almost invariably come in contact with a health or mental health professional. Clearly, all health care providers are strategically positioned to prevent violence, detect risk or victimization of vulnerable groups, and provide service to survivors and their families.

Health professionals' unique role derives from their numbers, their membership in one of the major domains of social life, the variety of their practice locations, and their contact with potential victims throughout the life cycle. Although every citizen can help eliminate the global plague of violence against women and children, the particular power of health professionals to make a difference on this issue cannot be overstated. Not only can health providers ease the profound suffering of victim-survivors, but their potential in violence prevention is enormous. For example, research documents that physical punishment of children not only is less effective than other forms of discipline but also lays the foundation for learning the acceptability of physical force as a conflict resolution tactic (Gil, 1970; Greven, 1990). Yet against all evidence, many adults believe in the necessity of such physical discipline; furthermore, nurses who conduct parenting classes rarely address nonphysical discipline, support for stressed parents as a primary prevention tactic, and laying foundations for preventing later violence by alienated youth.

Health professionals also have a powerful influence in the complex and controversial process of defining violence and abuse. The legacy of interpreting intimate partner violence as a private matter is compounded by the tradition in medical and psychiatric practice of imputing the "cause" of abuse to the purported psychopathology of the victim or her "provocative" behavior while excusing assailants on grounds of mental incapacity or as the inevitable outcome of aggressive instincts. These myths are still rampant despite research documenting violence and abuse as intentional social actions for which the perpetrator should be held accountable. Historically, violence has sometimes been excused as a "cultural norm." Today, however, violence is widely interpreted in psychosociocultural and feminist terms (International Council on Women's Health Issues, 1992): in other words, violence—in most instances—constitutes deviant behavior learned in a milieu accustomed to long-standing inequalities based on gender, age, ethnicity, and so forth and permeated with images of violence and physical force as the dominant modes of conflict resolution (see Dobash and Dobash, 1979; Hoff, 1990).

Violence consists of exerting physical force and power over another person with the intention of controlling or injuring the other. Though violent abuse has serious implications for physical and mental health, it is not in itself a medical phenomenon except in the few instances in which a person is found to be "insane"—a legal descriptor designating a person's mental incapacity (and therefore excusability) while behaving violently. Nor is violence merely a criminal justice phenomenon. Rather, it crosses the legal, ethical, and health care domains, as well as society's major institutions, thus rendering it a complex issue with moral, sociocultural, political, and personal ramifications. In all these areas, violence is universally condemned as wrong.

Physical violence is almost invariably accompanied by verbal abuse. For example, regular verbal threats of abuse or killing cause no immediate physical trauma but clearly strike terror in the heart of the intended victim. Today, most people recognize the damaging effects of verbal abuse, the particular traumas of racial or ethnic slurs, and the taunting of lesbians and gay men or individuals with disabilities, which is often followed by threats or acts of physical violence. Persistent psychological abuse, even without physical attack, can devastate a person emotionally and lead to serious health problems.

The terms *abuse* and *violence* are often used interchangeably, although abuse—especially sexual abuse—does not always entail physical injury. Thus, for example, an incest victim after several years of abuse may have no visible injuries but most assuredly has been "violated" and almost always suffers severe emotional trauma. As battered women often say, "It is easier to heal from the physical wounds than the emotional ones," though the two are linked. One way many cope is by excessive dependence on alcohol or psychotropic drugs, especially in the absence of access to comprehensive health care from trained professionals.

SOME CROSS-CULTURAL COMMONALITIES AND DIFFERENCES

Evidence from the 1985 and 1995 UN Conferences on Women, professional publications, and cross-cultural training outcomes reveals several common experiences with victimization among women worldwide. Survivors of abuse typically endure social isolation, lack of crisis services and safe refuges, the legacy of victim blaming that leads to self-blame, depression, suicidality, substance abuse, and various morbidities. Furthermore, educational and economic inequality leaves millions of women with few options but to remain with abusive partners. Another cross-cultural observation is the frequent attribution of a causal (versus contextual) relationship between substance abuse and violent behavior—this against evidence that alcohol and other drug use often serve as grounds for disavowing responsibility for violence. In societies where recognition of domestic violence as a public issue is more recent, patterns of addressing the problem are similar to those recorded, for example, in the United Kingdom, the United States, Canada, and Australia. Generally, child abuse is first in capturing national attention, followed by intimate partner abuse, sexual assault, and elder abuse. Currently, major attention includes the devastating effects on children who witness violence between their parents. Across cultures, however, victim-survivors themselves and their advocates have led the way in making public their plight and demanding better responses from criminal justice and health care sectors.

Globally, the world is getting smaller through technological developments that greatly enhance our opportunity to learn from one another cross-culturally. Given the urgency of the global epidemic of violence, societies that have only recently addressed it publicly and those advantaged with greater resources can benefit mutually from cross-cultural exchanges. Recognition of commonalities and commitment to collaborative rather than competitive approaches can be cost-effective in the time and money needed to enhance the effectiveness of health providers in addressing violence and its health sequelae.

While acknowledging common patterns in public and health providers' responses to violence, we must be sensitive to cultural differences in educational and practice settings. For example, shelters for battered wives are commonly accepted in Western societies but may be virtually meaningless and impossible to create in a rural African setting where extended family connections are primary sources of support. And indeed, even in Western societies, the very idea of establishing refuges for victims and their children, rather than holding centers for their assailants, symbolizes the reactive or quick-fix approach to a problem much broader in scope than the crisis needs of victims. Nevertheless, there is no question of the need for such life-saving shelters so long as assailants can slip through criminal justice loopholes, public tolerance of intrafamilial abuse prevails, and women and children are unsafe in their own homes.

The irony, albeit necessity, of shelters for abused women is this: after centuries of promulgating the message that a woman's "proper" place is in the home, when she is victimized and threatened with her life at home, the expectation has been that *she,* not her assailant, should leave. Usually this means living as a fugitive with her children in substandard housing on public support. Further, she has often been judged by friends, acquaintances, and professionals for *not* leaving the abusive relationship, without their giving any thought to the obstacles, including homelessness, she faces in attempting to do so. A more appropriate approach for professionals and whole societies would be to require assailants (rather than their victims) to leave the marital dwelling and learn how to live nonviolently with spouse and children. The cross-cultural lesson here is that societies without resources for sheltering battered women might focus more intensively on primary prevention rather than stopgap measures. However, it is safe to predict that refuges for abused women and their children will be necessary for perhaps another generation. That is the estimated time needed for a new generation of parents to learn nonviolent child rearing and a widespread public education campaign of zero tolerance of violence.

Another example illustrating cross-cultural differences concerns female genital mutilation (FGM), a procedure that the World Health Organization and other groups have declared a human rights violation. Physicians in the United States and Canada face professional discipline if, at the request of immigrant parents, they perform this procedure on daughters. Women from countries where the ritual is a cultural mainstay can claim political asylum in the United States or Canada on grounds of FGM as a human rights violation. Yet health professionals in Western countries caring for immigrants whose heritage includes this ritual must be sensitive to its cultural meaning, without "excusing" it as a cultural norm. Navigating such tumultuous terrain requires understanding of the wider context in which this procedure developed and still thrives—the social inequality of women, control of their sexuality in traditional roles, and the virtual loss of a respectable social role for a woman who has not undergone this "rite of passage" (Gullen, 1992).

Another instance of addressing violence in cultural context is its compounding by colonial policies calculated to oppress or eliminate entire cultures, as in the reservation system in the United States and Canada and apartheid in South Africa. The disproportionate rates of violence and self-destructive behaviors among First Nations and aboriginal inhabitants of North and South America, Australia, and New Zealand illustrate the toll taken on the human spirit and on the physical and mental health of generations of native peoples. The communal values characterizing traditional cultures are pivotal as the context for health services provided to members of these groups. While reempowerment is central to the healing of all who have been traumatized by violence, it is particularly important for mainstream health professionals to recognize that elders and spiritual healers are the key specialists for many members of native groups. Thus, for example, recent mandatory arrest laws in the U.S. are a new twist on the tradition among the Lakota Sioux in North America that if a man battered his wife, he had to leave, was forbidden to marry again, and couldn't lead or participate in a war party or a hunt, or own a pipe (Mousseau, 1989).

PROGRESS, GAPS, AND INTERNATIONAL EDUCATIONAL INITIATIVES

In 1985, U.S. Surgeon General C. Everett Koop convened a national interdisciplinary workshop on violence and public health. The 150 participants represented practitioners, activists, researchers, and educators concerned with violence against family members and acquaintances at all stages of life. Workshop topics included violence prevention and the evaluation and treatment of violence survivors. A major recommendation from this workshop was that all professionals should be trained and examined in the essentials regarding violence and health services for survivors as a condition of licensure (Health Resources and Services Administration, 1986).

In 1992, Health Canada convened nationwide interdisciplinary consultations to facilitate collaboration and team approaches to violence detection and the care of survivors. A major outcome of these sessions was the realization that formal preparation for interdisciplinary practice around violence was rare in health sciences curricula. The result was Health Canada's commissioning of an interdisciplinary curriculum guide for health professionals (Hoff, 1995).[3] In 1996, Health Canada supported a survey of five Canadian health sciences faculties and students to obtain baseline data about the knowledge, attitudes, and skills related to violence issues that are required by health professionals and to identify ways to develop discipline-specific and interdisciplinary curricula for the preparation of future health professionals. Results of this study ($N = 635$ students, 181 faculty) reveal considerable attention to the issue, especially child abuse and woman battering, with sexual assault, elder abuse, and interdisciplinary practice receiving less attention. Significantly, a very small percentage of students had planned clinical experience focusing on the detection, crisis response, and treatment of abuse survivors. Students who had had clinical practice opportunities with survivors said that the experience was coincidental rather than systematic or directed by faculty. One professor's comment illustrates a theme from this study: "Professors either are afraid of the subject or are undereducated about it."[4]

Results of this study coincide with surveys of all schools of nursing in the United States (Wootli and Breslin, 1996) and Canada (Ross, Hoff, and Coutu-Wakulcyzk, 1998) to ascertain the extent of classroom instruction and planned clinical experience on violence issues. Overwhelmingly, in both countries, though considerable curricular attention is directed to the issue, it is incidental rather than systematic.

Thus progress is evident in health professionals' awareness of violence as a major public health problem and the importance of including this content in formal curricula; however, much work remains across cultures in the challenging task of addressing it in health sciences curricula in a manner commensurate with its epidemiological significance. A marker of further progress will be, for example, medical and nursing curricula in which battering during pregnancy (with at least a 24 percent incidence rate) is considered as important a risk factor as gestational diabetes (with a 2 to 6 percent incidence rate).

A recent mark of progress in the United States is a 1999 position paper on violence content developed by the American Association of Colleges of Nursing (AACN, March 1999). This paper builds on the survey results noted here and other findings that underscore the urgency of systematic instruction of nurses in violence-related matters. Complementing this national effort by the AACN is a January 2000 commission to launch the Committee on the Training Needs of Health Professionals to Respond to Family Violence. This study is mandated by the U.S. Congress and funded by the Centers for Disease Control and Prevention of the U.S. Department of Health and Human Services.

Internationally, collaborators in the adaptation of Health Canada's interdisciplinary curriculum guide for health professionals on violence issues represent major regions of the world. A key element of this work includes illustrations of collaborative relationships between grassroots groups and health professionals. Besides technical knowledge and skills, health professionals need to present positive role models of collaborative (rather than conflictual) relationships in practice settings as one element of the healing process. The Power and Control Wheel—developed in Duluth, Minnesota, and widely used to illustrate the abuse of power in interpersonal relationships—is unfortunately sometimes mirrored in practice settings by the Medical Power and Control Wheel, which can compound a survivor's trauma.

Table 30.1 illustrates the essential interdisciplinarity of violence as a health and social issue. Unfortunately, there is more than enough work to go around. Today, millions of health providers recognize their enormous potential for making a positive difference to violence survivors. Yet their goodwill is often not matched with the formal preparation they need to respond adequately to survivors and their families. The table's illustration of complementary and discipline-specific func-

Discipline	Function
All Health Disciplines	▪ General understanding of and alertness to the issue in all facets of practice as background for detection, intervention, treatment, and/or referral for longer-term psychosocial counselling or treatment. ▪ Role modelling nonviolence in general behavior, and in clients/provider and interdisciplinary team relationships ▪ Advocacy for violence prevention and victim services in professional organization and community roles.
1. Medicine, Nursing (generalist roles)	Detection, assessment, diagnosis, crisis inervention, treatment, referral for follow-up counselling/treatment. Key roles at entry points in primary, secondary, and tertiary care settings. Nursing has key coordinating role in most settings.
2. Dental Hygiene, Pharmacy	Detection, immediate support and initial steps of crisis intervention, referral.
3. Dentistry, Physiotherapy	As in 2 above, plus treatment for maxillo-facial injuries (dentistry), and for chronic pain from injury (physiotherapy).
4. Occupational Therapy	As in 2 above, with more extensive role in community and mental health treatment settings.
5. Psychology, Social Work (clinical)	Frequently in liaison or consulting role to medicine and nursing; key role with families and follow-up counselling and/or psychotherapy across the spectrum of health and mental health services.
6. Graduate Specialists	Entry point and follow-up treatment or counselling. May include traditional mental health disciplines (clinical psychology, clinical specialist in psychosocial nursing, psychiatric social work, psychiatry); pastoral counsellors with clinical training; family medicine and women's health specialists; midwifery; nurse practitioners—various specialties.

Table 30.1. Categories and Functions of Particular Disciplines.

Source: From *Violence Issues: Curriculum Guide.* Health Canada. © Minister of Public Works and Government Services, Canada, 2000.

tions can address a common fear expressed by physicians and nurses when urged to inquire routinely about abuse during health assessments; that is, some fear that if they open the subject, they will be drawn into an extended counseling session that is untenable in terms of their time and skills. Training about boundaries and skills in linkage to follow-up sources are key to alleviating these fears.

A major goal for the international curriculum guide in process is its production in seven languages: Arabic, Chinese, English, French, Portuguese, Russian, and Spanish. Countries with few trained professionals to teach violence-related content currently depend heavily on consultants and trainers from the United States and Canada who do not speak their language and must rely on interpreters. Obviously, this is not ideal educational practice. Though necessary as an interim step, the goal is for health professions students to be taught in their own language.

These and related developments portend well for correcting the current situation of a temporary role reversal in the complementary but different missions of health *service* and *educational* institutions. Continuing education for practicing professionals on new health care issues is, of course, a requirement for relicensure. But because we have not yet met the goal of systematic (rather than incidental) preparation of health sciences students on violence issues *before* completion of their degrees, institutions whose primary mission is *service delivery,* not basic education of health providers, must currently divert a disproportionate amount of time and money to compensate for curricular deficits. This situation will continue for years to come, as only now is the systematic inclusion of violence content being addressed by health sciences faculties.

CONCLUSION

Now that national and international bodies have proclaimed violence as a grave public health issue and the health implications of violence are undisputed scientifically, a major question is this: How can future health professionals be prepared without a burdensome "add-on" approach to already crowded health sciences curricula? And what are the arenas for further collaboration between health professionals and their community-based counterparts? Violence prevention and the care of traumatized persons is everybody's business, while health professionals can be seen as "ritual experts" (complementing the wise elder or healer in traditional societies) whose task is to assist victim, assailant, and children in "contemporary rites of passage" to a violence-free life (Hoff, 1990). This implies solid grounding in the reality and complexity of the client's experience, that is, the "emic" approach—beginning with where the client is. Work toward delineating the individual and collaborative tasks to achieve this end is well under way through the efforts of educators, practitioners, researchers, and the governmental and other institutions that have diligently addressed this global epidemic.

Notes

1. See especially paragraphs 112–130 (United Nations, 1996a). Noteworthy at both UN conferences was the relative invisibility of health professionals and scant attention given to the direct linkages between women's health status and their victimization by violence in the context of family and war.
2. See also Rodgers (1994). This national survey is cited as one of the most comprehensive and scientifically sophisticated of its kind. Researchers at Statistics Canada can be contacted for replication or adaptation in countries wishing to establish an epidemiological database on violence. A special issue of *American Psychologist* (1999, vol. 54, no. 1), titled "International Perspectives on Domestic Violence," cites the need for such research as a base for improving advocacy and treatment programs for survivors.
3. This work is currently being adapted and expanded across cultures as an outcome of presentations and networking at the 1995 UN Conference on Women in Beijing.
4. Results of this study are being prepared for publication by principal investigator Margaret Ross and myself. The tool developed for this study has been used in the Philippines to survey schools of medicine and nursing.

References

American Association of Colleges of Nursing, 1999.

American Medical Association. "Violence Against Women: Relevance for Medical Practitioners." *Journal of the American Medical Association,* 1992, *267,* 3184–3189.

Dobash, R. P., and Dobash, R. E. *Violence Against Wives: A Case Against the Patriarchy.* New York: Free Press, 1979.

Gil, D. *Violence Against Children.* Cambridge, Mass.: Harvard University Press, 1970.

Greven, P. *Spare the Child: The Religious Roots of Punishment and the Psychological Impact of Physical Abuse.* New York: Knopf, 1990.

Gullen, J. *Report on the First International Study Conference on Genital Mutilation of Girls in Europe.* Ottawa, Canada: Family Service Centre, 1992.

Health Resources and Services Administration. *Report: Surgeon General's Workshop on Violence and Public Health.* Washington, D.C.: U.S. Public Health Service, U.S. Department of Health and Human Services, 1986.

Hoff, L. A. *Battered Women as Survivors.* London: Routledge, 1990.

Hoff, L. A. *Violence Issues: An Interdisciplinary Guide for Health Professionals.* Ottawa: Minister of Supply and Services Canada, 1995. (Available from National Clearinghouse on Family Violence, Family Violence Prevention Division, Health Programs and Services Branch, Health Canada, Ottawa ON K1A 1B5, Canada.)

International Council on Women's Health Issues. "Environment, Daily Life and Health: Women's Strategies for Our Common Future." In *Congress Statement.* Copenhagen: Danish Technical University, 1992.

Mousseau, M. *The Medicine Wheel Approach to Dealing with Family Violence.* Dauphin, Manitoba, Canada: West Region Child and Family Service, 1989.

Rodgers, K. "Wife Assault: The Findings of a National Survey." *Juristate Service Bulletin.* Ottawa: Canadian Centre for Justice Statistics, 1994.

Ross, M., Hoff, L. A., and Coutu-Wakulcyzk, G. "Nursing Curricula and Violence Issues." *Journal of Nursing Education,* 1998, *37,* 53–60.

Stark, E., and Flitcraft, A. *Women at Risk: Domestic Violence and Women's Health.* Thousand Oaks, Calif.: Sage, 1996.

United Nations. *The Beijing Declaration and the Platform for Action.* New York: United Nations, 1996a.

United Nations. *Report on the World's Women, 1995: Trends and Statistics.* New York: United Nations, 1996b.

U.S. Department of State. *Overview to Country Reports on Human Rights Practices for 1997.* Washington, D.C.: Bureau of Democracy, Human Rights, and Labor, 1998.

Wootli, A., and Breslin, E. "Violence-Related Content in the Nursing Curriculum." *Journal of Nursing Education,* 1996, *35,* 367–374.

CHAPTER THIRTY ONE

Terrorism

Jessica Eve Stern

Jessica Eve Stern, PhD, *is a Senior Fellow at the Belfer Center for Science and International Affairs and an Adjunct Fellow at the Council on Foreign Relations. She is the author of* The Ultimate Terrorists *(Harvard University Press, 1999).*

O ne of the challenges physicians worldwide can expect to face in the twenty-first century is an increase in the number of deaths and injuries caused by terrorists. Especially if terrorists or their sponsors escalate to nuclear, biological, chemical, or radiological (NBCR) weapons, physicians and other health professionals will play an important role in treating victims, preventing the spread of disease, and assuaging exaggerated fears.[1]

The number of deaths due to acts of terrorism varies from year to year, and different organizations report varying numbers of deaths and injuries (depending in part on whether domestic incidents are included). Nonetheless, we have seen a clearly increasing trend over the past quarter century. In 1998, international terrorists killed 741 people and injured 5,952 (U.S. Department of State, 1999). Although the number of international incidents is generally

---

The author would like to thank Darcy Bender for her valuable research assistance.

declining, terrorists are becoming more lethal: deaths and injuries continue to increase. Most assessments suggest that international terrorists target the United States more than any other country.

During the next century, terrorism is likely to become an increasingly popular mode of conflict or as a means to express religious or other grievances. Because of vast asymmetries in military might, the West invites covert retaliation whenever it involves itself in regional wars. In future wars between the West and minor powers, massive asymmetries in power and pain are bound to enrage the victims and may lead to covert attacks against Western targets. Some adversaries are likely to believe that covert attacks—including the use of NBCR weapons—are their only hope for taking on the West, given its staggering military superiority. "In today's world," Martin Van Crevald warns, "the main threat to many states, including specifically the U.S., no longer comes from other states. Instead, it comes from small groups and other organizations which are not states. Either we make the necessary changes and face them today, or what is commonly known as the modern world will lose all sense of security and will dwell in perpetual fear" (1996, p. 58).

Even actions taken directly against terrorists can have unforeseen and counterproductive consequences. The U.S. government accused Usama bin Laden of carrying out bombings at two American embassies in August 1998, which killed some three hundred people, many of whom were Muslim. When the United States retaliated by striking targets in Sudan, Afghanistan, and, accidentally, Pakistan, bin Laden's popularity rose among Sunni fundamentalists. In interviews, Pakistani mujahideen describe bin Laden as a "great hero" to the Muslim world. Also troubling was the U.S. decision to strike a pharmaceutical facility in Sudan, purportedly used by bin Laden to produce nerve agent. Secretary of Defense William Cohen's subsequent admission that he was unaware that the plant produced pharmaceuticals strongly suggested that the decision to strike was made in the absence of adequate intelligence. Those strikes, regarded by many observers as entirely unprovoked, only served to heighten bin Laden's stature among Sunni extremists throughout the region. U.S. and other Western officials claim that bin Laden is seeking to acquire nuclear, chemical, and biological weapons.

The U.S. policy of supplying arms to influence the outcome of regional wars has made Afghanistan, Angola, and parts of Central America a virtual arms bazaar, with destabilizing consequences not just for the affected regions but for the entire world. Perhaps even more disturbing, by financing and training the mujahideen in Afghanistan's war with the Soviet Union in the 1980s, the United States created what it now perceives as a significant threat to its own security: networks of violent extremist Islamist groups funded in part by Usama bin Laden. The "blowback" resulting from the decision to arm the mujahideen is affecting not just Afghanistan, as is widely known, but the stability of the surrounding region, especially Pakistan. It is also affecting Western interests worldwide.

Usama bin Laden, whom the CIA reportedly trained in Afghanistan (Venter, 1998), is calling for an international *jihad,* or holy war, against the United States. America's "crimes" against Saudi Arabia (by stationing troops near Islam's holiest sites), Iraq, and the other Islamic states of the region constitute "a clear declaration of war by the Americans against God, his Prophet and the Muslims. . . . By God's leave, we call on every Muslim who believes in God and hopes for reward to obey God's command to kill the Americans and plunder their possessions wherever he finds them and wherever he can," bin Laden wrote (Lewis, 1998, p. 15). To most Muslims, Islamic scholar Bernard Lewis explains, bin Laden's *fatwa,* or edict, is a "grotesque travesty of the nature of Islam and even of its doctrine of jihad" (p. 19). No basic Islamic texts support the murder of uninvolved bystanders, he explains. Another scholar, Edward Said, explains that "most Arab Muslims today are too discouraged and humiliated, and also too anesthetized by uncertainty and their incompetent and crude dictatorships, to support anything like a vast Islamic campaign against the West" (Said, 1996). Nonetheless, a small fraction of Muslims are ready to carry out bin Laden's distorted "religious" command.

Domestic terror groups inside America are also becoming increasingly violent. Anti-abortion activists have taken to terrorism. One activist, now on death row for killing an abortion doctor in 1993, said in an interview that he wouldn't rule out the use of chemical or biological terrorism against abortion clinics. Other activists predict an increase in anti-abortion violence of all kinds. A number of libertarian, militia, and neo-Nazi believers and groups have acquired chemical and biological agents or their precursors. Although these groups are unlikely to be capable of mounting catastrophic attacks employing these agents, even a small-scale attack could have profound psychological repercussions. Beginning in 1998, pranksters and terrorists have carried out hundreds of anthrax hoaxes. Even though hoaxes do not result in illness or injury, they can be costly to local communities because of the perceived need to respond overwhelmingly with emergency personnel.

THE SPECIAL CASE
OF NBCR WEAPONS

Government and academic analysts are increasingly concerned about the prospects that terrorists will escalate to NBCR weapons. A number of factors are increasing the risk. First, NBCR weapons are especially valuable to terrorists seeking to conjure a sense of divine retribution, to display scientific prowess, or to invoke horror. Terrorists motivated by goals like these rather than traditional political objectives are increasing in number.

Psychologists have found that fear is disproportionately evoked by certain characteristics of risks, for example, when exposure is involuntary and the effects are delayed or when long-term effects are difficult to predict or poorly understood. Risks that are invisible, unfamiliar, or mysterious or have the potential to lead to a spectacular catastrophe affecting many people invoke special fears. NBCR weapons are unusual in that they possess all of the characteristics that psychologists have shown to be conducive to disproportionate fear. And fear creates its own dangers: if victims panic and attempt to flee, they could spread contamination and disease still further. Moreover, disproportionate fear could influence public officials to overreact by revoking civil liberties, especially if they perceive themselves to have been caught unprepared. NBCR weapons could incite disproportionate fear even if a threat to carry out a major attack turned out to be a hoax or small numbers of people were affected. In summary, fear of NBCR weapons is important for two reasons: it increases the psychological impact of low-level NBCR attacks, and it makes counter-terrorists susceptible to implementing policies that adversely affect civil liberties.

Second, terrorists' motivations are changing. A new breed of terrorist—including ad hoc groups motivated by religious conviction or revenge, violent right-wing extremists, and apocalyptic cults—appears more likely than terrorists of the past to commit acts of extreme violence. Religious groups are becoming more common and are more violent than secular groups. Of eleven international terrorist groups identified by the Rand Corporation in 1968, none were classified as religiously motivated. By 1994, one-third of the forty-nine international groups recorded in the Rand–St. Andrews Chronology were classified as religious. In 1995, religious groups committed 25 percent of the international incidents but were responsible for 58 percent of the total number of fatalities (Hoffman, 1997).

Third, with the breakup of the Soviet Union, the black market now offers weapons, components, and know-how. Soviet nuclear security procedures were designed during the cold war to prevent Americans from stealing secrets, not to prevent theft by insiders. That inadequate system has largely broken down. Hundreds of tons of fissionable material (used for making nuclear weapons) are stored at vulnerable sites throughout the former Soviet Union, guarded only by underpaid, hungry, and disheartened people. A dozen or so cases of theft of nuclear-weapons-usable materials have been confirmed. Worse still is that the weapons themselves are vulnerable to theft or unauthorized launch. Since many of Russia's nuclear custodians and weapons scientists are now unpaid or entirely out of work, they may eventually give in to financial pressures by selling their expertise or their wares abroad. Russian biological weapons scientists acknowledged in interviews with two veteran reporters that at least five of their colleagues from the Soviet biological weapons program had left to work in Iran (Miller and Broad, 1998). Many scientists have reportedly disclosed Iran's recruitment efforts, specifically with regard to biological warfare.

Fourth, in a related development, chemical and biological weapons are proliferating. The U.S. State Department lists seven countries as sponsors of terrorism: Iran, Cuba, Iraq, Libya, North Korea, Sudan, and Syria. All are suspected of having acquired or attempted to acquire chemical or biological weapons. The situation in Iraq shows how difficult it is to prevent the proliferation of nuclear, biological, and chemical weapons. Preventive war did little to root out Iraq's illicit weapons, and the most intrusive inspection regime ever devised left inspectors guessing, especially about Iraq's biological weapons program. A prominent defector from the Soviet biological weapons program claims that the Soviets had put biological warheads on intercontinental ballistic missiles and that the program included work on genetic manipulation of smallpox to make it more virulent (Alibek, 1999).

Fifth, advances in technology have made terrorists with weapons of mass destruction easier to carry out. For example, the Internet allows terrorists to recruit from a larger pool of potential sympathizers and to communicate instantaneously. Advanced fermenting equipment makes it easier to optimize the growth of biological organisms, and new technologies for disseminating microorganisms make spreading biological agents less difficult.

Terrorism with NBCR weapons involves the most modern—and the most extreme—forms of random violence. These weapons are innately terrifying: in most scenarios; the radius of fear would dwarf that of injury and death. Their effects are also inherently random. It is impossible to aim at a particular target; only the most sophisticated militaries can use these weapons in open areas without putting noncombatants at risk. The radius of injury depends on conditions that are impossible to control or to predict with certainty. The movement of aerosols, the virulence of microorganisms, the susceptibility of victims, and the spread of fallout all depend on exogenous variables like meteorological conditions and terrain. Their fear-inspiring, all-encompassing, unpredictable nature is what makes these weapons consummate vehicles of terror. Despite these developments and the inherently terrifying nature of NBCR weapons, terrorism employing these weapons—especially to create mass casualties—is likely to remain rare. Few terrorists will be capable of using these weapons except in small-scale incidents, and fewer still would want to kill hundreds of thousands of people even if they could. Conventional terrorism is likely to remain far more common.

A danger that has been largely ignored is the prospect for terrorists to use commonly available industrial and agricultural chemicals, some of which are highly toxic. The leak of methyl isocyanate at Bhopal, India, in December 1984 and ensuing explosion illustrate their deadly potential. Union Carbide, the owner of the pesticide plant in Bhopal, concluded that a disgruntled employee caused the blast by deliberately adding water to a storage tank. The Indian government reports that nearly four thousand people died from exposure to the lethal gas, and approximately eleven thousand were disabled. Whether the leak was caused deliberately, as Union Carbide claims, or accidentally, this incident shows that industrial chemicals can be extremely dangerous; more people were killed in this chemical release than in any single terrorist attack to date. It would make sense for governments and private industry to think carefully about how to minimize such threats. Many plants are designed to withstand accident, but few are designed to withstand deliberate sabotage.

Public Health Aspects of the Threat

Though physicians and other public health professionals will be called on to respond to any major act of terrorism, their expertise will be needed most in the event that terrorists use biological weapons.

Attacks employing these weapons range from hoaxes and small-scale attacks of the kind that terrorists have perpetrated in the past to state-sponsored attacks involving aerosolized warfare agents. The latter—the least likely kind of biological attack—could result in hundreds of thousands or even millions of deaths. The Centers for Disease Control and Prevention estimates that the cost of responding to such an attack would be $26.2 billion per hundred thousand persons exposed (Kaufman, Meltzer, and Schmid, 1997).

Governments are adopting a number of policy remedies in response to their perception of a heightened threat of NBCR terrorism. Of particular importance is the need to upgrade the global system of monitoring of disease around the world, since biological attacks could be difficult to distinguish from natural outbreaks of disease. Such a policy has the virtue of being useful for improving public health in general, regardless of whether terrorists ever mount a biological attack. Detection technologies, medical countermeasures, therapeutic regimens, and knowledge of the relevant organisms all need to be improved. Governments need to ensure that dangerous pathogens are adequately secured and safely stored. This applies in particular to former Soviet states, whose biological weapons program was most advanced. Alternative employment must be found for scientists formerly engaged in weapons work, to minimize the risk of a continuing brain drain to Iran and other countries. And laws need to be updated to reflect new threats. In the United States, for example, although it is illegal to threaten to poison someone, stating in a letter that its recipient has already been poisoned is not explicitly forbidden, making it difficult to prosecute perpetrators of hoaxes. The challenge is to make sure that if NBCR terrorism occurs, governments are prepared to minimize loss of life, reduce public panic, and respond effectively, compassionately, and justly.

Note

1. Biological warfare agents are microorganisms that are intended to cause disease or death in humans, animals, and plants and depend for their effects on their ability to multiply in the victim. Toxins are poisonous substances usually produced by living organisms. Chemical warfare agents are chemical substances—gaseous, liquid, or solid—that are used for hostile purposes to cause disease or death in humans, animals, or plants and depend on their inherent toxicity for their primary effect. Radiological weapons are radioactive compounds deliberately disseminated to harm humans or animals.

References

Alibek, K. *Biohazard: The Chilling True Story of the Largest Covert Biological Weapons Program in the World.* New York: Random House, 1999.

Hoffman, B. "Viewpoint: Terrorism and WMD: Some Preliminary Hypotheses." *Nonproliferation Review,* 1997, *48,* 48.

Kaufman, A. F., Meltzer, M. I., and Schmid, G. P. "The Economic Impact of a Bioterrorist Attack." *Emerging Infectious Disease,* 1997, *3,* 83–94.

Lewis, B. "License to Kill: Usama bin Laden's Declaration of Jihad." *Foreign Affairs,* Nov.–Dec. 1998, 15.

Miller, J., and Broad, W., "The Germ Warriors." *New York Times,* Dec. 8, 1998, A1.

Said, E., "God has Ninety-Nine Names: Reporting from a Militant Middle East," (review). *The Nation,* 263, no. 5, 28.

U.S. Department of State. *Patterns of Global Terrorism, 1998,* Washington D.C.: U.S. Department of State, 1999.

Van Crevald, M. "In Wake of Terrorism, Modern Armies Prove to Be Dinosaurs of Defense." *New Perspectives Quarterly,* 1996, *13,* 57–58.

Venter, A. "America's Nemesis: Usama bin Laden." *Jane's Intelligence Review,* Oct. 1, 1998, 8.

CHAPTER THIRTY-TWO

Urban Health

Jeremiah A. Barondess

Jeremiah A. Barondess, MD, *is President of the New York Academy of Medicine and Professor Emeritus of Clinical Medicine at Cornell University Medical College, where he held the William T. Foley Distinguished Professorship in Clinical Medicine. Since Dr. Barondess's appointment to the presidency in July 1990, the New York Academy of Medicine has conducted its programmatic activities primarily in the areas of urban health, recruiting to the health professions, medical education, the medicine-science-society interface, and the health of the biomedical enterprise itself.*

Massive migration in recent decades has resulted in the progressive urbanization of humankind: at the turn of the twenty-first century, most of the world's population lives in urban areas, for the first time in history. The phenomenon of urbanization has been global, although irregularly distributed. The bulk of further urban expansion in coming decades will take place in developing countries—indeed, seventeen of the twenty-five largest cities in the world are already in developing countries, where urban populations, 25 percent of the total in 1970, reached 37 percent in 1995 and are projected to reach 49 percent in 2015. In the industrial countries, by contrast, 67 percent of the population was already urbanized in 1970, and the projected figure for 2015 is 79 percent. Urban growth rates, on the other hand, are expected to drop in upcoming decades (Harpham and Blue, 1997).

Urbanization carries with it not only concentration of populations but also social and infrastructure problems tightly bound to life expectancy, morbidity patterns, mortality rates, and health-related quality of life. Such linkages are largely mediated by poverty, which is increasingly concentrated in urban populations and has emerged as the most powerful predictor of health status among city dwellers, relating to health both in an immediate, direct sense and as an expression of chronic social and economic disparities. Poverty is linked not only to environmental contaminants, inadequate housing, polluted water, uncollected garbage, and in many cities exposure to raw sewage but also to inadequate education and illiteracy, factors of substantial importance in accessing health care and in personal behaviors that compromise health and related also to a number of crucial health outcomes, including, prominently, high infant mortality rates. Yet further, poverty is to an important degree self-perpetuating, related to unemployment not only as a cause but also as a result and associated also with great difficulties in maintenance of family units or indeed coherent social structures that extend beyond the family. Under these circumstances, social pathologies are superimposed on immediate disease risk: violence of a variety of sorts is epidemic, for example, and substance abuse is hyperendemic. Since poverty is the most powerful common denominator of the health problems of cities, policy responses to urban health issues must include efforts to deal not only with immediate medical problems, such as infantile diarrheas and respiratory infections, HIV infection and AIDS, childhood asthma, and malnutrition, but also with the determinants of diseases of high prevalence among the urban poor, such as substance abuse, alcoholism, cigarette smoking, unsafe sex, high-fat diets, sedentary lifestyles, and the like, and the determinants of such determinants, including crowding, deteriorating housing, poor air, water, and food quality, and, yet further, education, unemployment, isolation in deteriorating urban confines, and restricted opportunities for self-sustaining lives and engagement in the structure of the society. In other words, to be effective, urban health policy must take a very broad view of health and its complex relations to human life and social structures.

In the past fifteen years, the number of persons living in extreme poverty has increased, currently amounting to more than 20 percent of the global population, and the aggregate impacts on health are readily visible. In the developing world, for example, WHO studies indicate that up to 43 percent of children, some 230 million, are short for their age, and about 50 million children weigh too little for their height. An average individual in one of the least developed countries has a life expectancy at birth of forty-three years, but in one of the most developed countries life expectancy at birth is seventy-eight years. Strikingly, even within industrialized countries, similar disparities exist; a comparison in 1990 showed that survival rates for men in inner-city New York were lower than in Bangladesh, with approximately 40 percent alive at age sixty-five, at a time when the figure for white males nationally in the United States was about 75 percent. Other studies have demonstrated similar impacts in the developing world: children in the poorest areas of Accra, Ghana, have a threefold higher risk of dying from infectious diseases and a twofold higher mortality rate from respiratory conditions than their wealthier counterparts, while in São Paulo, Brazil, a far wealthier city than Accra, with the highest economic disparities in the developing world, both respiratory and infectious mortality rates for children under age five in the most deprived zone are four times greater than in the most privileged area (de la Barra, 1998).

The impact on health of social and economic status is thus powerful and pervasive, and these effects are glaringly expressed in cities: death rates for most major causes have been shown to be higher in the United States for persons in the lower social classes, and in Great Britain, a clear hierarchy of mortality ratios has been demonstrated for men, with the highest ratios among the unskilled and the lowest among professional workers (Fein, 1995). Such differences, as demonstrated in the Multiple Risk Factor Intervention Trial (MRFIT) in the United States, are explained to the extent of only about 25 percent to 35 percent by differences in smoking, obesity, sedentary lifestyle, high blood pressure, and high plasma cholesterol levels (Smith and others, 1996). Evidence from these and other studies suggests that chronic social disenfranchisement and wide discrepancies in income are both associated with a shortening of life expectancy. Although differences in health measures in comparisons of countries at similar levels of development are not related to per capita gross domestic product—for example, with regard to life expectancy at birth—there is a strong relationship between income inequality and mortality *within* countries. Life expectancy tends to be longest in nations with the smallest spread of incomes across the population and the smallest proportion of the population living in relative poverty. Thus countries such as Sweden, with relatively narrower disparities in wealth, have longer life expectancies than less equitable nations, such as the United States. Such data suggest not only that the relative socioeconomic position of the person is associated with health but also that chronic social and psychological stress are health-adverse factors of considerable power (Wilkinson, 1992).

At the national level, clear correlations exist between gross domestic product and health investment on the one hand, and a number of measures of health status on the other. Although disparities between urban and rural populations with relation to many morbidities are obscured by national-level data, such information highlights the health-related derivatives of national economic development, which tend to be concentrated in cities. Thus in the least developed countries, infant mortality rates averaged 109 per 1,000 live births in 1996, while in industrialized countries the corresponding rate was 13 per 1,000. Twenty-two percent of infants in least developed countries had low birthweights, while the corresponding figure in industrialized countries was 7 percent; and maternal mortality rates in the least developed countries averaged 1,100 per 100,000 live births, compared with 30 per 100,000 in the industrialized world. Further, malaria and tuberculosis rates are higher and immunization rates lower in less developed than in industrialized countries, and the availability of doctors and nurses is likewise strikingly asymmetrical, with the least developed countries averaging 14 physicians and 26 nurses per 100,000 population, compared with 287 physicians and 780 nurses per 100,000 in the industrialized world. Public expenditure on health varies to an extraordinary degree: in 1990, among all developing countries, 2 percent of GDP was spent on health; in the industrialized world 6 to 8 percent of expenditure on health was common, with the United States at the highest level, currently some 14 percent. Even the figures cited require refinement. Thus gross comparisons of urban and rural measures of health status, such as infant mortality rate, require separation of overall urban rates into rates for urban slums as opposed to the rest of city populations. In American cities, rates vary widely by census tract, with the highest morbidity and mortality rates and the lowest life expectancies concentrated in areas characterized by urban poverty, crowding, high unemployment, and attendant social deterioration. The same is true for malnutrition, infant mortality, and the frequency of low-birthweight infants (Human Development Report, 1998).

All these factors demonstrate that a rational approach to urban health can be mounted only if efforts are tightly tied to social and economic development, national health investment, and the socioeconomic infrastructure of cities. It is clear that the health of urban dwellers represents a final common pathway, a convergence of powerful social and contextual forces.

For the future, a comprehensive approach to urban health problems must be broad enough to involve agencies concerned not only with clinical care and standard public health practices but also with the condition of the environment, social services, housing, education, communication, and social support programs. Prevention of disease must be a high priority, since in terms both of human welfare and economic development, preventing disease is infinitely to be preferred. Disease prevention must be understood in terms that include not only appropriate childhood and adult immunization programs but also attention to personal behaviors corrosive of health, such as smoking, substance abuse, unsafe sex practices, and violence, as well as broad efforts oriented around prenatal care, sanitation, and personal hygiene. Broader efforts at prevention, such as reduction of exposure to environmental lead, control of air quality, and the purity of the food and water supply fall largely to departments of urban government, dependent for their budgets on federal and regional sources. In this sense, the health of each urban inhabitant is a reflection of national policy and health investment.

Going forward, effective systems for tracking the health status of urban inhabitants will be vital, since interventions must be not only evaluated but also targeted so that they will have the greatest possible impact. Conventional indicators, such as life expectancy, mortality, and morbidity are available at national levels, and gross targets have been established by the Global Strategy for Health for All by the Year 2000 (WHO, 1981), including, at the global level, life expectancy at birth greater than sixty years, infant mortality rate below 50 per 1,000 live births, and under-five mortality rate below 70 per 1,000 live births. While there has been progress along these vectors, they are not sufficiently refined to allow for the development of effective urban programs. City-level data and comparisons of important health measures are needed to place urban health data in perspective and to facilitate analysis of underlying morbidity and mortality trends in the social context of cities. Even in the United States, there is no national system in place for compiling city-level data, and the few measures for which such data are available are not commonly presented according to relevant demographic categories such as gender and race or ethnicity. Refinement of such measures to the urban level will be a necessity.

The health prospects of urban populations in the new century will continue to be determined largely by social and economic inequalities and the consequences of poverty; in terms of dominating disease patterns, cardiovascular and malignant diseases are likely to lead in the developed world and infectious and parasitic diseases will remain primary in the least developed countries, with some tendency toward erosion of their primacy as control mechanisms become more effective. As is pointed out in Harpham and Tanner (1995), planning and implementation of programs addressing urban health issues will of necessity involve further devolution of significant degrees of responsibility to the urban level. At the same time, as noted earlier, governmental health establishments by themselves cannot effectively address the multifaceted issues underlying the health of urban populations: agencies concerned with food and water safety, housing, sanitation, education, communication, pollution control in the energy and industrial sectors, and control of occupational hazards, as well as community development for health promotion and increasing community involvement, will all have to be further engaged, and their activities will have to be coordinated. In addition, connections between these population-oriented programs and the clinical enterprise will need to be developed to a far greater degree than obtains at present. There are already effective collaborations between the clinical and public health sectors, as has been extensively documented for the United States by Lasker (1997); these collaborative efforts connect clinical services oriented around individuals with population health planning and programs. An important element of public health research for the decades immediately ahead, perhaps particularly with regard to urban populations, lies in exploring and developing further such collaborative strategies.

Educational programs are likely to offer particularly rich opportunities for enhancing the health of urban populations. School-based health education programs can provide broad, graduated curricula beginning in the earliest grades and provide entree as well to the families of pupils and through them to community organizations and the wider community. In this sense, schools are a particularly useful potential vehicle for the promulgation of community-based health programs and allow for the construction of effective interactions between municipal governments and urban populations. Beyond educational programs specifically targeted at health issues, literacy itself, as noted earlier, is a key component of personal and family health.

The intimate relationships between the health of urban populations, especially disadvantaged, inner-city populations, and the social and economic environment in which they live must be framed by government at every level as a set of challenges to be addressed more effectively if progress is to be made. Urban ecology, broadly construed, is a frame of reference that should lead to coordinated programs that recognize the stresses that underlie the vulnerability of individuals to health threats of a variety of kinds, some extrinsic to the individual and some arising in biological and psychological processes, many as yet poorly understood. In this construct, the margins between health investment and investment in social support systems and the urban infrastructure are highly ambiguous, and programmatic boundaries are likely to be counterproductive.

References

de la Barra, X. "Poverty: The Main Cause of Ill Health in Urban Children." *Health Education and Behavior*, 1998, *25*, 46–59.

Fein, O. "The Influence of Social Class on Health Status: American and British Research on Health Inequalities." *Journal of General Internal Medicine*, 1995, *10*, 577–586.

Global Strategy for Health for All by the Year 2000. Geneva: World Health Organization, 1981.

Harpham, T., and Blue, I. "Linking Health Policy and Social Policy in Urban Settings: The New Development Agenda." *Transactions of the Royal Society of Tropical Medicine and Hygiene*, 1997, *91*, 497–498.

Harpham, T., and Tanner, M. (eds.). *Urban Health in Developing Countries: Progress and Prospects.* London: Earth Scan 1995.

Harpham, T., and Tanner, M. "Urbanization and Health in Developing Countries—A Review of Source Trends." In Harpham, T. and Tanner, M. *Urban Health in Developing Countries: Progress and Prospects.* London: Earthscan Publications, Ltd., 1995, 1–8.

Human Development Report, 1998. United Nations Development Programme. New York and Oxford: Oxford University Press, 1998, 156–159.

Lasker, R. D. *Medicine and Public Health: The Power of Collaboration.* New York: New York Academy of Medicine, 1997.

Smith, G. D. and others. "Socioeconomic Differentials in Mortality Risk Among Men Screened for the Multiple Risk Factor Intervention Trial: I. White Men." *American Journal of Public Health*, 1996, *86*, 486–496.

Smith, G. D., and others. "Socioeconomic Differentials in Mortality Risk Among Men Screened for the Multiple Risk Factor Intervention Trial: II. Black Men." *American Journal of Public Health*, 1996, *86*, 497–504.

Wilkinson, R. G. "National Mortality Rates: The Impact of Inequality?" *American Journal of Public Health*, 1992, *82*, 1082–1088.

CHAPTER THIRTY-THREE

Biomedical Research in the Next Century

Bruce Alberts

Bruce Alberts, PhD, *President of the National Academy of Sciences in Washington, D.C., is known for his work in both biochemistry and molecular biology. He chaired the Department of Biochemistry and Biophysics at the University of California, San Francisco, before moving to Washington in 1993 to head the National Academy and its operating arm, the National Research Council.*

One needs to be very bold to try to predict the future of science and technology in the twenty-first century, considering our striking inability to predict the major advances of the past hundred years. Even after a revolutionary new technology emerges, the experts often fail to appreciate its impact. Witness the often quoted 1978 statement by the CEO of Digital Equipment Corporation that he could not imagine why anyone would want a computer in his home or the claim by one of the early critics of the Human Genome Project in 1987 that it is "a ploy to raise money . . . justified for its public relations value, not its scientific value" (Burris, Cook-Deegan, and Alberts, 1998). Both of these remarks were made by unusually wise and accomplished people, pioneers in the relevant technologies. Our past difficulty in predicting the future should give us pause.

Nevertheless, because new knowledge in science is built through combinations of old knowledge, it does seem safe to anticipate that the pace of scientific discovery will continue to accelerate throughout the twenty-first century, with unpredictable new technologies arising periodically to greatly facilitate the research process. I also believe that we will see a dramatic acceleration in the speed of translating progress at the laboratory bench into progress at the bedside, due to an enormously increased number of transient, rapidly established collaborations between small groups of researchers and clinicians who have complementary expertise.

In this chapter, I begin by expanding on the two predictions I just made, using some examples from my own experience. In the process, I suggest a few changes in our traditional mode of operation that would seem to be warranted if we are to exploit to the fullest the vast opportunities before us in biomedical research. Last but not least, I shall try in a small way to fulfill what I suspect was meant to be my main task: to forecast one promising new area of biomedical research with profound implications for human health.

AN ACCELERATING PACE OF DISCOVERY

I began my career as a research scientist in the summer of 1959, just before my senior year at Harvard College. This was only six years after the discovery by James Watson and Frances Crick of the DNA double helix and six years after the demonstration by Fred Sanger that a protein is formed from a unique sequence of amino acids. I have therefore been active as a researcher throughout a period when incredible advances have been made in our understanding of how cells and organisms work at the molecular level. In 1983, when the first edition of *The Molecular Biology of the Cell* was published, my coauthors and I felt that we could include nearly all of the critical information then known about cells in the twelve hundred pages of this advanced undergraduate textbook. In fact, so little was known then about how things actually worked that we often felt forced to guess at possible mechanisms. As I write this article, we are in the midst of preparing the fourth edition of the same textbook. So much is now known that the most difficult decisions concern which large sets of well-studied mechanisms are to be left out so as to avoid producing an encyclopedic volume that is undigestible for most students.

My own research focused on the molecular mechanisms that cells use to replicate their chromosomes. In 1961, when the critical point of action was discovered to be a DNA replication fork, this Y-shaped structure was drawn with a fig leaf over the Y, in recognition of our ignorance of what was going on beneath it. Today, we know that an incredibly efficient, tiny protein machine makes the DNA at a replication fork, and scientists have even worked out where the atoms are in the three-dimensional structures of nearly all of its many protein parts. This striking progress is the result of studies carried out by thousands of scientists, each building on the knowledge accumulated by their predecessors and published in scientific journals. The knowledge needed came from many different fields of investigation, and it was often combined in unexpected ways to produce a significant advance. Some of this progress involved the development of new methods, which in turn greatly increased the speed and power of the science that followed.

Figure 33.1 presents a highly schematic comparison of the early progress of my field (left side) with the much more rapid progress that is being made today (right side). The pace is accelerating primarily because of a large increase in the total pool of relevant scientific knowledge that can be combined in new ways to create new knowledge. Mathematically, there is an explosive increase in the possibilities: for example, 100 units of knowledge can be combined in 1,000 times more ways than 10 units of knowledge can. Even scientists seem surprised by the modern explosion of scientific progress. Could the root of this surprise be our failure to appreciate fully the counterintuitive power of combinatorics?

THE COMBINATORIAL PRINCIPLE
APPLIED TO RESEARCH LABORATORIES

So far I have expanded on the first of my two general predictions about the future of biomedical research. My second main point is a corollary of the first: our biomedical knowledge is now so extensive, with so many specialized new methods and scientific approaches, that no single laboratory can hope to master all of the techniques that can usefully be brought into play in a particular scientific investigation. Nor can laboratories with a specific expertise or technology hope to be able to apply that expertise to the most important biomedical problems without outside collaborations.

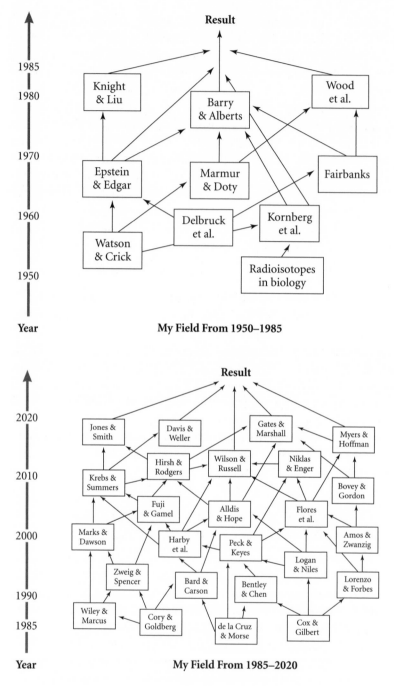

Figure 33.1.   The Accelerating Pace of Biomedical Research.

In 1985, I pointed out the benefits of a laboratory group in biology that is limited to ten or so researchers, led by a scientist who is fully involved in the research process (Alberts, 1985). That article was based both on my personal experience in trying to run a larger laboratory and on a sense that there had been a decrease in the innovation and creativity of most of my colleagues once the laboratories they led became too large. As an extension of the arguments made there, I emphasize the great advantage to be gained from a research tradition in which two such laboratory groups form transient, opportunistic collaborations that exploit the unique skills of each—if you wish, the power of the combinatorial principle when applied to biomedical research laboratories.

Today, such collaborations are perhaps most common when one laboratory is expert in a highly specialized technique, such as X-ray crystallography, and the other laboratory provides the biological material to be analyzed by that methodology. But in the future, some type of interlaboratory collaboration is likely to become the standard practice for nearly all biomedical investigations. As an especially important example, if we are to bring modern biomedical science to bear much more effectively at the bedside, we will need to find better ways of promoting highly productive collaborations between MDs carrying out clinical studies and laboratories headed by PhDs skilled in fundamental biomedical research. Today, this must be viewed as an "unnatural act," but one that has tremendous future potential. The reason for the potential is clear: we have finally reached a stage in our understanding of cell biology and immunology (and in the development of powerful, highly sensitive analytical technologies) where an effective, intelligent attack can be made in understanding, and then ameliorating, almost any human disease. But this will happen only if the special expertise of clinicians and basic scientists can be brought together in much more vigorous ways than are generally feasible today.

NEW EXPERIMENTS IN SCIENCE POLICY

My former colleagues in the basic science departments of research universities seem to be busier than ever; they work nights and weekends and still seem to be always behind. How can they hope to keep up with the exploding amount of biomedical knowledge, much less to explore new collaborations with clinical scientists in those areas of human biology where their expertise could be especially valuable? The natural path for an individual scientist to take as the amount of knowledge explodes is to drill deeper in one ever-narrowing area of biomedicine. Will we eventually be giving PhD degrees in departments of ribosome function or departments of membrane transport, rather than in departments of cell and molecular biology? I certainly hope not; but it will take a concerted effort from our scientific leadership to counteract the strong tendency to overspecialize.

What kind of leadership makes sense? We are fortunate that the explosion of scientific knowledge has been accompanied by a computer and telecommunications revolution. This revolution now provides biomedical scientists with powerful, no-cost ways of finding relevant knowledge through electronic searches (for example, see PubMed at http://www.ncbi.nlm.nih.gov). It also enables free access to valuable databases of genes, gene sequences, chromosome maps, protein structures, mutations, and many other research resources on the World Wide Web, along with relevant computing tools. The next step in this revolution would be to make the full electronic text of all biomedical publications freely available to researchers around the world at their desktop, as recently proposed by Harold Varmus, the director of the National Institutes of Health (Marshall, 1999).

An ability to immediately access all of the relevant literature in this way—going instantaneously from one journal abstract in PubMed to a list of related articles (available today) or from a journal article to the full text of any of its citations (available tomorrow)—should greatly facilitate the broadest possible cross-fertilization of ideas between biomedical scientists, as needed to optimize scientific progress. It should also speed progress at the bedside by improving the connections between clinical and basic researchers.

What can we do to make this valuable knowledge resource fully effective? Experience shows that researchers in different fields are unlikely to start a collaboration, unless they have first met each other face to face. I propose that this be done in special workshops, organized as a series of "mixers," each carefully designed to bring together scientists whose differing expertise might be profitably combined at some future time.

Some of us first became aware of the power of such settings when we were brought together in a 1994 workshop in Seattle focused on the brain tumor known as glioma. We were there because of a common friend, the scientist Harold Weintraub, who was dying of this disease. We spanned the gamut from molecular biologists working on gene regulation in bacteria to cell biologists to clinicians treating the disease. During two days of intensive discussions, it became clear to all of us that this important subfield of cancer research would benefit from a much more intensive, ongoing interaction between clinical and basic researchers.

The same could be said for many other areas of biomedical research. Scientists often attend seminars and scientific meetings, but these are generally so specialized that we often fail to benefit from the broader types of cross-fertilization that can produce real innovation. As an experiment, small meetings focused on catalyzing specific types of collaborations in areas with important medical implications could be regularly sponsored by the National Institutes of Health, each cochaired by a distinguished clinician and a distinguished basic scientist. The attendees at the meeting might be invited to compete in pairs for a modest catalytic research grant that would give equal status to a clinician and a basic scientist, both of whom serve as principal investigators (PIs). (Currently, there can only be a single PI on a grant, with a collaborator serving as a co-PI.) If skillfully arranged, I am convinced that some powerful new types of biomedical research would emerge.

When promoting these new connections between scientists, we must admit to a cultural problem. Medical schools are organized into departments of two different kinds: the so-called basic science departments like physiology, microbiology, and biochemistry and the clinical departments like medicine, pediatrics, and surgery. The two types of departments have very different traditions, the basic science departments containing mostly PhDs and the clinical departments almost all MDs. The faculty and students in each type of department naturally seek to emulate the most prestigious individuals in their professions, who are PhDs or MDs, respectively. Young scientists are constantly being evaluated as individuals so that the best can be selected for leadership positions, and for this reason cooperative work is discouraged. And yet it is precisely these scientists—the postdoctoral fellows and assistant professors—who one hopes would start new research laboratories at the interface between clinical and basic research in biomedicine.

In my opinion, our present system strongly discourages innovation and risk taking among young scientists. Far too many of the most successful young scientists go on to establish a research program that simply extends the work that they did in their mentor's laboratory. As a result, large numbers of scientists are competing with each other by working on an unnecessarily narrow range of research problems, while many important, newly accessible opportunities at the interface between conventional disciplines remain largely unexplored and unexploited. Finding a solution is a critical task for the twenty-first century—and a challenge to our universities, our charitable foundations, and our government funding agencies.

A MAJOR ROLE FOR GROWTH FACTORS IN THE TREATMENT OF DISEASE

I now come to part of the chapter where I stick my neck out and risk future embarrassment. Here I shall extrapolate from my eight years of experience as a volunteer scientific adviser to the Scleroderma Research Foundation, run and inspired by a woman with the disease, Sharon Monsky. I have learned that there are many debilitating human diseases, of mysterious origin, that lead to the degeneration of a specific tissue, or set of tissues, and often result in death. These diseases eventually cause an abnormal immune response, and for this reason they are often classified as "autoimmune diseases."

However, treatments that suppress the immune response have no effect on the fundamental course of many of these diseases, suggesting that a production of specific self-antibodies is an effect, rather than a cause, of a disease like scleroderma. What, then, is the cause of the progressive tissue degeneration?

At this point, I enter the realm of speculation, based on what we know about the mechanisms that individual cells use to decide how to behave in the functional cell cooperative that we call a tissue (muscle, bone, or skin, for example). The cells in tissues are constantly sending sets of signals to each other by producing special proteins that are loosely called "growth factors." These are either displayed on the cell surface of the sending cell or secreted into its surroundings. When they contact a receiving cell, the growth factors bind to specific receptors embedded in the cell's plasma membrane that transmit a message to the cell interior, generally by regulating enzymes called protein kinases that change the state of phosphorylation of selected proteins in the receiving cell. The cells in a tissue are both senders and receivers of multiple signals, and each cell has been programmed during its development in the embryo to interpret each of the many combinations of signals it will receive so as to either remain quiescent, multiply, differentiate further, or commit suicide (the last cell function is called apoptosis, and its importance in tissue maintenance has only recently been recognized).

It is this complex signaling system that makes multicellular life possible by ensuring that the cells in our body cooperate rather than compete, and there is much that remains to be learned about it. The first complete genome sequence obtained for any multicellular organism is that of the tiny nematode (worm), *Caenorhabditis elegans* (*C. elegans* Sequencing Consortium, 1998). Among the nineteen thousand proteins encoded in this worm's genome are a large number specific to cell signaling, including more than four hundred protein kinases and many growth factors, as I have broadly defined them. And for humans, DNA sequencing studies have already revealed many hundreds of growth factors, a number that is certain to rise considerably when most of the human genome sequence is completed in the next few years.

We already know that these signaling pathways contain many feedback loops, and in such a complex system, pathologies can develop in which the network becomes altered in a way that causes abnormal amounts of signaling molecules to be produced. This could in turn profoundly perturb the structure of a tissue. One such pathology is well known—cancer, in which inappropriate signals cause a clone of cells to multiply without the usual restraints and produce tumors. But many other types of pathologies are to be expected, in which signals go awry so as to cause inappropriate cell differentiation, a deficit of cell proliferation, or excess cell death. This type of problem, one suspects, is the underlying cause of scleroderma and numerous other degenerative diseases whose cause is presently mysterious (see, for example, Liu and Connolly, 1998).

Because each growth factor has an effect on cells that depends both on the cell type and on the other growth factors present, the combinatorial use of these powerful reagents and their agonists and antagonists should provide medicine in the new century with a precise and powerful new tool for controlling cell behaviors in a wide variety of different human diseases. The analyses of a particular pathological tissue for growth factor anomalies may eventually require that the levels of perhaps a thousand different proteins be measured routinely and cheaply—including all of the growth factors, their receptors, and perhaps selected other signaling molecules. Thus the mass production of the appropriate low-cost probe arrays, containing a thousand nucleic acid probes to test for levels of gene expression or a thousand antibodies to test for protein levels, for example, would seem to be warranted (Brown and Botstein, 1999). And I predict that the pharmaceutical industry will be investing heavily in the production of growth factors and their antagonists in the years ahead as a major market develops for them in the treatment of human disease.

References

Alberts, B. "Limits to Growth: In Biology, Small Science Is Good Science." *Cell*, 1985, *41*, 337–338.

Alberts, B., and others. *The Molecular Biology of the Cell*. New York: Garland, 1983.

Brown, P. O., and Botstein, D. "Exploring the New World of the Genome with DNA Microarrays." *Nature Genetics*, 1999, *21*, 33–37.

Burris, J., Cook-Deegan, R., and Alberts, B. "The Human Genome Project After a Decade: Policy Issues." *Nature Genetics*, 1998, *20*, 333–335.

C. elegans Sequencing Consortium. "Genome Sequence of the Nematode *C. elegans*: A Platform for Investigating Biology." *Science*, 1998, *282*, 2012–2018.

Liu, B., and Connolly, M. K. "The Pathogenesis of Cutaneous Fibrosis." *Seminars in Cutaneous Medicine and Surgery*, 1998, *17*, 3–11.

Marshall, E. "Scientific Publishing: NIH's Online Publishing Venture Ready for Launch." *Science*, 1999, *285*, 1466a.

CHAPTER THIRTY-FOUR

The Role and Potential of Health Services Research

Gordon H. DeFriese

Gordon H. DeFriese, PhD, *is Professor of Social Medicine, Epidemiology, and Health Policy and Administration and Director of the Cecil G. Sheps Center for Health Services Research at the University of North Carolina at Chapel Hill. He is a former president of the Association for Health Services Research and was the editor of the association's official journal,* Health Services Research, *from 1983 to 1996.*

There is no question that the global and political context within which health services research takes place has dramatically changed, in both developed and developing countries, since the early 1980s. In most countries of the world, the formal systems for the delivery of health services have encountered substantial difficulties regarding the financing and organization of basic health care at every level of service, and many new diseases and health conditions associated with changes in the sociodemographic profiles of these countries have brought forth enormous pressures for system change and adaptation.

Health services research has been conceptualized and developed very differently in developed and developing countries, but in most there has been an increasing emphasis on the measurement of outcomes, the effectiveness of program interventions, and the assurance of value for money invested in health care services. One of the most important areas of health services research from which important contributions to global health have emerged has to do with efforts to measure inequities in the distribution and accessibility of personal health services.

THE CENTRAL QUESTIONS FOR HEALTH SERVICES RESEARCH

Over the course of the coming decade, the field of health services research will have to confront at least five principal sets of questions or issues in nearly every country. In large part, these relate to the measurement of the structural properties and the performance of health care delivery systems, but they also include important issues pertinent to the epidemiology of health needs and the social and behavioral epidemiology of factors known to influence important health outcomes. The five sets of issues are as follows:

1. Measurement of objective and subjective health care needs

2. Description and evaluation of the impact of various approaches to the organization and financing of personal health care services

3. Geographical and socioeconomic variations in health care resource allocations and levels of service use, including issues of equity in access to care

4. Measurement of health care system performance (or effectiveness)

5. Definition and measurement of health care outcomes

Together, these five sets of issues represent an enormous challenge and an indication of what this field may contribute to the effort toward the realization of health care goals for all nations in the new century.

MEASUREMENT OF HEALTH CARE NEEDS

The planning of effective and appropriate health care services cannot take place without a foundation of reliable and valid information on the health status and health care needs of the population to be served. This should include comprehensive statistical reporting systems for disease incidence and prevalence, as well as population-based statistics on the use of specific types of health services. The importance of measuring patterns of consumer use of health care services, as well as the psychosocial predictors of use, has been well recognized for most of the past century. What is problematic in these studies is the difficulty of distinguishing between levels of *need* for such services and their effective *demand*. In estimates of the requirement for health care resources (such as health care personnel), demand-based approaches are like self-fulfilling prophecies: they will always define services that are *used* as services that are *needed*. They measure only the current performance of a delivery system, taking into account numerous barriers to the receipt of care. Yet if estimates of staffing requirements are based on the judgment of health professionals as to what level and volume of health services *should be* consumed, these estimates will generally overshoot actual health services consumption patterns.

Among the most important aspects of the literature of health services research are those dealing with the determinants of personal perceptions of health need and the patterns of individual reaction to symptoms of ill health, which may lead to episodes of health care use. Interest in this area of research has increased since the mid-1970s in the developed countries of North America, western Europe, the United Kingdom, and Scandinavia as more attention has been focused on the prevention of disease and the promotion of positive, health-enhancing lifestyles.

In many countries of the world, especially the developing countries, important transitions are occurring in the social role of women that have important implications for the future need and demand for health care services. The realization is growing that women constitute an important, if not the most important, influence on the health and life prospects of children and families. Yet interventions that target adult women miss a critical set of opportunities for influencing the future health status of women. The reproductive health of women is influenced by such factors as nutrition, education, and understanding of sex roles and practices, which are acquired as part of socialization in childhood and adolescence.

Moreover, it is now recognized that women determine (or mediate) the potential impact of health care interventions and technologies in many developing countries. In many areas of the world, women are victimized by the proletarianization of the agricultural labor force and through the sociological phenomenon of divorce, separation, or desertion, which leaves them the sole providers for their households.

These socioeconomic changes in the life situation of women in many areas of the world make clear the need for health services research to determine what those forces have meant for the health status, and therefore the health care needs, of women.

ORGANIZATION AND FINANCING OF HEALTH CARE SERVICES

Just as issues related to the organization of health care delivery systems have given the field its distinctive niche among other aspects of health-related research, so these issues are expected to continue as the mainstay of the field. Without an understanding of the way health care systems are structured, the way they bring resources together into organizational arrangements to deliver needed services and access to technology, and the way in which the funds to support health care flow into and through those systems, one cannot begin to formulate a sound approach to health policy appropriate for the future. Among the issues of concern to the organization and financing of health care are the facilities within which these services are provided, the personnel who perform the essential clinical and administrative maneuvers of which these services consist, the arrangements through which differing levels of service are classified and through which persons seeking these services are triaged or processed, the interorganizational relationships among units or structures offering these services, and alternative approaches to payment for care within particular service delivery systems.

Efforts to describe and measure the structural and processual aspects of health care organization will be of considerable interest over the coming decade in both the developed and developing nations. Only a few of the developed nations have yet to establish universal systems of health care financing guaranteeing all citizens access to essential health care. There remain significant questions in each of the developed nations with regard to such issues as how to control the expansion of the supply of health care facilities and personnel, how to monitor and effectively plan for the acquisition and use of health care technology, how to ensure the availability of basic primary health care in rural areas, and how to assure the most effective linkages among differing levels of health care services, facilities, and providers. Just as the concern over the shortage of needed health care personnel and other resources is a major issue wherever such shortages exist, there are also problems with a sudden and unexpected growth in the supply of health care personnel. Oversupplies in the developing world can lead to increased pressure for emigration of health personnel brought to bear on the developed nations.

Another issue of considerable importance in many of the developing nations of Africa, Asia, and the formerly socialist countries of central and eastern Europe is the transformation of national health care systems coupled with the privatization of health services. These trends have brought about tremendous change in the structure of health care systems and altered the basic relationship between client-patient and health care professionals.

RESOURCE ALLOCATION AND USE OF SERVICES

Separate from the questions pertaining to the organization and financing of health care are those related to national priorities for the distribution of health care resources and controls on the level of health services use. Every health care system must confront issues related to the acquisition, diffusion, use, and control of access to health care technology. Moreover, fundamental issues are related to the reasons for variations in health services and technology use among populations within the same general systems of care that cannot be explained by a differential burden of illness. The underlying analytical challenge in these studies is to determine the factors responsible for variations in the use of specific diagnostic tests or therapeutic procedures within small geographical areas of a state or country. For example, when the rate of "major surgical procedures" varies among hospitals in a given region or country from seventy to five hundred per hundred thousand population, it is important to examine the reasons for these procedures being performed in each hospital and to determine whether scarce health care resources are being used ineffectively or inappropriately and whether they might be better directed toward accomplishing national health care goals, such as the provision of basic primary health care.

MEASUREMENT OF HEALTH SYSTEM PERFORMANCE

The measurement of critical indicators of health system performance or effectiveness has taken on a higher level of importance in recent years as the financial demands of health care have put increasing pressure on national economies. Now more than ever, there are expectations that any health care service, whether a surgical or diagnostic procedure or a routine immunization program, will demonstrate a favorable ratio of benefits to cost and that the expenditure of resources will address specific target conditions effectively and efficiently. For this reason, the techniques of cost effectiveness analysis and cost-benefit analysis have been widely advocated as analytical strategies for the assessment of health care technologies and clinical and public health strategies for addressing the health care problems and needs of defined populations.

The critical and evaluative perspective once directed toward expensive diagnostic and therapeutic procedures is now increasingly used to assess the potential impact of public health interventions such as immunization programs, risk factor counseling, and primary care clinical screening maneuvers for extant disease. Basic questions are being asked about the advisability and cost effectiveness of screening for such diseases as hypertension, diabetes, anemia, cervical cancer, colorectal cancer, glaucoma, and phenylketonuria.

DEFINITION AND MEASUREMENT OF HEALTH CARE OUTCOMES

As emphasis has begun to shift from inputs to outputs in health systems research, there has been a corollary interest in the development of better measures of health care outcomes. These measures have proved essential to the evaluation of alternative approaches to the organization and financing of personal health services. Criteria for the evaluation of health care quality now include not only measures of the structural and processual aspects of care but also measures of the end results of care. These measures give emphasis to two critical outcomes of medical care: functional status and well-being (or quality of life).

Among the most important areas of research over the coming decade will be the continuation of research on the measurement of health status, involving both subjective and objective assessments. Two major problems we face in the measurement of health status are defining the concept of "health" in a way that facilitates its operational measurement and distinguishing health care *use* from health status *assessment*.

In the coming decade, we may expect that health services research will give even greater attention to the measurement of personal valuations of clinical services and procedures in terms of their impact on self-esteem and self-concept, a general sense of well-being, the convenience of the services used, functional status, pain, and discomfort. In other words, an increasing degree of attention will be given to the measurement of individuals' satisfaction with care.

Measures of satisfaction with health care and with providers are intentionally subjective indicators designed to measure a different aspect of care than other measures of health care quality. They give an indication of the way in which patients respond to care, a dimension of care that cannot be directly observed.

Underlying the increasing concern for the measurement of outcomes such as quality of life is the view that health care should improve (or contribute to) both the *quantity* and the *quality* of life. Work in this vein has produced a series of measures, both generic and disease-specific, by which the individual's current heath and well-being are measured with respect to a number of dimensions of fundamental importance to the everyday experience of living. In measuring quality of life as part of the assessment of health care outcomes, it is important that the dimensions being measured are indeed ones that may logically be expected to be affected by medical care. The economic evaluation of medical care in recent years has facilitated the development of quantitative estimates of the value of one year of life free of disease or disability or pain. The so-called quality-adjusted life year (QALY) is now a common measure; its value is determined through a series of questions designed to ascertain the relative utilities of different health states in relation to others. From these studies, it has been possible to determine that a year of life with a handicapping condition is often valued as less desirable than the risk of undergoing a surgical procedure with some limited probability of eliminating the handicap or the pain, discomfort, or inconvenience associated with a present level of disability.

CONCLUSION

In summary, the future of health services research, in both the developed and the developing world, will see far more emphasis given to such questions as "Do available treatments really work?" and "Do the people who experience these treatments associate different values with specific outcomes?" The scarcity of resources available for application in the provision of health care services and the increasing empowerment of consumers of these services—which has led to heightened expectations and demands for quality, accessibility, and reasonable cost of these services—has created an environment (more evident in some countries than in others) that places a greater burden on health systems research to assist in achieving a measure of accountability to both the people who receive health care services and the people who pay for them. Our measurement tools are still in a stage of infancy with respect to some of the questions now being raised.

In the future, better means of communication among health services researchers worldwide should lessen the informational and methodological gap between developed and developing countries. And through this process, we will, ideally, come to visualize the generic concerns of our field as those associated with the assurance of minimum basic health care for all.

CHAPTER THIRTY-FIVE

Reinventing Medicine and Public Health

Kenneth I. Shine

Kenneth I. Shine, MD, *is President of the Institute of Medicine, National Academy of Sciences, and Clinical Professor of Medicine at the Georgetown University School of Medicine. Dr. Shine's research interests include metabolic events in the heart muscle, the relation of behavior to heart disease, and quality of health and health care. Dr. Shine is the author of numerous articles and scientific papers in the area of heart physiology and clinical research.*

I t has been estimated that human life expectancy during the time of the Roman Empire was approximately twenty-eight years. In 1900, this life expectancy had been extended only nine years, to an average of thirty-seven years throughout the globe. In 1990, global life expectancy had increased to sixty-five years (Preston, 1977, 1995, 2000). Significant variations still exist among countries or even within countries, depending on the particular group being studied. However, the advances in life expectancy in the twentieth century were remarkable by any standard. Although many factors contributed to this enhanced life expectancy, by far the largest proportion of the increase occurred as a consequence of decreased maternal and infant mortality. (Only in the last part of the century did *adult* life expectancy begin to increase significantly.) Improvements in housing, sanitation, and water supplies contributed to these improvements, particularly during the early part of the century. Probably the greatest contributing factor was the control of infectious diseases. Advances in public health made much of these advances possible.

THE ROLE OF PUBLIC HEALTH

The first explicit definition of public health's mission arose from the Shattuck report of 1859, issued by the Massachusetts Sanitary Commission, which declared "the conditions of perfect health, either public or personal," to be the goal of public health. Emphasis was placed particularly on response to epidemic crises, with prevention, prolongation of life, and organized community activities regarded as central to the role of public health (Preston, 1995). Sanitation and the control of communicable diseases were an important part of this effort, but the organization of medical and nursing services for early diagnosis and effective treatments of diseases were also part of the charge. To the extent that public health focused on environmental, social, economic, and occupational determinants of health and disease, it became increasingly involved in social activism. The Institute of Medicine defined the mission of public health as "the fulfillment of society's interests in assuring the conditions in which people can be healthy." (Waterfall [ed.], 1988)

Physicians and surgeons played key roles in solving many of these public health problems. John Snow, who applied epidemiology to the London cholera epidemic in 1854, was a surgeon and anesthetist who administered chloroform to Queen Victoria at the birth of Prince Leopold. Edward Jenner, who introduced the use of cowpox to infect humans in order to protect them from smallpox, was an English surgeon. D. A. Henderson and William A. Foege, both of whom contributed extraordinary leadership to the elimination of smallpox, are physicians. Semelweiss and Lister were physicians who recognized that the transmission of infectious disease in pregnancy and in other clinical conditions could be dramatically reduced with hand washing and other preventative measures.

Many nonphysicians contributed to these advances as well. Edward Chadwick, who led the sanitary reform movement, was a lawyer. Lemuel Shattuck, John Griscom, Dorothea Dix, W. T. Sedgwick, Theobald Smith, and Charles Chapin were among the great leaders of the public health movement. Into the first part of the twentieth century, medicine and public health were largely inseparable. Physicians were intimately involved in their community, and although they focused primarily on individual patients, they often made observations that related to public health. Public health maintained epidemiology, population medicine, and prevention as a central part of the medical agenda.

THE GROWING DICHOTOMY

As the twentieth century proceeded, a growing dichotomy between public health and medicine occurred. In the United States, the division had its origins particularly in economics and control. The development of insurance systems in the 1930s focused on payment for the treatment of disease. Public health practitioners became increasingly concerned about the care of the poor and individuals with special illnesses and so set up public health clinics, which many physicians regarded as direct competition. The increasing focus on the individual, rather than the population, and the emphasis on disease cure versus prevention became fundamental differences between the orientation of medical professionals and public health professionals. The 1930s introduced the first truly effective nonsurgical therapies, followed by an explosion of new technologies during and after the Second World War. Payments for care became increasingly focused on technology and specialization.

REALIGNING MEDICINE AND PUBLIC HEALTH

Why is it critical to examine the interface between medicine and public health as we enter a new century? There are at least three major reasons:

1. The increasing importance of population medicine to health care systems
2. The increasing importance of biology to public health
3. The necessity to find the most cost-effective interventions to maintain health in the face of rising health care costs

These developments are important not only in developed countries such as the United States but in the developing world as well. The tendency for health professionals in developing countries to be trained in the developed world has often resulted in the transportation of the medicine–public health dichotomy to developing countries. It is critical to wealthy nations, struggling with cost containment, to balance public health approaches more effectively with medical ones. It is at least equally important to developing countries to find a proper balance for their societies.

EVOLVING HEALTH CARE SYSTEMS

Many countries around the world are experimenting with a variety of health care delivery systems. Few, if any, countries provide a single form of health care. Despite the existence of a national health service, as much as 10 to 15 percent of health care in Great Britain is provided on a fee-for-service basis outside of the national health care system. In Russia, patients must pay for timely services in the health care system, even though such payments are often illegal. As state ownership of enterprises has diminished, the Chinese have become even more dependent on fee-for-service medical and hospital care. Fifty percent or more of health care expenditures in China are for medications, which are purchased from physicians who use the income for their own support. In attempts to control costs, many countries are experimenting with market strategies. In some developing countries, this is accompanied by a systematic decrease in the amount of direct public expenditures for health. The United States has experienced a dramatic shift from fee for service to forms of managed care.

Regardless of the setting, fee for service favors the wealthy and the well-off, thereby perpetuating a multiple-class system of health care. When a third party pays the fees, as has been the case in the United States for the past fifty years, fee for service leads to overuse of services, which rewards the providers with more fees. Managed care experiments, which have attempted to encourage competition, are characterized by underuse of services, as providers attempt to operate within limited budgets and generate net income. In the for-profit sector, this means profits to shareholders, and in the not-for-profit sector, it means net income for further capital investment and expansion.

EVIDENCE-BASED MEDICINE
AND INFORMATION SYSTEMS

Until very recently, health care was provided by professionals who used science extensively in practice but did not apply science to medical practice itself. In addition to the intrinsic resistance to being measured, health care providers have been notoriously slow in developing and applying information systems, including computerization, to care. However, this technology is now developing rapidly, from computerization of patient records to systems for measuring risk-adjusted mortality and morbidity for particular services. The result has been an increasingly corporate form of medical care in which individual providers practice as part of a body of providers. Although doctors and patients used to the autonomy of individual practice may resent this change, the development of the corporate practice of medicine for the first time offers real opportunities for investments in information systems and the collection of data, allowing us to assemble evidence as to what works and what does not work in health care. This is evidence-based medicine. In the United States, the response to these kinds of data in some areas has been remarkable. Immunization rates in managed care organizations have risen sharply in comparison to previous levels and to those achieved in the fee-for-service arena. Regular publication of the results for coronary artery "bypass" surgery in the state of New York has led to the lowest surgical mortalities among the fifty states in a process of continuous quality improvement in surgical care.

POPULATION-BASED HEALTH CARE

These developments arise out of the introduction of the concepts of public health to health care. For the first time, in the corporate practice of medicine, there is concern about defined populations. The health of those populations becomes important to the health care provider. Although capitated care (annual payment of a fee per person for the provision of health services) has not grown as rapidly as expected in the United States, it does offer significant incentives to promote health as opposed to treat disease. If one can diminish the burden of illness in a population, for which capitated fees are provided, the organization can develop net income to extend and elaborate its services. Clinical epidemiology can now be applied to these populations of patients. This extends not only to rates of preventative services but also to such questions as the level of hypertension control in the population or the frequency with which cost-effective agents such as beta blockers or aspirin are used in the treatment of myocardial infarction.

In a population-based system designed to maximize the health of a group, issues of health care effectiveness become increasingly salient and recognizable. Epidemiology, biostatistics, cohort studies, cost effectiveness analysis, evidence-based practice, and preventive services are all intrinsic features of public health now brought to the practice of medicine. The extent to which this is recognized among countries around the world varies substantially. In North America, for example, the American Medical Association has active programs to engage health professionals in smoking cessation and substance abuse programs. In some other countries, health professionals still do not accept that smoking cessation or other similar preventive programs are in the province of medicine but instead rely on the public health community for this purpose. As recently as the mid-1980s, the British Heart Fund saw prevention and public education of heart disease as a function of the press and not of the Heart Fund or health professionals.

BIOLOGY AND PUBLIC HEALTH

Molecular biology and genetics have revolutionized thinking in medicine, but these advances, as well as other developments in biomedical science, stand to revolutionize public health. It is now possible to predict the likelihood of a drug's toxicity by knowing the genetic phenotype of the recipient in terms of the pathways available for drug metabolism. Similar phenomena can occur with industrial exposures to chemicals and drugs. Hepatitis C is a public health problem in many countries of the world. The etiological agent was identified by a remarkable process of genetic subtraction of the genetic makeup of normal liver cells from those of liver cells infected with the hepatitis C virus. Biology and fundamental science will have much to contribute in the next century to environmental and occupational health, infectious diseases, and the study of chronic illnesses in populations. Information systems that are important to health care are equally important to the public health system. Communication between information systems developed in the public health community and the health care community will be crucially important in identifying new illnesses. It will also be critical in identifying antibiotic-resistant organisms, drug-resistant malignancies, and a host of other phenomena, which are susceptible to medical and public health monitoring.

OPPORTUNITIES FOR SYNERGISM

These developments do not argue that the intellectual bases of medicine and public health ought not continue to develop in schools of medicine and schools of public health. However, they do argue that research, education, and care must increasingly include elements of both medicine and public health in every country of the world. Whether a developed or developing country, each nation seeks to control its costs and understand the nature of the burden of illness among its citizens and to strive toward preserving and maintaining health.

Research in health care can benefit significantly from collaborative efforts between experts in epidemiology, biostatistics, environmental and occupational health, prevention, and related fields. In this context, public health researchers have strategies and methodologies that are valuable in assessing the health care system. At the same time, medicine can further introduce into public health consideration of the individual within the community. The role of genetic and other biological variations within population studies and the impact on developments on bioscience are relevant to the public health agenda. Education of medical and public health professionals will also benefit from joint experiences, including the opportunity to examine real-world cases jointly but from the perspective of the various disciplines. Opportunities for alliances between public health, medicine, preventive services, health promotion and disease prevention, and disease therapy can be substantially expanded. The public health community is concerned about tobacco use, family violence, and environmental injury. The formation of alliances with health care providers offers opportunities for individual counseling about tobacco use, which reinforces public education activities. Tax policy, advertising policies, and so on, offer a level of reinforcement to individual smokers.

REINVENTING RELATIONSHIPS

The opportunities to reinvent the relationships between medicine and public health can be seized on in important aspects of health professional education, health sciences research, and the care of populations and individuals.

Increasingly, health professionals should be exposed to teachers who can provide both public health and medical approaches. Medical students, interns, and residents can benefit from expanded instruction in clinical epidemiology, evidence-based practice, continuous quality improvement, cost-effective risk analysis, cohort and population studies, and strategies for health promotion and disease prevention. Students in public health will require expanded understanding of developments in biology, including genomics, genetics, toxicology, and the organization and development of health care. Opportunities for students in public health and medicine to study together will facilitate the use of these various disciplines to solve problems of mutual interest. Environmental and occupational health and systems for health care delivery are good examples of areas in which a joint learning activity will enhance the experience of all the students.

Research programs will similarly benefit from the expertise of medicine and public health collaborating, analyzing, and interpreting events together. With the growth of evidence-based medicine, quality improvement, and ethics, medicine is developing substantial expertise in medical economics, population analysis, statistics, and legal and ethical issues associated with health care delivery. For these research capabilities to develop entirely independent of public health when many of these research skills are well developed in schools of public health would be to miss significant opportunities for synergism in an enhanced research outcome.

The creation of health care delivery systems that focus on populations provide real opportunities for expertise from public health to join with that of medicine to examine the nature of databases, data collection, information systems, and analysis. The opportunities to develop cost-effective strategies for prevention as part of the health care delivery system are substantial and will grow as penetration of managed care and information systems expand. Purchasers, public or private, will increasingly wish to understand the value of the services they are purchasing. Value will be defined by the relationship between financial expenditures and quality of services. Combined efforts of public health and medicine to enhance this analysis of value will have increasing importance in the medical marketplace, public or private.

RELEVANCE TO DEVELOPING COUNTRIES

Of particular importance for developing countries will be the challenge to seize on the best that is available from the developed world, rather than repeating many of its costly mistakes. Individuals from developing countries who are educated in the developed world often attempt to reproduce in their own country the systems in which they were trained. For this reason, some developing countries expend substantial resources in tertiary and quaternary health care activities for the wealthiest part of their population while losing the opportunity for introducing maximally cost-effective treatments or preventive measures. As this synergism between medicine and public health evolves, it will be increasingly important for the leadership of public health and medicine in developing countries to work together for precisely the same reasons that are relevant in the developed world. The role of aspirin and beta blockers for secondary prevention of myocardial infarction or the rational development of diets that minimize cardiovascular disease and cancer are both examples of areas in which health professionals and public health professionals in the developing world must be encouraged to work closely together. Dealing with the expanding scourge of tobacco in the developing world is another area that too often health professionals perceive not as central to their activities but rather as a problem for public health when in fact both must work closely together to resolve the issues for their societies. AIDS presents a similar challenge.

Both medicine and public health have long traditions of great accomplishment of which both can be very proud. Neither will lose its identity by virtue of collaboration, cooperation, and synergy. The benefits to society from these interactions can and will be substantial. Reinventing the relationships will be a critical part of global health for the next century.

References

Preston, S. H. "Mortality Trends." *Annual Review of Sociology*, 1977, *3*, 163–178.

Preston, S. H. "Human Mortality Through History and Prehistory." In Simon, J. (ed.), *The State of Humanity*, London: Blackwell, 1995.

Preston, S. H., personal communication, 2000.

Additional Reading

The Future of Public Health. Washington, D.C.: National Academy Press, 1988.

Carl Haub, Population Reference Bureau, communication.

Rosenkrantz, B. G. *Public Health and the State*. Cambridge, Mass.: Harvard University Press, 1972.

CHAPTER THIRTY-SIX

Integrative Medicine

Andrew T. Weil

Andrew T. Weil, MD, *is Director of the Program in Integrative Medicine at the University of Arizona College of Medicine. He is the author of seven books, including the best sellers* Spontaneous Healing *and* Eight Weeks to Optimum Health.

These are extraordinary times for medicine. Throughout the world, medical costs have risen to the point where health care systems are strained and the latest therapeutic advances cannot be delivered to the many people who need them because the treatments are too costly. In the United States, hospitals are going bankrupt, even large, established, academic teaching hospitals. The out-of-control spiral of medical costs in America has produced a logical reaction: managed care, which represents the corporate takeover of medicine by managers whose only interest is profit. Managed care has made the lives of both doctors and patients miserable. It has taken away the autonomy of physicians so that many now find they can spend only minimum amounts of time with patients and can only recommend certain approved protocols of treatment. It has angered patients by greatly intensifying the impersonality of contemporary medicine and making them feeling shortchanged.

Why has modern medicine become so expensive? The answer is not simple. In industrialized nations, victories over infectious disease in the early twentieth century left doctors treating much more chronic, degenerative illness, by nature more stubborn and more costly to manage. Improved public health, better nutrition, and better treatments for common diseases have also resulted in greater life expectancy in developed countries. In the West, the baby boomers are now in middle age and soon will create an unprecedented "demographic bulge" of old people. As populations age, their use of medical services increases, and the diseases they develop become more difficult and more expensive to treat. In addition, the treatments favored by modern doctors depend heavily on technology, which is inherently costly.

This last contribution to cost deserves more comment. At the end of the nineteenth century, Western medicine made a conscious decision to become scientific, to employ scientific methods to determine causes of disease, and to discriminate between useful and useless treatments. Along with Western culture as a whole, it became enamored of technology, turning its back on most of the simple, natural, inexpensive methods of maintaining health and treating disease used by previous generations and by indigenous cultures. Throughout the first half of the twentieth century, this course of development produced great advances in our understanding of diseases and our ability to treat them, the isolation of antibiotics in midcentury being one of the most significant and most popular. During this period, most people viewed technology as an unmixed blessing with the potential to end all varieties of human suffering.

Around 1960, this fantasy began to fade as people came to see that technology creates as many problems as it solves. In medicine, the problem created was expense. The economic disaster that has engulfed modern medicine in America and will engulf it in other countries has not come out of the blue. Its roots go back to the philosophical turn that medicine took a hundred years ago.

As the twentieth century came to a close, another economic force was taking its toll on medicine, one completely unforeseen and also long in developing. That was the rise of a worldwide consumer movement toward so-called alternative medicine. First dismissed as a fad, this movement has by now clearly shown itself to be a sociocultural trend of vast proportions. In the United States, surveys show consistently that between 30 and 40 percent of people are now going to alternative providers. These visits outnumber visits to primary care physicians, and the money spent on them exceeds the money spent on primary care. And the numbers are growing. Clearly, this is a market force to be reckoned with, especially at a time when conventional medical institutions are facing economic collapse.

The usual definition of alternative medicine is all modalities of treatment not currently taught in schools of conventional (allopathic) medicine. These include formal systems like homeopathy, traditional Chinese medicine, and Ayurvedic medicine, along with specific interventions like hypnotherapy and other mind-body techniques, botanical medicine, nutritional medicine (encompassing the use of dietary supplements), various forms of ethnomedicine, systems of body work and manipulation, and forms of energy medicine. This is obviously a very mixed bag, containing theories and practices that make sense and are useful, others that are silly and useless, and some that are dangerous.

Conventional medicine has usually distanced itself from all of this, lumping it all together as unscientific and antirational. Spokespersons for the medical establishment argue that there is no such thing as alternative medicine, only medicine that has been proven and medicine that hasn't. Proven, in their view, means confirmed by randomized, double-blind, placebo-controlled trials; other sorts of evidence for safety and efficacy are inadmissible.

This narrow-minded view relegates all of Chinese medicine and its myriad herbal remedies, some of which are highly bioactive, to the wastebasket of superstitious nonsense, ignoring the fact that it has served a very large population very well for a very long time. Doctors with this attitude refuse to look at the vast amount of uncontrolled clinical data suggesting therapeutic efficacy of many alternative interventions, and they insult the intelligence of all those consumers who find, from their experience, that alternative medicines work.

I believe the challenge we face is to sort through that mass of theories and practices to determine which are useful and which are not, using scientific methods and good sense, prioritizing those therapies that should be subjected to randomized, controlled trials (RCTs), while being open to other kinds of evidence than that produced by RCTs. We can immediately begin integrating those therapies that appear safe and useful into conventional practice. This is one of the aims of the new system of integrative medicine that I am helping to bring into existence at the University of Arizona Health Sciences Center.

Integrative medicine is not synonymous with alternative or complementary medicine; its goals go beyond simply adding new tools to the physician's black bag. Above all, integrative medicine seeks to reestablish a healing orientation in medical education, practice, and research. It teaches that the body has intrinsic mechanisms of self-regulation, repair, and regeneration and that when treatments produce successful outcomes, they do so by activating or unblocking the organism's natural healing potential. The best treatment, therefore, is the least—the least invasive, the least expensive—that produces a maximum healing response. (From this viewpoint, placebo responses are not curiosities or nuisances to be ruled out but healing responses from within, elicited by the power of belief and in many ways central to good medical practice.)

Both doctors and patients need to know when and when not to use the drastic and expensive methods of conventional medicine. In general, those methods are good for managing crises and emergencies, disease involving vital organs, fast-moving disease, and very serious disease. If doctors would save them for those cases when they were really indicated, we would not now have the economic crisis in health care that we do. The problem is that since doctors are not taught alternatives, they know only to use the drastic methods, and they use them as the first line of intervention for everything. If there is not an emergent or very serious threat to health, it is often possible to use gentler, less expensive treatments first. If they fail to work, one can then go to stronger measures.

Integrative medicine also regards human beings as more than physical bodies, taking account of their mind and emotions, their spirit, and the communities in which they live. It empowers patients by charging them with responsibility for the maintenance of health through wise choices of lifestyle and encourages them to enter into partnerships with physicians rather than into dependent roles. The primary role of physicians should be to teach people how not to get sick in the first place, and a main method of teaching should be by example. In other words, doctors should model health for patients and thus inspire them to make better choices about how to eat, how to exercise, how to deal with stress, and how to protect and enhance the human body's capacity for self-healing.

The consumer tide flowing toward alternative medicine indicates great dissatisfaction with standard medicine. It is clear that a gulf exists between what patients want and expect from doctors and what they get. Patients want doctors who can take the time to explain to them the nature of their problems, who will not just push drugs and surgery as the only solutions, who are conversant with nutritional influences on health, who can answer questions about dietary supplements, who are familiar with the most important botanical remedies, who are sensitive to mind-body interactions, who understand that people are more than physical bodies, and who will not laugh at them for inquiring about Chinese medicine or chiropractic. Those strike me as eminently reasonable expectations, but it is also clear that this is not the kind of physician our medical schools are producing.

Therefore, a fundamental goal of integrative medicine is reform of medical education. It is in no way sufficient to offer medical students elective courses that survey various alternative therapies. Basic information about healing, nutrition, lifestyle medicine, mind-body medicine, botanical medicine, and the strengths and weaknesses of major alternative therapies must be required subjects. Furthermore, medical training must not actively thwart the development of a future physician's own healthy lifestyle. At the moment, it is an unusual man or woman who can come through the process of medical education with habits that can inspire patients to improve their lifestyles.

The movement toward this change is gathering momentum, propelled now by the powerful economic forces mentioned earlier. Hospitals facing bankruptcy and health maintenance organizations operating in highly competitive markets cannot afford to ignore the market trend. The limiting factor in offering integrative care is the dearth of physicians trained to provide it. As this becomes clear, medical schools are beginning to explore ways of changing curricula to integrate the missing material. On their own, many physicians in practice are seeking opportunities to educate themselves in areas their schooling did not cover, including the nature of the therapies so many of their patients are using.

The benefits of these changes can be far-reaching. An immediate result will be restoration of public confidence in the medical profession and a reversal of the exodus from conventional medical offices and institutions. Another will be a widening of medical horizons to include ideas and interventions now excluded from consideration, thus increasing effectiveness. For example, increasing numbers of patients present with poorly understood, often debilitating conditions for which standard medicine has no effective treatments, such as chronic fatigue syndrome, fibromyalgia, and environmental sensitivity. An integrative approach has much to offer here.

Despite decades of research on the interaction of mind and body and the ability of interventions like hypnosis, biofeedback, and progressive relaxation to influence physiological processes, use of these therapies remains low. Yet for many ailments, including common dermatological and gastrointestinal disorders, these interventions are safer, cheaper, and more effective than commonly prescribed pharmaceutical drugs. In other conditions like cancer, where allopathic interventions may be required, an integrative approach may permit lower doses of drugs to be used, may mitigate the toxicity of drugs and other treatments, and may improve general health and quality of life.

By emphasizing prevention and lifestyle and attending to all the factors that influence health, integrative medicine can help patients reduce risks of diseases, especially of the preventable diseases that now cause so much premature death and disability and account for such a high percentage of health care costs. Thus in various ways, integrative medicine should halt the escalation of medical expenses.

It can also help validate traditional healing methods of other cultures, which have often been held in contempt by Western scientists. Clearly, allopathic medicine is too expensive to be delivered to large populations of the Third World. If research can establish the safety and efficacy of particular herbal remedies and other indigenous treatments, that will be a very practical accomplishment that might help build bridges between medical doctors and traditional healers. Given the shortage of doctors worldwide, it would be useful to augment their services with those of other practitioners respected by local people. One model for this kind of cooperation or integration exists on the Navajo Reservation in the American Southwest, where the government-run Indian Health Service and traditional medicine men work together on many cases.

In summary, integrative medicine is one line of development for health care in the twenty-first century. People want it, and medical institutions have no choice than to offer it. Integrative medicine promises reductions of medical costs by providing less expensive alternatives to interventions that require costly technology as well as by promoting wellness and preventing illness through attention to lifestyle. Integrative medicine neither rejects conventional medicine nor accepts alternative medicine uncritically, and although it calls for an expanded scientific paradigm and a variety of ways of collecting and analyzing evidence for the safety and efficacy of treatments, it relies on scientific methods and the accumulated experience of the profession. In many ways, integrative medicine is what good medicine has always been and should always be, trying not to cause harm and always working to help the body heal itself. If it flourishes in the new century, as I believe it will, a sign of its success will be that we can drop the word *integrative.* I will be the first to do so.

CHAPTER THIRTY-SEVEN

Health Promotion, Health Education, and Disease Prevention

Lawrence W. Green, C. James Frankish

Lawrence W. Green, DrPH, *served for eight years as Director of the Institute of Health Promotion Research and Professor and Head of the Division of Preventive Medicine and Health Promotion, Department of Health Care and Epidemiology, at the University of British Columbia, and is currently Distinguished Fellow and Visiting Scientist in the Office on Smoking and Health at the Centers for Disease Control and Prevention in Atlanta. He served as the first Director of the U.S. Office of Health Information and Health Promotion and received the American Public Health Association's Distinguished Career Award and Award of Excellence.*

C. James Frankish, PhD, *is Acting Director of the Institute of Health Promotion Research and Assistant Professor in Health Care and Epidemiology at the University of British Columbia. He was selected as a B.C. Health Research Scholar and has contributed widely to health promotion development in Canada, the United States, and Australia through his research, writing, and lectures.*

H ealth promotion arose in the fertile delta produced by the converging streams of health education, the self-care movement, public health, social and preventive medicine, the women's movement, and various rumblings in the professions and disciplines concerned with health. It drew inspiration from remnants of the community development and participatory traditions of public health programs in developing countries, the New Society and New Frontier legislation of the 1960s in the United States, and the cost containment and decentralization of the 1970s and 1980s in North America, Europe, and Australasia. It was swept inexorably by the emergence of chronic diseases as the dominant causes of death, displacing communicable diseases, and the recognition that lifestyle and conditions of living shaping people's lives from early childhood were the important determinants of health.

It blossomed with the rich fertilization of behavioral and social science research blended with the soil of the earlier sciences of public health: epidemiology, biostatistics, health administration, and policy analysis. Further tilling with increasingly sophisticated and rigorous health services research and program evaluation methods weeded out the less productive health education methods and programs. It began to call into question some of the conventional medical and public health approaches to the emerging chronic diseases and injury issues that were displacing the communicable diseases central to earlier approaches. Health promotion's first rays of nourishing spring sunshine came almost simultaneously with the 1973 U.S. President's Committee on Health Education report and the 1974 Lalonde Report, *A New Perspective on the Health of Canadians.*

Both health education and health promotion have helped distinguish preventive medicine from other specialties of medical practice, along with emerging technologies of prevention available for applica-

---

This chapter was prepared while Dr. Green was Director of the Institute of Health Promotion Research and Professor of Health Care and Epidemiology at the University of British Columbia. Parts of this chapter were presented to the Strategic Planning meeting of the University of Alberta Health Promotion Studies Centre, May 1999, and the Healthtrac Foundation Lecture at the Society for Public Health Education, Washington, D.C., November 1998. The twentieth-century background for each of the "lessons" discussed can be found in Green (1999).

tion in medical practice settings, such as new vaccines for primary prevention and new screening methods for secondary prevention. Disease prevention other than that defined by preventive medicine and health promotion has consisted largely of public health measures applied to environments affecting whole populations. These have included reducing the exposure of people to health-threatening organisms, toxic chemicals, and injury-producing agents and increasing their protective agents, such as fluoride and chloride in the water supply, seat belts in cars, bicycle helmets, thermostats on water heaters, and iodine in salt. Even these interventions for disease prevention have depended on health education for an enlightened electorate to support the regulations and interventions required and on health promotion to mobilize organizational and community support for their enforcement.

We concentrate our global look at the twenty-first century, therefore, on health promotion and health education, for these will be the initiating and implementing arms of new technologies that might arise in disease prevention and injury prevention. The new technologies for prevention will likely increase the scope and effectiveness of vaccines, the accuracy of screening and diagnostic tests that permit earlier detection of controllable diseases, and the efficacy of methods for engineering safe environments and products and enforcing regulatory reforms. The most widely discussed disease prevention possibilities at the end of the twentieth century—genetic screening and biotechnology—are unlikely to go as far as many people imagine, for reasons geneticists, ethicists, and legal scholars have explored anxiously (Omenn, 1996). Whether the disease prevention technologies of the future are medical, genetic, or engineering advances, their development and implementation will require a growing degree of public acceptance, assent, or tolerance, because the public has become more cautious about the promises of technology. These imperatives of democratic, increasingly informed publics will make health education and health promotion increasingly important to disease prevention.

TEN LESSONS FROM THE TWENTIETH CENTURY

The professional and scientific literature of the last years of any decade or century is predictably replete with speculative articles on what the next decade or century might hold. The Y2K transition was all the more so because it was a millennium marker as well. National commissions and international conferences (see, for example, World

Health Organization, 1997) have declared positions on what the twenty-first century should hold. We venture more cautiously with our crystal ball, taking a retrospective-prospective approach to project the lessons from public health's experience with health education and health promotion from the twentieth into the twenty-first.

Lesson 1: The Educational Imperative

With few exceptions, the scientific and technological advances from the bacteriological decades of the early part of the twentieth century failed to produce the absolute protections or eradication of problems that they seemed to promise. The projection for the twenty-first century is clear enough: the technological fixes in the offing now for public health problems will fall short of their expected effects to the degree that societies inadequately support health education and health promotion in their tasks of advocacy, dissemination, education, training, and other forms of public mobilization and capacity development. Besides the implementation failures, however, the twenty-first century will face expectation failures. In the middle of the twentieth century, René Dubos (1958) described "the mirage of health"—the elusive image of a utopian human condition that keeps evaporating and reappearing on another horizon as we raise our expectations. Sir Godfrey Vickers's frequently quoted definition of the history of public health as "a record of the successive redefinings of the unacceptable"(Vickers, 1958) also applies here. Both the causes and effects of ratcheting up public expectations involve public education, particularly health education in its broadest interpretation.

Lesson 2: The Accountability Imperative

The acceptance of health education and health promotion in public health policy appears to depend on its presentation of concrete, specific, achievable, evidence-based objectives for which it can be held accountable. Redefining the unacceptable to write new objectives as the world discovers new possibilities makes projection to the distant future impossible. In the shorter term—in the early decades of the twenty-first century—health promotion and disease prevention will do well to continue the relatively newfound formula for success of the last two decades of the twentieth century of articulating its goals and targets in quantifiable ten-year objectives. Programs that can be monitored in relation to progress in achieving goals have greater staying power and standing in policy (especially through transitions in government) than those that stand on practitioner principles, rhetoric, or ideology alone.

Lesson 3: The Ecological Imperative

The drift of medicine in the flow of science toward increasing ability to measure and explain disease and health in submolecular units also swept epidemiology toward the same reductionist tendencies, emphasizing individual risk factors over social determinants of health. The rediscovery in the last decade of the twentieth century of more distal determinants of health that disease prevention and health promotion must address predicts a twenty-first century in which these fields will use health education more for policy advocacy and community mobilization than for individual behavior change alone.

Lesson 4: The Technological Imperative

The late twentieth century was marked by successful efforts to put technological resources more at the disposal of people seeking greater control over their own lives and less dependency on professionals, technicians, and large, impersonal institutions. Occasional successes by professional associations and growing medical care institutions to beat back these tendencies notwithstanding, we can project an acceleration of personal control in areas where people want to exercise it, thanks especially to computer and other information technologies.

Lesson 5: The Participatory Imperative

The public and professional responses to the technological and economic blessings of the late twentieth century resulted in calls for more participatory, socially responsive, environmentally friendly approaches to scientific and professional practices in health. The populations affected by a health issue in the twenty-first century will participate more actively in health promotion research, in developing relevant policy, and in planning and evaluating programs (Raeburn and Rootman, 1998). Participatory research in health promotion has demonstrated that nonexperts can contribute to the design, implementation, and evaluation of programs and policies (Cornwall and Jewkes, 1995;

Green and others, 1995). This will be even more imperative when those policies call for changes in environments or social institutions that will rebound on other aspects of their lives.

Lesson 6: The Biomedical Imperative

Another lesson from the late twentieth century is that research funding for health promotion, when based in biomedical peer review traditions, tends to favor psychological models and measures over sociological, cultural, and political models; behavioral change measures over broader lifestyle or social measures of change; and proximal over more distal determinants of health. The peer review systems of the mid-twentieth century remain largely intact at the beginning of the twenty-first century, and they are inherently conservative in their effect on public health research (Daniel, Green, and Sheps, 1998). For disease prevention and health promotion, this perpetuates an emphasis on self-responsibility, a worthy component of a comprehensive strategy but one that tends to dominant at the cost of attention to the broader determinants of health (Blane, 1995).

Lesson 7: The Evidence-Based Imperative

Another lesson of the late twentieth century is that the concept of "best practices," when imported from biomedical research on human organisms to population health circumstances, does not hold the same constancy across the more varied social, cultural, and political circumstances in which public health and lifestyle issues operate. To understand causal complexity in the twenty-first century, health promotion and disease prevention will have to examine distal causal relationships as chains or linked sequences involving multiple short-term effects or operations (Logan and Spencer, 1996). Although health-related behavior is often a "proximal" cause of ill health, researchers, practitioners, and policymakers need to take account of the complex causal pathways along which these proximal causes lie and allow for the infinite variations that arise in each locality and era. Health promotion interventions will place particular emphasis on the educational functions of enhancing local ability to assess needs and resources and building capacities at the several levels of individual, family, institution, and community (Green and Kreuter, 1999; Hamilton and Bhatti, 1996; Trickett, 1997). The "evidence" in evidence-based practice will be as much the locality-specific social evidence as the generalizable biomedical, epidemiological, and evaluative research evidence from afar.

Lesson 8: The Intersectoral Imperative

The twentieth century ended with growing skepticism about the potential of the health sector acting alone or any sector acting by itself to influence complex lifestyles and social trends without engaging wider social forces. Health professionals in the twenty-first century face the need for integrated, multifaceted health promotion and disease or injury prevention interventions that link specific health promotion strategies (for example, creating supportive environments and healthful public policy) across multiple levels of society (individual, family, community) and across time (Nutbeam, Smith, Murphy, and Catford, 1993). They will employ concepts from systems theory (interdependence, homeostasis, feedback) (Green, Richard, and Potvin, 1996; Stokols, 1996). They will thus be able to apply health education principles such as situational specificity, multiple methods, individualization, relevance, feedback, reinforcement, and facilitation that recognize the interdependence of the individual and his or her environment (Frankish and Green, 1994).

Lesson 9: The Institutional Imperative

The twentieth century also tells us that the decisions on priorities and strategies for social change affecting the more complicated lifestyle issues can best be made collectively as close to the homes and workplaces of those affected as possible. Although the intersectoral imperative of Lesson 8 suggests a multi-institutional, communitywide strategy for the twenty-first century, the need will grow for institutions such as families, schools, workplaces, clubs, churches, and informal groups to play a pivotal role in mediating between broader social policies and individual preferences in lifestyle and health. The twentieth-century ideal of "community" was a throwback to the nineteenth-century North American and Australian traditions of frontier communities in which people were interdependent and community-oriented because they had few of the institutional supports they had left behind in the big cities. That ideal persisted into the late twentieth century because it was a cultural icon of American, Canadian, and

Australasian history that seemed to replace community with neighborhood in the suburbanization of their cities and rural towns. The twenty-first century seems to hold a future in which people will relate more to their workplace than to their neighborhood, more to their primary and secondary membership groups—including virtual groups on the Internet—than to their larger geopolitical community. Institutions or membership organizations will need to bridge the gap between the necessary policymaking at broader regional levels necessitated by global interdependence and the rank individualism made possible by global economies. Most of the evidence that will support health education, health promotion, and injury and disease prevention strategies is based in such institutions.

Lesson 10: The Interdisciplinary Imperative

Finally, the contextual health promotion and disease prevention strategy suggested in the first nine imperatives will call for a more aggressive commitment to multidisciplinary approaches to developing and implementing healthful public policies and practices. It recognizes that various disciplines each bring epistemologies and research methodologies that can be of value. Moreover, these multidisciplinary approaches must become more interdisciplinary, blending and integrating knowledge and evidence from different fields of study, as well as the collaboration of local stakeholders to help contextualize the generalized knowledge from research elsewhere.

CONCLUSION

Health education and health promotion seek, on behalf of public health and disease and injury prevention, to affect the behavior of individuals and their social environments of family, groups, organizations, and communities. They are concerned with life conditions and life chances as well as with lifestyle. Their strategies in the twenty-first century will be concerned as much with social, economic, and environmental change as they were in the twentieth century with altering behavior or lifestyles.

Drawing lessons from the history of health education, health promotion, and disease and injury prevention in the twentieth century, population health promotion in the twenty-first century will operate in and with expanded numbers and varieties of settings, participants, sources of evidence, support, disciplines, and professions. Health promotion interventions that begin with inadequate resources, vague objectives, and rigid notions of "best practices" that do not have local evidence or support from those affected by the targeted problem and that fail to recognize the social construction of knowledge will create interventions of diffuse, ill-fitting, and questionable quality. The use of inappropriate or unrealistic objectives, outcome measures, and time frames will only perpetuate the perception in some quarters of the failure of health promotion, health education, and disease and injury prevention.

A contextual, participatory, interdisciplinary approach views promoting the health of populations and preventing disease and injury as fundamentally collectivist, interdisciplinary pursuits. It recognizes that power *with* rather than power *over* is a necessary principle of future research, practice, and policymaking. It is concerned with a future in which a dramatic reduction or elimination of health inequities is seen as the preferred end state of population health promotion.

References

Blane, D. "Social Determinants of Health: Socioeconomic Status, Social Class, and Ethnicity." *American Journal of Public Health,* 1995, *85,* 903–905.

Cornwall, A., and Jewkes, R. "What Is Participatory Research?" *Social Science and Medicine,* 1995, *41,* 1667–1676.

Daniel, M., Green, L. W., and Sheps, S. "Paradigm Change and Uncertainty About Funding of Public Health Research: Social and Scientific Implications." *Journal of Health and Social Policy,* 1998, *10*(2), 39–56.

Dubos, R. *The Mirage of Health.* New York: Doubleday, 1958.

Frankish, C. J., and Green, L. W. "Organizational and Community Change as the Social Scientific Basis for Disease Prevention and Health Promotion Policy." In G. L. Albrecht (ed.), *Advances in Medical Sociology,* Vol. 4: *A Reconsideration of Health Behavior Change Models.* Ipswich, Conn.: JAI Press, 1994.

Green, L. W. "Health Education's Contributions to Public Health in the Twentieth Century: A Glimpse Through Health Promotion's Rear-View Mirror." *Annual Review of Public Health,* 1999, *20,* 67–88.

Green, L. W., and Kreuter, M. *Health Promotion Planning: An Educational and Ecological Approach.* (3rd ed.) Mountain View, Calif.: Mayfield, 1999.

Green, L. W., Richard, L., and Potvin, L. "Ecological Foundations of Health Promotion." *American Journal of Health Promotion,* 1996, *10,* 270–281.

Green, L. W., and others. *Participatory Research in Health Promotion in Canada.* Ottawa: Royal Society of Canada, 1995.

Hamilton, N., and Bhatti, T. *Population Health Promotion: An Integrated Model of Population Health and Health Promotion.* Ottawa: Health Promotion Development Division, Health Canada, 1996.

Lalonde, M. A. *A New Perspective of the Health of Canadians.* Ottawa: Ministry of National Health and Welfare, 1974.

Logan, S., and Spencer, N. "Smoking and Other Health Related Behavior in the Social and Environmental Context." *Archives of Disease in Childhood,* 1996, *74,* 176–179.

Nutbeam, D., Smith, C., Murphy, S., and Catford, J. "Maintaining Evaluation Designs in Long-Term Community-Based Health Promotion Programmes: Heartbeat Wales Case Study." *Journal of Epidemiology and Community Health,* 1993, *47,* 127–133.

Omenn, G. S. "Comment: Genetics and Public Health." *American Journal of Public Health,* 1996, *86,* 1701–1704.

Raeburn, J., and Rootman, I. *People-Centered Health Promotion.* New York: Wiley, 1998.

Report of the President's Committee on Health Education. New York: Public Affairs Institute, 1973.

Stokols, D. "Bridging the Theoretical and Applied Facets of Environmental Psychology." *American Psychologist,* 1996, *51,* 1188–1189.

Trickett, E. "Ecology and Primary Prevention: Reflections on a Meta-Analysis." *American Journal of Community Psychology,* 1997, *25,* 197–205.

Vickers, Sir G., "What Sets the Goals of Public Health?" *New England Journal of Medicine,* 1958, *258,* 12.

World Health Organization. *Jakarta Declaration on Leading Health Promotion into the 21st Century.* Geneva: World Health Organization, 1997.

CHAPTER THIRTY-EIGHT

The Role of Communication and Advertising

Thomas P. Lom

__Thomas P. Lom__ is Executive Vice President and Worldwide Account Director at the Saatchi & Saatchi advertising agency. He has been active in health care advertising for twenty-five years, both in the United States and globally. He has developed numerous communication programs with companies like Johnson & Johnson, Glaxo, Merck, and Hoffman-La Roche. He has been at the forefront of consumer health care communication and is considered a leader in the field.

Never before in human history have we been blessed with such a constant stream of medical advances as we are today. Medical science allows us to understand the human body as never before. We understand what makes our body tick and what makes it stop ticking. The science of medicine is discovering new therapies that can cure many diseases and slow the progression of others. Yet as encouraging as the progress is, there remains the enormous challenge of making people aware of this innovation and turning that awareness into positive health behavior.

To meet this challenge, communication has a crucial, even obligatory role to play. It may take the form of journalism (broadcast, print, and Internet) or advertising (paid and public service). In the United States, advertising spending on prescription medicines in 1998 reached $1.3 billion, compared to a mere $12 million in 1989. Medical journal advertising of prescription medicines to health care professionals increased 42 percent between 1995 and 1998 (Medical Advertising News, September 1999, p. 18). And in consumer magazines, the number of editorial pages devoted to health care increased 19 percent between 1995 and 1998. The disease states covered by this explosion ranged from traditionally discussed ones such as arthritis pain, hypertension, and diabetes to newly discussed conditions such as depression, Alzheimer's, and impotence (Hall's Magazine Reports).

The explosion of information has had two benefits critical to our health. The first is that both the public and the physician are now aware of new and improved therapies that can save lives or improve the quality of life. People with HIV can have longer, better lives; people with migraine headaches can get relief; people with neurological disorders can more easily cope. The second benefit is that much of the information explosion has led to proper diagnosis of diseases previously undiagnosed or misdiagnosed and therefore untreated. We are now more aware of the symptoms of depression; we now know the possible benefit of hormone replacement therapy; we now know that chemotherapy can cause anemia that can be treated. As a result, we feel more empowered and better prepared to discuss our health with a physician.

Beyond disease treatment, communication encourages disease prevention or at the very least early diagnosis. Journalistic coverage especially has increased awareness that certain kinds of cancers are far less deadly if caught early. Frequent and early screenings for breast, prostate, and colon cancer have led to a significantly improved prognosis for millions of men and women. The link between cholesterol and heart disease is well communicated and is leading to improved management of hypercholesterolemia through lifestyle changes and drug therapy. The link between calcium and osteoporosis is also well communicated and leading to much more proactive behavior in the form of dietary changes and calcium supplementation. Of particular note, these behaviors are happening at an earlier age.

The motivation for the dissemination of all this information is driven by a convergence of public policy and public health interest with private sector commercial interests. In fact, in a highly developed country such as the United States, it is the private sector that drives the process.

The biggest private sector influence is the pharmaceutical industry. The industry is consistently investing in new drug development. In 1998 alone, the top ten companies invested $17 billion (Medical Advertising News, November 1999, p. 1) in research and development. From 1994 to 1998, the U.S. Food and Drug Administration approved 172 new drugs. Is it any wonder, then, that this industry also invests heavily in educating people about these medicines?

The first investment is in physicians. For years, drug company sales representatives have been calling on physicians to inform them of the clinical story behind a wide array of drugs. In fact, the number of such representatives has grown substantially since 1995. This has accelerated the process of diffusion of innovation. So, too, has the investment in industry-sponsored education for physicians. Be it in large medical conventions or smaller local meetings, physicians can review pharmaceutical science in more depth. Even if the science is commercially driven, good science is good science from any source.

As we look into the new century, this science will be even more broadly and more quickly available via the Internet. Company-sponsored Web sites will proliferate as a tool for physicians to gain access to clinical data. This will no doubt be supplemented with editorial comment from scientific opinion leaders. It will also be supplemented by commentary from practitioners as to their experience in clinical practice. Another trend that will accelerate is that information about experience with experimental drug trials will be shared over the Internet. This is already happening in such areas as oncology and antiviral treatment where specialists can't wait to learn about promising new options.

The second investment is in patients. And this comes at a time when Americans especially are becoming much more proactive about their health care. There is a broad trend in American society toward self-reliance. We see it all around us. We do more of our own financial planning. We buy stocks on-line, not through a broker. Home improvement is driven by do-it-yourselfers. Health is no exception to this trend. Americans are not shy about offering their physician opinions about diagnoses and helpful suggestions about treatment.

The pharmaceutical industry is only too happy to fuel this trend. Nowadays, when a new drug is introduced, a substantial patient-directed ad program almost always supports it. There is no better or faster way for new therapies to work their way into the public consciousness. It is especially valuable in encouraging patients to identify themselves as having certain symptoms and to initiate discussion with a physician. It also helps remove the stigma associated with certain diseases. Among the most notable of these is depression. Advertising has started many people on the road to a more normal life.

Another industry is joining the party of health education: the food industry. More and more is being learned about the positive health value of mainstream food, from calcium to oat bran. And new foods are being developed with clinically proven benefits derived from newly discovered natural ingredients (like plant sterols for cholesterol reduction). People are eager to learn about nature's solutions for living healthier, and the food industry is providing that information. A third industry, dietary supplements, is also providing educational stimulus in much the same way.

In the twenty-first century, the consumer education process will only grow. Mass media like television, magazines, and newspapers will continue to be heavily used, and targeted media will become even more important. The decade of the 1990s saw major advances in the sophistication of techniques that can get patients with specific diseases to identify themselves. Once that identification happens, targeted and specific educational material can be sent to that patient. The Internet will also be a tool of enormous value as every drug can have its own interactive Web site. Questions can be answered with an immediacy that used to require a doctor visit. New professional experts can be accessed via the Web.

Manufacturers are not alone in fueling the public demand for health information. Books, newspapers, and magazines have also been major forces. Visit your local bookstore and notice the substantial health section filled with "guides" of all sort. Visit your local newsstand and notice the magazine titles and cover stories devoted to health. And notice that almost every newspaper has a weekly health section. Health sells.

As we look forward, all of these media will have Web sites to complement the printed word. This wide array of information sources will collectively take on a new role as the resource patients increasingly turn to. And medical institutions will participate in this trend, whether it's a nationally recognized name like the Mayo Clinic or the local hospital.

The public sector has also played an increasing role in the diffusion process by way of not-for-profit patient advocacy organizations.

Although these have existed for many years, their number has grown. They have always been aggressive in "spreading the word" on new treatments. However, today the Internet gives enormous numbers of people immediate access to this information, not just in the United States but around the world. And with Internet connectivity, these Web sites will increasingly steer people to a myriad of related sites on related topics. All of this fuels our tendency toward self-reliance.

The U.S. public sector also has a valuable tool in the Ad Council. The Ad Council is a clearinghouse for public service messages of all kinds. They range from social issues to ecological issues to health issues. Perhaps the best-known health message is the antidrug message sponsored by Partnership for a Drug Free America. In 1998, Ad Council messages received $1.2 billion worth of free media space and time. When the Ad Council puts its weight behind an issue, the message gets heard, and positive behavior change usually follows. This is also the case when the federal government uses its "bully pulpit" to educate, as it has, for example, on the perils of cigarette smoking.

In addition to physicians and patients, a third stakeholder has assumed increased prominence in the communication process—payers. Insurance companies, managed care organizations, and governments have an important stake in keeping people healthy in the most cost-effective way possible. Increasingly, they are using communication to encourage appropriate behaviors such as screenings, early diagnosis, and proactive wellness activity. Payers recognize the financial cost of bad health. And they have a special incentive to promoting good health. As long as they don't abuse access as a tool for financial cost containment, their influence should be very positive.

Health care communication abounds in the United States. To what extent can the U.S. communication paradigm be a constructive model elsewhere? That requires a review of participants and roles and depends on the state of economic development involved.

In other developed countries, where the populace has the interest and means, the private sector is likely to take a dominant role. Just as in the United States, the pharmaceutical industry is well motivated commercially to invest in educating about new drugs. Companies will want physicians to be educated and patients to be aware in the same way. Similar dynamics will be at play ensuring that the diffusion of scientific innovation occurs.

Where Europe and Japan differ from the United States is in the regulatory environment. Regulations there do not allow for the kind of direct-to-consumer advertising permitted in recent years in the United States. However, since the Internet is giving consumers access to the information anyway, governments are being forced to reconsider their regulations. Both directly and indirectly, the Internet will accelerate globalization of the education process.

Journalism will also be a powerful force if these national populations follow the trend toward self-reliance—and all indications are that they already have. The consolidation of media companies and the growth of the European Union have contributed to this. As in the United States, health sells wherever people can take action to improve their health and have the financial means to do so.

This brings us to payers. Many developed countries have some form of nationalized health system. These systems place constraints on how much is spent on new and sometimes costly health care innovation. New diagnostic tools, new drugs, new treatments, and new surgical procedures all have a cost. How national health systems deal with that cost will have a substantial impact on how proactive the private sector will be. Private sector communication expenditure will be in proportion to the commercial incentive.

In less developed countries, the public sector will have to take more of the lead in health care communication. Where populations are poor and literacy rates are low, the dynamics are quite different. National governments must make communication a major part of public policy. The health care issues will be more elementary. The media will be more grassroots. The workplace, schools, and clinics will be more important. Access to technology will be limited, so the utility of the Internet will be lessened. Some physicians will benefit (more and more as the century progresses, I hope), as will the general public (libraries will provide access for the public). Unfortunately, public sector activity won't add much to the critical mass of educational activity, as it does, for example, in the United States.

Though there are differences around the world, as we look to the twenty-first century, one central reality is common around the globe: no matter what the country or region, public policy is focusing on health, individuals are focusing on health, and commercial enterprises are focusing on health. At the same time, the new century will see even more progress in medical science. And communication will continue to explode to allow for an optimal diffusion of this wealth of medical advance. It will be a remarkable time.

CHAPTER THIRTY-NINE

Effective Communication as the Path to Ideal Health

Scott C. Ratzan

Scott C. Ratzan, MD, MPA, *is Senior Technical Advisor, Center for Population, Health, and Nutrition, U.S. Agency for International Development. He is also editor in chief of* the Journal of Health Communication: International Perspectives *and holds faculty appointments in the Department of Family Medicine and Community Health at Tufts University School of Medicine and the Department of International Public Health at George Washington University Medical Center. His publications include the* Mad Cow Crisis: Health and the Public Good *and* AIDS: Effective Health Communication for the '90s.

Though many authors in this book point to great successes in the twentieth century, there are even greater challenges ahead for the six billion people that inhabit the planet today. Health is clearly the common currency for humankind, but its attainment is convoluted. There is great promise that the twenty-first century will be a new era of communication. However, with new communication technologies come the risks of developing a new poverty, a so-called digital divide.

I intend to show how we can maximize our effectiveness in communicating health. Ethically employed communication strategies can advance our ability to promote a healthier public who can obtain, interpret, and understand health information to make appropriate decisions. In short, I hope to present how effective communication can be ideal medicine.

First, I will suggest that we select a path in global health that maximizes our progress with scientific prowess. Subsequently, I will explore the potential use of communication technology that can inform and motivate each of us with ideas and actions.

Prior to her election as Director-General of the World Health Organization, Dr. Gro Harlem Brundtland aptly described the challenges that the world faces: "As the century closes, the rate of change outstrips the ability of scientific disciplines and our current capabilities to assess and advise. This frustrates the attempts of political and economic institutions, which evolved in a different world, to adapt and cope."

Dr. Brundtland's prescient prediction can help guide leaders in health. Realistically, we have three choices: (1) we can say that the problems we face in global health today are far too difficult to resolve and so rely on a lowest-common-denominator approach to public health, (2) we can wait for "scientific" discoveries to lead us to biomedical approaches with incremental success, or (3) we can strive to overcome widespread health illiteracy and communicate health in a way that affects public health policy to build a scientific and humanitarian society.

THE STATE OF OUR HEALTH TODAY

In a world where communication has replaced armies as a source of power, we have not treated communication as a determinant of health. Nonetheless, we have created "communicated disease"—diseases that are not promulgated by a microscopic infectious agent (virus or bacterium), environmental factors (cosmic radiation), or genetic predisposition. Communicated diseases are advanced through a variety of channels and vehicles such as the news and entertainment media, advertising, or the new telecommunications media that affect culture, society, and ultimately our individual health behavior. Many twentieth-century communicated diseases relate to nutritional disparities and sedentary lifestyle habits, but the most important communicated disease is tobacco.

What does this problem mean for those of us advancing global health—dedicated to preserving our greatest resource, the viability of the human species? How can we learn from those who communicate ill health to develop true health instead?

The ideals to seek the "truth" were promulgated by Plato well over two thousand years ago, and modern-day health science has built on the writings of Plato and Hippocrates. In the twentieth century, "truth" was systematized with the invention of the randomized clinical trial and evidenced-based medicine. Countless studies now examine variables termed "risk factors" as predictors of disease and its magnitude. Among such "progress" is a proliferation of information with over twenty-five thousand medical and health journals printed annually, which may not actually translate science-based findings into behavior change.

Concomitant with the volume of medical studies, popular health and medical news stories have multiplied in print, in television broadcasts, and on the Internet. At the end of the twentieth century, fads included functional foods (for example, split pea soup fortified with St. John's wort and cholesterol-busting margarine) and pharming (impregnating vaccines in cow's milk), along with other genetic modifications.

Despite great medical progress, the diffusion of health innovations for the global citizen has been uneven and limited. Even with all of the discovery and "new" information and knowledge this produced, most people rely on an organized health system—rather than themselves—to manage their health.

The fact that in communication we have a powerful intervention that could reach everyone means that in the twenty-first century, we can deliver health to the billions of people who had little access during the twentieth century, despite the "progress" made by biomedical science.

DEVELOPING A HEALTH LITERACY THROUGH COMMUNICATION

"The new communication" is often taken to mean the Internet, associated with the use of computers. Though a majority of the world's population does not have direct access today, soon the Internet will be ubiquitous, accessed via television, land-linked and cellular phones, satellites, radio, kiosks, watches, and other new ways. The "wearable

Web" or "e-device" will be a multidirectional gadget with the potential to monitor physiological components and to communicate with providers of instant feedback, advice, and recommendations. Eventually, it will also overcome the reliance on English and the twentieth-century forms of written language.

Although we can imagine a twenty-first century with information everywhere, our overarching goal should be the effective delivery of health information. In short, it means getting the right message to the right people, at the right time, with the intended effect. It requires an understanding of the science and art of communicating health.

New communication opportunities can help individuals be more involved in their own health decisions and treatment. With appropriate access, the new communication technology can create a health-literate public. Such a public would know the consequences of health-related individual and community behaviors and choose accordingly among self-care options, access the health system when necessary, seek information to make the best decision based on a reliable knowledge base, and demand healthy public policy.

HOW CAN INFORMATION TECHNOLOGY BE USED?

We can imagine the inevitable progression of the technological use of medical information in the modern-day hospital—instantaneous laboratory results, X-rays, oxygen levels, and so on—via a handheld computer at the patient's bedside. In a wireless world, e-devices could be developed to assist in the decision-making process so that people with chronic diseases (such as diabetes) can titrate interventions (insulin, sugar intake) within an acceptable range for blood sugar, cholesterol, and blood pressure.

With the increased bandwidth, speed, and reach of the Internet, new branded health channels can cross language and cultural divides. Such sites attempt to develop the hope and hype of how the Internet could deliver tailored health information for individual consumers. Physician practices, health delivery systems, and new media sources will have access to personalized information (for example, diagnosis, treatment, and the latest breakthroughs on daily healthcasts) salient to the individual based on the person's age, sex, medical history, and genetic makeup, among other factors. With the interactivity built in to the system, the physician can communicate synchronously (Webcast, worldwide radio, satellite lecture, voice-activated interfaces, audioconferences, and so on) and asynchronously (e-mail, store and forward technology) with all of the diabetic patients in the physician's medical practice, health plan, or geographical region. Furthermore, the diffusion of discoveries to practitioners with the integration of images, audio, and live video can speed the adoption process throughout the world.

The implications of new technologies to collect, store, share, and interpret data cannot be overstated. With the translation of data into knowledge, a health care provider can examine benchmark data with practice guidelines and ideal population-based approaches. On the other hand, a patient will have the opportunity to compare his or her profile with others throughout the world, as well as to obtain or provide psychological support and data sharing. For example, a woman newly diagnosed with breast cancer can begin interacting (asking questions, receiving information and, potentially, misinformation) with thousands of others. At every level of the health care enterprise, new technologies can help manage information in order to maximize the appropriate health impact.

While the new technologies present an opportunity for interactive communication, they can also provide information unmediated by human decision making. Artificial intelligence and decision systems can offer diagnoses and treatment options based on large population databases. Other devices, such as a "nano-implant" (subcutaneous semiconductor chip smaller than a grain of rice), could track blood pressure, cholesterol, cardiac parameters, fat and sugar levels, and other relevant data. Information could be transmitted to a device that interprets information or tells the individual how to vary his or her behavior (alter food or liquid intake, take a drug supplement) or even have a calibrated response from another implant (electrodefibrillation, antibody release, vasodilator, insulin or glucose infusion, and the like).

Other individuals who wish to be "in control" of their health can seek tailored information on the latest discoveries related to their genetic makeup and predisposition or current disease. Each of us could control our personal computerized health record by encrypting it on a handheld computer device, a microchip, or a personal health "Web page" that we share with our health providers. Given twentieth-century measurements and know-how, such a basic record would have blood pressure, body mass index, cholesterol levels, vaccination records (against influenza, tetanus, hepatitis B, and so on), cancer screenings (Pap smears, mammograms, prostate-specific antigen, and the like). It would instantaneously remind both the consumer and health provider over existing (phone, postal service, e-mail) and new channels (programmed alarm clock alerts, digital radio or wristwatch devices) of the need for vaccinations, preventive health checkups, and medication refills. Such an approach can advance the ideals of shared decision making to enhance one's control of one's health.

APPROACHING INTERACTIVE HEALTH COMMUNICATION

Though all of the aforementioned new technologies—principally the Internet, devices, and decision-support systems—have unlimited promise, they will not automatically lead to a healthier world. We must view them realistically. The twenty-first century will require a new way of thinking in that we may have to look beyond the individual as being able to control "risk factors." Individuals will also have opportunities to select diagnosis and treatment options based on their demographic, psychographic, genographic, environmental, and immunological markers. Susceptibility and identification of disease will be more precise, with the identification of causative factors and with ideal treatment based on validated data. New customized treatments, such as tailored designer antibiotics or antibodies to certain pathogens and genetic therapeutics will be available.

HEALTH HEGEMONY: COMMUNICATION FOR BETTER PUBLIC HEALTH

As the world globalizes, the frontier of cyberspace creates an opportunity to place health high on everyone's agenda. In the United States, an Institute of Medicine committee (1999) recommended the creation of "leading health indicators" to identify components that best predict the health of the U.S. population. Ideally, these indicators could become common vernacular, adapted by the news and the new media, so that every consumer could be aware of individual, community, and public health developments. Even in the global marketplace of medicine, health is local. Leading health indicators could be localized to prioritize policy and to galvanize health action. Indicators could be related to the individual environment, disease patterns, or social structure.

We also need to harness the prevention message with simple interventions that could translate the jargon of primary, secondary, and tertiary prevention. Strong global health leadership could help advance health literacy through communication. New communication technologies could provide the tools so that every global citizen could answer three simple questions: (1) What do we do to keep ourselves well? (2) If we are getting sick, how can we detect and treat these conditions early? and (3) If we are sick, how do we get the best medical care?

In addition to using the World Wide Web to gather information and to provide expert collaboration, new and traditional media will continue to educate the public by delivering health and medical content. Even with globalization, the localization of messages and approaches will help health systems develop interactive channels in one's home for health on demand, with "customized" information from "your doctor." Health delivery will devolve from hospital to home, from cure to self-care, and from schools to desktop TVs. The increasing demand of people who wish to be healthy will help provide health information that "matters," moving beyond traditional conferences or printed reports.

By increasing supply *and* demand for health information, new health communities will develop as the twenty-first century's accessible and user-friendly cyberlibrary becomes ever more widely available. "Collaboratories" for common community initiatives (to exchange information, hold virtual meetings, and share materials and best practices) will develop, along with lifelong learning opportunities for contacting local and national experts, directories of health resources, local health services, and other community information. Literacy on health issues should be ensured in the home, in school, over the airwaves, and via the Internet.

Of course, scientific discovery has an important role in advancing health. But scientific breakthroughs are incremental, and people are less apt to change their behavior if they are led to believe that science will provide a magic bullet. In the twenty-first century, we must not only strive for new medical discoveries but also seek to translate such knowledge into actions for a healthier society. Communicating health accurately will require understanding the context and choosing new media technologies that reach everyone, especially underserved, minority, and disabled populations.

HEALTH LEADERSHIP

Finally, leadership position should be advanced, not only in publications and media channels via hospitals, health care facilities, and academic health centers but also in the marketing milieu. Individuals can become health advocates to ensure that appropriate health issues are on the political agenda. A highly credible organization like the World Health Organization or professional organizations and governmental agencies can provide accurate, trustworthy data for public consumption. Developing health leadership could be the most important advance made possible by communications technology.

Consider the age-old ideal of an individual as an "island" in making personal decisions about health. This perspective is unrealistic, given the disparities of health services, environment, and financial challenges. Communication, however, can harness knowledge and power to advocate health change at the community, region, national, or multinational level. For example, if health data were translated into understandable decision-making briefs for policymakers, opinion leaders, and community champions, more appropriate decisions regarding health and economic outcomes would be made. Choosing to invest in vitamin A fortification, folate and fluoride supplementation, tobacco taxation, immunizations, seat belt laws, insecticide-impregnated bed nets, and other technological innovations could be a crucial contribution of the communication function. Furthermore, the diffusion of such innovations based on sound science via new communications technologies can connect similar groups around the globe. These communication tools can help us create decentralized data-based, decision-making systems to advance the health of individuals who lack training or access to data on benefits from health policy changes.

CONCLUSION

Could a future be envisioned in which an individual would elicit an accurate, up-to-date interpretation of scientific results that translates "health as we know it" into real-life daily activities? Could we communicate well enough to individuals so as to develop health "news you can use"?

Though many observers are optimistic that we can create a new health "as it ought to be," health as we know it today might prevail—

a world with disparities of income, health and human rights, gender, and environmental justice. In the twentieth century, market forces dominated, as in the marketing of tobacco and alcohol products—drugs that result in ill health. We have identified the latest frontier as cyberspace, yet 75 percent of the world's population has never made a telephone call. Many of these people smoke. Clearly, our ability to reach people for profit supersedes the humane ideals of promulgating prosperity through health. As we begin the twenty-first century, we have an unparalleled opportunity in the communication age.

Nearly seventy-five years ago, John Dewey presaged our potential as an "organized articulate public." He believed that the "highest and most difficult kind of inquiry and a subtle, delicate, vivid, and responsive art of communication must take possession of the physical machinery of transmission and circulation and breathe life into it" (Dewey, 1954, p. 184.)

We have the power to create, deliver, and access appropriate interactive health communication to enhance the health of all six billion humans in today's world. We must attempt to use communications technology to "do the right thing," to educate people at all levels to make ideal health decisions for themselves and their communities.

As a physician, my primary concerns remain the prevention of disease and the promotion of health and the overall quality of life for all people. My hope is that we can all maximize the effectiveness of communication to deliver successfully an ethical, daily dose of health to make a difference in everyone's lives.

References

Dewey, J. *The Public and Its Problems*, Ohio: Swallow Press, 1954. (Originally published 1927.)

Institute of Medicine. *Leading Health Indicators for Healthy People.* Washington, D.C.: National Academy Press, 1999.

CHAPTER FORTY

Changes Associated with Aging

Knight Steel

Knight Steel, MD, *is President of the American Federation for Aging Research and is the University of Medicine and Dentistry of New Jersey and is Endowed Professor of Geriatrics at the New Jersey Medical School. He is also Director of The Homecare Institute, Hackensack University Medical Center. Previously, he was in charge of the Health of the Elderly Programme, World Health Organization, Geneva.*

This chapter was adapted in part from presentations delivered at the World Health Organization International Symposium on Aging and Health in Kobe, Japan, and at a meeting of the American Clinical and Climatological Association in Sea Island, Georgia. The author acknowledges the valuable participation of the following contributors: Palmi V. Jónsson (Iceland), Jean-Noel Du Pasquier (Switzerland), Ruedi Gilgen (Switzerland), John Hirdes (Canada), Marianne Schroll (Denmark), Gunnar Ljunggren (Sweden), Iain Carpenter (United Kingdom), and Jan Bjørnson (Norway) on behalf of interRAI.

The author is supported in part by grants from the John A. Hartford Foundation, the Elizabeth and Stephen Bechtel Jr. Foundation, and the Hunterdon Health Fund. He would also like to thank Brant Fries and John Morris for their suggestions.

As Director-General Gro Brundtland of the World Health Organization noted in her speech to the fifty-first World Health Assembly in Geneva on May 13, 1998; "We have another transition, the transition from the communicable to the noncommunicable diseases." She also pointed out that an appropriate degree of attention to acute infectious illness is not at odds with a special emphasis on chronic conditions and the consequences of chronic disease. In her words, "They cannot be seen as competing tasks. They are complementary. We need to fight both. The burden of disease is the burden of unfulfilled human development." Nowhere is this viewpoint more important than in the prevention of frailty and the design of systems of care for the frail elderly so as to maximize function and quality of life. All persons in all countries endorse these goals for themselves, their elders, and even their children. This changing direction at WHO reflects both the change from acute to chronic illness worldwide and the dramatic demographic shift as almost all countries witness the aging of their populations. As noted by Kinsella and Taeuber (1992, pp. 92–93), "In 1991 the net balance of the world's elderly population grew by more than 800,000 each month. Projections for the year 2010 suggest the net monthly gain will then be in excess of 1.1 million elderly people."

Over the past several decades, the phenomenon of aging has been separated out from the multiple pathological processes that so frequently accompany this process. After Hayflick published his sentinel paper in 1965 demonstrating that cells in tissue culture will not divide indefinitely, a series of researchers published reports on sequences of nucleic acids known as telomeres, which are progressively "chopped off" with each cell division. Thus a mechanism was discovered whereby cells could be ordered along a continuum from young to old (Hayflick, 1996; Bodnar and others, 1998).

At the same time, any number of investigators of organ systems began to dissect away the changes that are associated with disease from those that might be attributed solely to aging. Thus, for example, the resting cardiac index does not appear to change significantly with age in men (at least until very late in life) and changes only very modestly in women, although there do appear to be age-related decrements associated with exercise (Fleg and others, 1995). Dementia has come to be viewed as an illness rather than "senility," with the most important consequence that risk factors, preventive measures, and therapeutic interventions are being sought in Alzheimer's disease. Similarly, research is increasingly being directed to the causes of a long list of other age-related illnesses, such as osteoporosis, late-onset diabetes mellitus, and osteoarthritis. At the level of the individual, the older person is increasingly viewed as reflecting certain fundamental changes associated with aging, which generally are not very limiting until very late in life, on which there are likely superimposed multiple diseases that individually and collectively diminish function.

Assuming increasing importance are preventive measures targeted to diminishing the deleterious effects of aging and modifying or even eliminating disease. Thus, for example, health professionals are detailing the benefits of exercise to maintain muscle strength and balance as well as to normalize glucose tolerance and cardiac function. They are publicizing the benefits of influenza vaccine to diminish the risks of morbidity and mortality associated with this illness, which requires renewed attention on an annual basis as the virus alters its appearance, thereby evading last year's defenses. Whether morbidity can be compressed progressively into fewer and fewer years at the very end of a long life remains a subject of debate, but regardless, ever larger numbers of elders with varying degrees of functional impairment will require an array of individualized services (Vita, Terry, Hubert, and Fries, 1998). Although the image of families and communities caring for their older members without significant assistance from private agencies or government programs is the traditional, often idealized view of elder care, the demographic changes are so dramatic that strictly "informal" support, as family care is termed, will soon no longer be an option for much of the world. Thus, for example, in 1950 in Japan, there were ten individuals sixty-five years of age and over for every one hundred persons aged twenty to sixty-four, the age group of most caregivers. By 2025, there will be almost fifty older persons for every one hundred persons in the caregiver age bracket (Kinsella and Taeuber, 1992). Furthermore, as women join the paid workforce, there will be still fewer persons at home to provide those health care functions traditionally assigned to women.

Indeed, in the developed world especially, it is already increasingly common to find women in their sixties, some of whom may have significant disability themselves and many of whom are employed full time, caring for or arranging the care of a parent. The parent support ratio, the number of persons eighty years of age and over per hundred persons in the fifty to sixty-four age range will continue to increase throughout much of the world; for example, it will rise from eleven to nineteen in Argentina, from nineteen to thirty-eight in Sweden, and from six to twelve in the Republic of Korea between 1990 and 2025 (Kinsella and Taeuber, 1992). This dramatic aging of the older 40 percent or so of the world's population reflects not only a truly gargantuan increase in the numbers of old-old and frail elders but also a diminishing number of individuals in the next younger generation who are capable of providing either personal or economic support to their parents. Thus no matter how much they may desire to do so, many families can no longer be expected to care for their elders without significant "formal" support.

To meet this need, an array of services has sprung up around the world, which, regrettably, are usually poorly integrated with each other. Thus home nursing and physical therapy may be provided in some locations, as may even more technologically sophisticated programs that offer cardiac monitoring, intravenous therapy, enteral feeding, or end-of-life care. Social support programs, often funded totally separately, including housekeeping services, meals on wheels and shopping, volunteer programs that arrange for visits to shut-ins, and even home repair services, may be provided in a given locale. Each is likely to exist less because of a measured need than because of the availability of government support or the well-intentioned efforts of an individual or small charitable group. Some services may be offered to those in their own home, and others may be available only to individuals who reside in institutions of considerable variability with respect to medical sophistication and the availability of support services.

How each nation chooses to address the problem of the design and implementation of a program for frail elders will likely reflect not only need but also local economic and political realities. As is apparent, the care of elders, especially those who are frail, requires an exceptionally complex and multifaceted conglomeration of services. Unlike the majority of disease-targeted illnesses or the care of most younger persons, a mix of medical and social interventions is frequently required if maximal function and quality of life are to be achieved. The difficulty lies in determining exactly what services, both medical and social, are required and in what quantity.

In keeping with the Director-General's directive, as articulated later in her address (Brundtland, 1998), there is a need to base our decisions about systems of care for frail elders on data so as to facilitate the identification of needs both for the elders and their families and to target interventions. Further, such a data-based approach will allow for the evaluation of interventions, be they strictly medical, more social service in nature, or a combination thereof. All nations must come to have the ability to assess outcomes, allowing for evidence-based decisions about elder care policies and even discrete medical and social programs. Finally, it should be emphasized that as virtually all nations are aging, the ability to learn from each other is not only wise but also efficient.

The importance of this data-driven direction to the design and implementation of care systems for the frail elderly cannot be gainsaid. Without viewing with precision the data defining the need and various interventions, the health care system for the frailest segment of our population will continue to be unsound. For example, what passes for a nursing home in one country may bear very little resemblance to a long-term care institution in another. As Ribbe and colleagues (1997) have noted, at present, long-term care resource development bears little resemblance to the aging status of a nation or even to patient need. Even in developed countries, rehabilitation programs that foster discharge from a long-term care facility to a community setting are highly variable, being reported to be well developed, for example, in the Netherlands and very limited or essentially absent in Denmark, the United Kingdom, and Italy. At least one such "system" to collect and analyze data to assist individual programs and nations facing these most difficult decisions is under development.

All health care professionals would agree that if care for the individual is to be exemplary, a comprehensive assessment is required. Similarly, if care is to be provided to populations in a cost-effective manner, a standardized assessment of need is necessary so that data can be grouped, risk factors for disease and frailty uncovered, outcomes of interventions measured, and quality of care addressed on a continuing basis. These points deserve emphasis because an abundance of resources is not a prerequisite for many effective health care polities. What is required is the avoidance of waste. This can be achieved only by determining an individual's needs with precision and using targeted interventions. On a more global basis, we must learn from other nations, thereby avoiding costly interventions that have already been shown to be wasteful or not effective. It must also be appreciated that standards for quality of health care are always evolving as science introduces new technologies, drugs, and systems of care, which require repeated evaluation (Steel, 1997).

During the period 1989–1992, under contract with the federal government in the United States, a group of investigators designed a standardized assessment of elders' instrument for use in skilled nursing facilities (Hawes and others, 1997). The Resident Assessment Instrument (RAI), as it is known, was field-tested, tested for validity and reliability, and ultimately mandated for use in all 1.7 million nursing home beds in the country. Computerization of the data is now mandated throughout the United States, and both the province of Ontario, in Canada, and Iceland have recently adopted it as well. Seven million completed assessments from many nations on more than 3.5 million individuals, including longitudinal data on large numbers of them, are on file with the University of Michigan Assessment Archive Project (UMAAP).

A few years ago, an international group of more than thirty researchers was formed under the auspices of a not-for-profit corporation, interRAI, dedicated to research and policy development in elder care. At present, researchers from sixteen countries—Canada, the Czech Republic, Denmark, Finland, France, Germany, Iceland, Italy, Japan, Norway, the Netherlands, Spain, Sweden, Switzerland, the United Kingdom, and the United States—participate in this initiative, which is made possible because even definitions and training are comparable across national borders. Its "fellows," as they are known, and their local collaborators direct their attention most especially to the frail elderly population. They began by translating the RAI into eleven languages, thereby allowing for its use in a large number of nations. This permitted each to have a better appreciation of the unique needs of that country in the long-term institutional setting as well as the opportunity to compare its requirements and its systems of care with those of other nations. Furthermore, by having data at hand, a process of prioritization by nations was made possible. For example, a relatively inexpensive intervention applicable to the needs of a large number of individuals could be chosen rather than an expensive intervention directed to the needs of just a few.

The investigators at interRAI have developed or are designing assessment tools for use in multiple other sites of care, including the home and the community, the hospital, the assisted living setting, and the mental health facility. These forms have many items and domains that are identical or nearly so to the original RAI. These assessment tools "cross-talk" and will, when completed, make possible a person-specific rather than a site-specific assessment of need and care planning (Steel, Sherwood, and Ribbe, 1997). This will in turn optimize the capability of making a directed needs-based series of decisions in the care of a unique person and of grouping data elements to allow for effective targeting of specific interventions to groups and subgroups, especially the frailest elderly, across settings.

As Hirdes, Zimmerman, Hallman, and Soucie (1998) noted, outcome measures have been developed for use with the RAI instruments. They include the Cognitive Performance Scale (Morris and others, 1994), the Resource Utilization Groups (RUG-III) (Fries and others, 1994), and the Index of Social Engagement (Mor and others, 1995). Longitudinal studies are under way in several countries to assess both the mental health and the quality of life of nursing home residents. The adoption of an RAI series of instruments by many if not most nations, and the associated outcome measures, will allow for the rational design of systems of care for the frail elderly and analysis to support the best possible outcomes for the least expenditure. For example, the RUG-III developed by Fries and colleagues allows for the explanation of 55 percent of the variance in resource use in long-term care facilities. Carpenter and others (1997) from the United Kingdom have illustrated that the RUG resource use case mix system explains how nursing time is distributed among residents of long-term care facilities in the same way, although characteristics of the services and the amount and training of staff varies enormously. The clinical characteristics of the individuals served determines resource use regardless of which country these persons reside in.

In addition, care plans that warrant review and revision may be identified by any number of mechanisms. Simple comparisons of populations of countries may highlight important issues that require more detailed consideration. For example, Ljunggren, Phillips, and Sgadari (1997) reported marked variation in the use of patient restraints in nursing homes. Fewer than 9 percent of the persons in long-term care settings in Denmark, Iceland, and Japan are restrained, in contrast to 15 to 17 percent of those in France, Italy, Sweden, and the United States and almost 40 percent of individuals in Spain. These differences persist even when populations are adjusted for physical and cognitive abilities.

One of the most important potential uses of RAI data is likely the initiative developed by Mor and colleagues at Brown University in Providence, Rhode Island. They have meshed drug use data with data provided by the RAI describing patient characteristics. This enterprise, known as the Systematic Assessment of Geriatric Drug Use via Epidemiology (SAGE), allows for the matching of patient need with drug intervention (Bernabei, Gambassi, and Mor, 1998). Not long ago, this group reported that a very significant number of persons in nursing homes in the United States with a diagnosis of cancer who complain of pain daily fail to receive adequate analgesia or even any analgesic agent at all (Bernabei and others, 1998). This study was subsequently reported on the front page of the *New York Times* and *USA Today* and covered by CNN and a number of other worldwide television networks. It was commented on in an editorial in the *Wall Street Journal* and, perhaps most significant of all, a *Doonesbury* cartoon strip, widely read in the United States and throughout much of the developed world. A detailed analysis of pain management in several nations is now in process. Thus RAI instruments designed by an international group of investigators can be used to uncover issues of considerable importance in a single nation and others that are common to many nations. It may even draw the public's attention to these issues and effect change.

As all of us age, we stare frailty in the face. Nations will be required to address the needs of tens of millions of us everywhere in the world who are approaching this stage of life. They will be required to do so in the most cost-effective manner if they are to do what they must to be great nations who assure all their citizens the opportunity to achieve the highest quality of life over a span now approaching a century in duration. Each nation shares this endeavor with all others by talking the same language and desiring the same ideals even as programs and policies are adapted to the individual cultures that sprinkle the globe. Each nation's goals will be achieved by collaboration on an international level never before possible but now readily available. Such collaboration will allow all nations to share in the successes of their neighbors throughout the world, allowing each to be not only an effective provider of care at home but also a partner in the care of all humanity.

References

Bernabei, R., Gambassi, G., and Mor, V. "The SAGE Database: Introducing Functional Outcomes in Geriatric Pharmaco-Epidemiology." *Journal of the American Geriatrics Society,* 1998, *46,* 250–252.

Bernabei, R., and others. "Management of Pain in Elderly Patients with Cancer." *Journal of the American Medical Association,* 1998, *279,* 1877–1882.

Bodnar, A. G., and others. "Extension of Life-Span by Introduction of Telomerase into Normal Human Cells." *Science,* 1998, *279,* 349–352.

Brundtland, G. H. Address to the 102nd session of the Executive Board of the World Health Organization, Geneva, May 18, 1998.

Carpenter, G. I., and others. "RUG III and Resource Allocation: Comparing the Relationship of Direct Care Time with Patient Characteristics in Five Countries." *Age and Ageing,* 1997, *26* (suppl. 2), 61–65.

Fleg, J. L., and others. "Impact of Age on the Cardiovascular Response to Dynamic Upright Exercise in Healthy Men and Women." *Journal of Applied Physiology,* 1995, *78,* 890–900.

Fries, B. E., and others. "Refining a Case-Mix Measure for Nursing Homes: Resource Utilization Groups (RUG-III)." *Medical Care,* 1994, *32,* 668–685.

Hawes, C., and others. "Development of the Nursing Home Resident Assessment Instrument in the USA." *Age and Ageing,* 1997, *26* (suppl. 2), 19–27.

Hayflick, L. "The Limited In Vitro Lifetime of Human Diploid Cell Strains." *Experimental Cell Research,* 1965, *37,* 614–636.

Hayflick, L. *How and Why We Age.* New York: Ballantine Books, 1996.

Hirdes, J. P., Zimmerman, D., Hallman, K. G., and Soucie, P. S. "Use of the MDS Quality Indicators to Assess Quality of Care in Industrial Settings." *Canadian Journal of Quality in Health Care,* 1998, *14,* 5–11.

Kinsella, K., and Taeuber, C. M. *An Aging World II.* Washington, D.C.: U.S. Bureau of the Census, 1992.

Ljunggren, G., Phillips, C. D., and Sgadari, A. "Comparison of Restraint Use in Nursing Homes in Eight Countries." *Age and Ageing,* 1997, *26* (suppl. 2), 43–47.

Mor, V., and others. "The Structure of Social Engagement Among Nursing Home Residents." *Journals of Gerontology and Psychological Sciences,* 1995, *50,* 1–8.

Morris, J. N., and others. "MDS Cognitive Performance Scale." *Journal of Gerontology,* 1994, *49,* 1117–1182.

Ribbe, M. W., and others. "Nursing Homes in 10 Nations: A Comparison Between Countries and Settings." *Age and Aging,* 1997, *26* (suppl. 2), 3–12.

Steel, K. "Research on Aging. An Agenda for All Nations Individually and Collectively." *Journal of the American Medical Association,* 1997, *278,* 1374–1375.

Steel, K., Sherwood, S., and Ribbe, M. W. "The Future. A Person-Specific Standardized Assessment Instrument." *Age and Aging,* 1997, *26* (suppl. 2), 119–125.

Vita, A. J., Terry, R. B., Hubert, H. B., and Fries, J. F. "Aging, Health Risks, and Cumulative Disability." *New England Journal of Medicine,* 1998, *338,* 1035–1041.

CHAPTER FORTY-ONE

The Relationship Between Oceans and Human Health

James D. Watkins, Anwar Huq

Admiral James D. Watkins, U.S. Navy (Ret.), *after serving as Chief of Naval Operations under President Reagan and Secretary of Energy under President Bush, became President of the Joint Oceanographic Institutions (JOI) in 1993. He concurrently serves as President of the Consortium for Oceanographic Research and Education (CORE), a large group of public and private oceanographic research institutions he helped bring together in 1994 to provide an effective and unified voice, at the national level, in support of expanded ocean research. These institutions make up most of the U.S. ocean science and technology community.*

Anwar Huq, PhD, Associate Professor at the University of Maryland Biotechnology Institute and Director of its UNESCO-sponsored Microbiology Resources Center, is an authority in cholera transmission and is currently working on the use of remote sensing in determining human health and cholera relationships to climate change. He has written more than sixty articles and has worked in close collaboration with Dr. Rita Colwell, Director of the U.S. National Science Foundation (NSF), on methods for cholera detection and intervention.

Recent discoveries in ocean science and medical research have shown that these two areas of science are pervasively and powerfully linked. The oceans drive the earth's climate and influence global warming, with the potential to generate major natural disasters via hurricanes, tsunamis, and El Niño–related storms. Anthropogenic and climate-related events have also been implicated, directly or indirectly, in harmful algal blooms that can endanger human health by production of potentially lethal toxins in coastal waters and contaminating seafood resources. Yet new biochemicals and pharmaceuticals from the sea have been discovered, with new findings occurring at a rapid rate involving compounds that hold promise in the fight against some of the worst diseases afflicting humankind, such as leukemia and other forms of cancer. Marine organisms are attractive models and excellent tools for medical research because they can provide novel ways to improve the public health and welfare.

The connection between the oceans and human health has received significant attention; several conferences have highlighted advances in molecular marine biology and biotechnology. At one meeting, "Global Perspectives on the Health of Ocean Resources," held at Woods Hole, Massachusetts, in 1996, Admiral James Watkins, one of the authors and President of the Consortium for Oceanographic Research and Education (CORE), presented a "road map" to the untapped wealth offered by the oceans for human health, citing their role in the global climate and its predictability, coastal weather forecasting, and marine biomaterials, among other things. Historically, none of the topics mentioned by Admiral Watkins has found a place on the national science and technology agenda for the United States. However, we strongly feel that each is long overdue for enhanced resource allocation by the U.S. government.

Dr. Jonathan Patz of Johns Hopkins University and his collaborators at the University of Maryland, University of South Florida, Pennsylvania State University, University of Delaware, and several overseas research institutions have been studying the relationship between human health and climate change (Seas and others, 2000). Dr. Rita Colwell, Professor of Microbiology at the University of Maryland and currently Director of the U.S. National Science Foundation (NSF), has demonstrated a close relationship between sea surface temperature and cholera cases in Bangladesh, in collaboration with colleagues at the Johns Hopkins University and the NASA Ames Laboratory and in several countries, including Bangladesh, India, Mexico, and Peru (Colwell, 1996; Lobitz and others, 2000). But the issue of global climate and world health goes well beyond disease and epidemiology. Consider the impact of major floods or drought on regional agriculture, particularly food production and availability. The El Niño phenomenon, characterized by a weakening of the easterly trade winds and increased sea surface temperatures in the eastern Pacific, is linked to extensive crop damage in Indonesia, Australia, Africa, and North and South America. By the same token, longer-term effects may have occurred several years ago when summer flooding of the Mississippi and its tributaries occurred in the midst of the growing season in the Midwest, the U.S. breadbasket.

To the extent that public health depends on the nature and variability of climate, either in controlling disease vectors and their geographical spread or affecting crop yield, it is clear that understanding and predicting ocean dynamics is a key but relatively unrecognized factor in need of development. Similarly ready for development is the more precise forecasting of coastal weather. Unlike the prediction of global climate, weather prediction is focused on scales that are very short in time, with localized geographical impact. Nonetheless, with more than half of the U.S. population residing in coastal areas, the impacts of coastal hazards on the economy and public health are daunting. Some forecasters suggest that in fifty years, 75 percent of the world's population (which may well be half again as large as it is today) will live within 90 miles of a coastline (UN Conference on Environment and Development, 1992). We have only to look at the consequences of hurricanes like Agnes, Hugo, Andrew, Georges, and Mitch to see the immediate and devastating impact of such events on public health and economic well-being. The utility of coastal weather forecasting, however, goes well beyond knowing when and where a hurricane or tsunami will strike.

Consider what is now standard operating procedure for many of the Norwegian salmon farmers. As they regularly feed and harvest their fish crops, they simultaneously monitor the coastal ocean, using a national ocean observatory that reports a wide range of physical, biological, and chemical properties of the ocean along their coast. With this information in hand, the salmon farmers can decide when to move their stocks up into fjords to avoid abnormally warm or toxic incoming waters. Extending this cost-effective concept of accurate coastal weather forecasting not only helps with preparatory measures for hurricanes and tsunamis but also adds new environmental parameters that can be used to prevent epidemics of disease for fish as well as for humans (National Academy of Sciences, 1999).

Recent studies have shown a strong correlation between cholera outbreaks and adjacent coastal ocean conditions (Ramamurthy and others, 1993; Tauxe and others, 1994). Most of the major epidemics that have occurred around the world have originated in coastal areas, including the 1991 cholera outbreak that originated in the coastal region of Lima, Peru, and devastated Latin America. The satellite imaging of sea surface temperature (SST), sea surface height, and plankton has been instrumental in establishing the link between appearance of cholera bacteria in coastal waters and cholera epidemics in Bangladesh. An important finding, established over a twenty-year period of research by Colwell, Huq, Lobitz, and others (Colwell and Huq, 1994; Huq and Colwell, 1996; Lobitz and others, 2000) made it possible to link the sporadic nature of cholera epidemics with climate and climate events, such as El Niño. Zooplankton are known to harbor the bacterium, and zooplankton blooms follow phytoplankton blooms. Thus remote sensing can be employed to determine the appearance of zooplankton and of cholera outbreaks with ocean color, which is a measurement of chlorophyll content. Sea surface temperature data obtained through remote sensing has been found to be directly correlated with the occurrence of cholera in Bangladesh. From clinical data and satellite imagery, it was observed that when the temperature of the sea surface rises, cholera cases are recorded.

By combining data gathered on SST, phytoplankton, zooplankton, and clinical cases of cholera, a correlation of selected climatological and oceanographic factors is being used to develop a global model for predicting conditions conducive to cholera outbreaks. The disease can be addressed effectively by intervention and prevention efforts if a better understanding can be obtained of the complex factors governing the survival and persistence of *Vibrio cholerae* in the environment. The key to this understanding lies in improved monitoring, as well as better knowledge of the interactions among global climate, ocean currents, coastal weather, and disease.

There is an entirely different set of resources for which we should turn more aggressively to the sea. These resources are made up of the class of materials, including natural products, that either derive from or mimic those occurring naturally in marine organisms. Many biotechnological applications of biometabolites, natural biopharmaceuticals from the ocean, have generated significant interest in the search for novel therapeutics for many diseases such as cancer, AIDS, cardiovascular disease, and central nervous system disease. It is estimated that marine organisms are in fact the source of 50 percent of all potential cancer drug discoveries. The diversity and abundance of biomedicines from the sea is enormous. For example, organisms living at temperatures ranging from 25 degrees to 400 degrees Celsius in deep-sea hydrothermal vents contain unique proteins that play a role in the survival and reproduction of these organisms in such hostile environments. What can we learn from these organisms and chemical compounds, and how can we capitalize on them? Nature has also developed unique capabilities for attaching unlike materials, such as mussels to rocks. Research on the applicability of these potentially powerful resources to medical needs has already proved to be commercially productive. By the same token, nature has developed extraordinary fouling-resistant materials that could, undoubtedly, be applied to biomedical research. The question is simple: What is there about organisms living without sunlight, under high pressure, in the extreme cold or intense heat, and in a very salty environment, the latter virtually identical to that of human blood, that could be of value to the medical community? Future discoveries, without doubt, will be made from studies of these sea creatures.

To establish a new baseline of reference for enhancing molecular marine biology and biotechnology research, the U.S. National Academy of Sciences and its Institute of Medicine established a joint committee in May 1997 to develop an integrated research strategy to address the wide-ranging, ocean-driven issues affecting human health. A workshop titled "The Ocean's Role in Human Health" was held subsequently by an expert panel, including members of both the medical and marine sciences communities. Connections between the ocean and human health were examined, and the state of knowledge of these links was assessed. Furthermore, current and future strategies to predict and respond to future health needs and threats were presented. The report emanating from this workshop (National Academy of Sciences, 1999) summarized the discussions and conclusions and gave an excellent overview of the issues and future needs with regard to oceans and human health. Some of the significant findings follow.

The oceans, through the interplay of currents, tides, and human activities, now threaten public health by distributing viruses, bacteria, protozoa, and algal toxins present in or discharged from these bodies of water. Human exposure occurs through direct contact with seawater, ingestion of contaminated seafood, or aerosol intake. Nutrient loading from runoff poses a serious threat to coastal waters by promoting algal growth and oxygen depletion. Commercially important filter-feeding organisms, such as oysters, crabs, and clams, are particularly vulnerable to marine pathogens and sewage contamination and pose a danger to human health. Transport via the seafood trade and in the ballast waters of ships can also introduce and spread new pathogens that can cause ecological, economic, and health problems. The report recognizes the health threats posed by severe climate and weather events related to the ocean, including tsunamis, hurricanes, storm surges, flooding, high winds, and El Niño. Accelerated global warming may increase the severity and frequency of intense storms, cause greater incidences of disease, blooms of harmful algae, and extreme episodes of heat, threatening the availability of food and fresh water. The report also emphasizes the important contribution of marine biodiversity to biomedical resources. With the need for new drugs to combat antibiotic-resistant bacteria, the sea offers a wealth of potentially new and urgently needed pharmaceuticals. However, many challenges need to be overcome for collecting, testing, and replicating marine compounds. Marine organisms are already being used as models for basic research on biological and disease processes. For example, the unusually large diameter of the giant axon in the squid neuron is already facilitating the study of the nerve physiology. Using marine models, scientists expect to learn more about diseases such as diabetes and cancer, as well as fundamental biochemical processes within the human body.

A strategy for improved understanding of the role of the oceans in human health should include several key components: a historical baseline of high-quality ocean and health observations; new technologies, such as satellite oceanography and molecular probes, and improved older methods in drifting and moored sensors, biological measurements, DNA probes, and antibody and toxin detection tests; and increased exploration for new drugs and pharmaceutically active compounds, with better understanding of natural marine toxin biology, development of new culturing techniques, and encouragement of training and research to expand our knowledge of marine organisms.

To address these challenges, the newly enacted National Oceanographic Partnership Program (NOPP) can be employed to help in the integration of U.S. federal ocean science and technology investments among the nine federal research agencies, approximately sixty academic institutions, and other state and private sector entities that have a stake in ocean science and technology. In the first two fiscal years of its existence, 1997–1998, around $100 million (in addition to the base of about $500 million across all federal agencies) has been provided equally by the U.S. Congress and private sector sources to carry out cross-cutting ocean research initiatives through NOPP. This marked the first real growth in ocean science research in fifteen years. NOPP is governed by the high-level National Ocean Research Leadership Council, representing each participating Federal agency, and is chaired by the Secretary of the Navy, with the NOAA Administrator as its Vice Chair. This council is advised by the Ocean Research Advisory Panel, made up of prominent scientists, public policy officials, state representatives, marine industry leaders and nongovernment stakeholders. The permanent Interagency Working Group from within all the participating federal agencies is responsible for the day-to-day implementation of the program as directed by the Leadership Council.

Having defined the need for a new understanding of ocean and human health issues and having fixed a new process with which to manage an integrated national and international partnership to satisfy the need, one should now ask what mechanism is to be employed to gather, assess, and provide access to all necessary scientific data. The scientific community can benefit most from ocean observations synthesized into a modern, sophisticated, quality-assured, and accessible database and a global, integrated ocean-observing system. Continuous data gathering on the nature and variability of the world's oceans will be critical for accurate weather forecasting, sensible coastal zone management, sound and sustained development of fisheries, oil and gas recovery and transportation, recreation, and defense of national interests.

Members of the U.S. Congress during the 1998 International Year of the Ocean said, our nation must "integrate existing and new ocean observing systems into a coherent, single system to address national needs." With few exceptions, the U.S. national agenda for ocean observation is composed of separate, short-term, focused scientific studies. But the United States has no national, comprehensive, long-term, continuous commitment to ocean observations. A serious and dedicated effort is now under way, in coordination with industry and the international research community, to develop such a capability, building on, but not impeding the progress of, our existing national system for oceanographic research and development. A preliminary plan sets the foundation for long-term ocean observations to meet research and operational requirements. Implementation will require an interdisciplinary approach to systems concept, design, and construction. Better climate change predictions, with all that this implies for sustained economic prosperity globally, can be realized and could be one of the twenty-first century's greatest achievements.

References

Colwell, R. R. "Global Climate and Infectious Disease: The Cholera Paradigm. *Science*, 1996, *274*, 2025–2031.

Colwell, R. R., and Huq, A. "Environmental Reservoir of Vibrio Cholera: The Causative Agents of Cholera." In M. E. Wilson, R. Levins, and A. Spielman (eds.), *Disease in Evolution, Global Changes and Emergence of Infectious Diseases.* Annals of the New York Academy of Sciences, 1994, 44–54.

Huq, A., and Colwell, R. R. "Vibrios in the Marine and Estuarine Environment: Tracking of Vibrio Cholerae." *Journal of Ecosystem Health,* 1996, *2*, 198–214.

Lobitz, B. L., and others. "Climate and Infectious Disease: Use of Remote Sensing for Detection of V. Cholerae by Indirect Measurement." *Proceedings of the National Academy of Sciences*, 2000, *97*, 1438–1443.

National Academy of Sciences. *From Monsoons to Microbes: Understanding the Ocean's Role in Human Health.* Washington, D.C.: National Academy Press, 1999.

Ramamurthy, T., and others. "Emergence of Novel Strains of V. Cholerae with Epidemic Potential in Southern and Eastern India." *Lancet,* 1993, *341*, 703–705.

Seas, C., and others. "New Insights on the Emergence of Cholera in Latin America During 1991: The Peruvian Experience." *The American Journal of Tropical Medicine and Hygiene*, (submitted).

Tauxe, R., and others. "The Latin American Epidemic." In K. Wachsmuth, P. Blake, and O. Olsvik (eds.), *Vibrio Cholerae and Cholerae; Molecular to Global Perspectives.* Washington, D.C.: American Society for Microbiology Press, 1994, 321–344.

United Nations Conference on Environment and Development, Agenda 21, Chapter 17.

CHAPTER FORTY TWO

Careers in Public Health and Medical Care

Alexander H. Williams III

Alexander H. Williams III *is a shareholder in the executive recruiting firm of Witt/Kieffer, Ford, Hadelman, and Lloyd. He is Director of the firm's physician executive recruiting practice. He is also Chairman of the Board of the Educational Commission on Foreign Medical Graduates. Previously, he had a long career in the management of health care organizations and associations.*

A career is the accumulation of a lifelong set of professional experiences. Early career choices focus on a discipline, such as medicine, nursing, public health, management, law, or engineering. Careers begin with specialized education and training and require mastery of an ever-expanding body of knowledge. Careers advance along responsibility and leadership axes. Individuals begin their careers on specific tasks. Mastery of tasks or jobs leads to increased responsibility and a broadened point of view. This in turn leads to greater influence. Greater influence places one in leadership positions.

Successful careers are seldom predictable, and successful people are highly flexible and adaptable in what they choose to do. They use their professional training, their experience, and the knowledge they accumulate to ferret out opportunities. They allow their imaginations free reign to grasp the possibilities, and they are ever alert to their changing environment. These traits will be crucial in the twenty-first century as the pace of technological and social change accelerates.

Initial career choice and subsequent career decisions require individual judgment about both need and demand. What are an individual's skills and aptitudes? What opportunities exist to fulfill a need, and will there be sufficient economic support to make the opportunity a reality?

SOME ASSUMPTIONS ABOUT HEALTH IN THE TWENTY-FIRST CENTURY

The discussion in this chapter is based on several underlying assumptions about the environment of the twenty-first century.

- Wide economic, social, and developmental gaps will persist between rich and poor societies as well as between rich and poor within the same society.

- The acquisition, storage, and retrieval of information on a massive scale will lead to new approaches to health on every level and will enable growth and development in technology and biomedical research.

- The pace of technological change will accelerate in every conceivable way, and much of the focus of that development will be health-related. Some technological changes will have unanticipated health consequences, both positive and negative.

- Biomedical research will continue to achieve dramatic and far-reaching results and will continue to attract significant public and private resources.

- Barriers to international travel and communication will continue to disappear.

- The human race will continue to be its own worst enemy, and there will be no shortage of aggression and intolerance, along with infectious diseases and natural disasters.

- New problems will arise as the unanticipated consequence of progress.

THE INTERNATIONALIZATION OF PUBLIC HEALTH AND MEDICAL CARE CAREERS

American professionals, particularly physicians, have not seen time spent on international assignments as career-enhancing or relevant, but other nationals have understood that a career is defined by what one does, not by where one does it, and so they avidly seek opportunities wherever these may occur.

The increasing realization that only a global approach to health problems can be successful will change insular attitudes. Instantaneous communication and access to worldwide data will force people who want successful careers to have a worldwide focus. The action will be global, the need for specific talent will be great worldwide, and opportunities to tackle key problems will not respect national boarders.

Especially for careers that focus on caregiving, barriers to achieving true internationalization exist, including these:

• Lack of comparability between professional training programs in different nations

• Inconsistent credentialing and licensure requirements

• Political barriers erected to prevent "brain drain" or to restrict entry into high-paying professions

• Language and cultural barriers

Nevertheless, the language of science is universal, and important forces are at work to eliminate or minimize the barriers.

CAREER OPPORTUNITIES IN PUBLIC HEALTH AND MEDICAL CARE

The following discussion will focus on broad areas for careers rather than on specific jobs or professions. Disciplines cut across all careers, and inevitably the barriers between disciplines will shift and blend.

One way to think of the array of potential career opportunities is to consider the target populations. A helpful analogy is wholesale versus retail. Public health planners and policymakers operate on the wholesale level, focusing their efforts on the widest possible populations. At the other end of the scale, caregivers focus on individual needs. Somewhere in the middle are epidemiologists, public health educators, and others.

Leadership and Management

Leadership and vision will be even more indispensable in the twenty-first century than they were in the twentieth. Good leaders combine their disciplinary training, the expertise they gain early in their career, and the wisdom they gather with experience. Leadership will come from individuals who have earned the responsibility of leadership through their lifelong success.

Management is an overarching function that uses special skills to bring together people, financial resources, information, planning, and communication into effective organizations. Like practitioners in any other discipline, managers need specialized education and training. Both public health and medical care will require strong management at all levels. Career managers in public health and medical care will be people who combine the detailed knowledge of specific disciplines and situations with management skill and training.

Information Management

The critical underpinning of all careers is information management, which is a career in itself. The twenty-first century will be the age of information. What we know is the basis of all we do, but as the available information increases exponentially, it has the capacity to both paralyze us and liberate us. How information is acquired, stored, analyzed, made available, and interpreted is the work of many specialists. Decisions about resource commitments, the education of the end users about the possibilities and limitations of information tools, and the integration of informatics into the fabric of all other careers will be the work of senior leaders in information management.

Public Health Monitoring and Evaluation

The worldwide monitoring of health and the dissemination of this information in ways that allow rapid and accurate responses will be an important career track.

Careers in public health monitoring will begin at the data gathering, analysis, and program design level and will culminate at the international policy and leadership level. The basic training required will be in one of the professional disciplines, especially medicine, nursing, and public health.

Monitoring is an important tool for evaluating the severity of problems and the effectiveness of the response. Individuals who have a balanced view and are capable of providing information in a nonjudgmental way will assume leadership.

Environmental Protection

The need to protect and enhance the environment will create many career opportunities. The most successful and influential careers will be those that focus on both problems and solutions. For example, many approaches to increasing the world's food supply have negative environmental consequences. Yet world hunger is a major public health issue. Careers in agronomy, including research and education in agricultural methods, water protection, and food storage and distribution, will have a large impact on world hunger.

A career in environmental matters will require basic training in a scientific discipline coupled with a strong grounding in specific environmental issues. Because of the need for effective interaction with many diverse disciplines, leaders in environmental protection will have broad-based points of view and the ability to balance and evaluate the competitive benefits of different policy approaches.

Health Promotion and Education

Traditional health care disciplines engage in health promotion and education all the time, either specifically or as a by-product of their caregiving and public health activities. But health promotion and education are legitimate career tracks in and of themselves. These careers will attract people from an eclectic group of disciplines.

Collaboration between health content experts and individuals with expertise in information management, communication, media, and the culture and lifestyle of target populations will have the most beneficial impact. This collaboration will create new careers, resulting in health education and promotion products that are problem- and population-specific.

Communicable Diseases

The world will continue to be at risk from communicable disease in the twenty-first century. Careers in the prevention, surveillance, and control of communicable disease will continue to be important, challenging, and lifelong. They will require political as well as scientific leadership, not to mention the courage to deliver messages no one wants to hear. Though traditionally the province of biomedical research, epidemiology, and infectious disease, individuals in many other disciplines will be attracted to this area, including health educators, environmentalists, engineers, sociologists, information managers, and health caregivers at the most basic levels.

Occupational Health

The twenty-first century will produce new occupational health problems related to stresses of increased individual productivity and nontraditional work styles. The widespread use of telecommuting is one example.

Occupational health will provide exciting career opportunities not only in traditional workplace prevention and caregiving but also in areas like psychosocial research. The steady stream of stories of workplace violence suggest that there is much we do not know about how and why different individuals react under stress, and we can be sure that the twenty-first century will produce new ways to stress us all.

Occupational health will increasingly become a function of top management, reflecting the importance of these issues to the success of the enterprise. Organizations will be increasingly willing to commit resources to making the workplace and the work experience positive, safe, and healthy. Research that studies and anticipates workplace problems will be indispensable. For example, the occupational health problems in space laboratories will be just as important and infinitely harder to solve than the logistical problems of getting the laboratories into space in the first place.

Research

Research is the engine that drives creativity. Careers in research have always been fundamental to health, and the twenty-first century will be no different. In a way, careers that have change as their focus are the very careers most protected from change.

The scope of research relevant to health will broaden as we tackle the health consequences of various social dysfunctions. For example, the numerous disciplines in the engineering profession will have much to contribute to solutions in housing, workplace safety, transportation safety, adjustment to disabilities, food production, waste disposal, and water quality and distribution.

Biomedical research at the basic science and clinical levels has attracted the best and the brightest in many disciplines and will continue to do so. But research in health services, the economics of health care delivery, and the problems of specific populations will contribute in increasingly important ways and will represent new opportunities for careers.

Caregiving

Careers that focus on the health problems of individuals will be important and satisfying in the twenty-first century, but different. Medicine, nursing, and the allied health professions will continue to treat individuals, but the focus and styles of those careers will change dramatically. Acute care will be greatly affected by technology in all specialties, with the net result being less and less institutionally based care and many fewer encounters between caregivers and their patients.

In the industrialized world, caregivers and their careers will be affected by two growing trends. The first is the rapidly increasing cost of caregiving. Although different societies devote greater or lesser portions of their gross domestic product to health care, the rising cost is a major public policy issue everywhere. Caregiver careers will be profoundly affected by twenty-first-century solutions to the issue of cost. At a minimum, there will be continued downward pressure on incomes and upward pressure on productivity. Functions will shift from higher-income professionals to lower-income professionals. "Alternative" medicine will grow and thrive. New technology will improve the speed of diagnosis, increase caregivers' productivity, and reduce the need for personal intervention through improved monitoring techniques. The basic solution, however, to the high cost of caregiving is to reduce the need for it—hence the emphasis in this chapter on careers that are oriented toward public health rather than caregiving.

The second trend is the aging of the population in the industrialized world. The demand for specialized caregivers for the elderly will grow, as will the need for specialized research and product development. The allied health professions, including nontraditional providers, will be in the forefront of caregiving to the elderly and the chronically ill. Nursing will also be a profession in continuing demand, and independent nurse practitioners will see their role and status grow, especially in health maintenance and patient education. Most primary care physicians will practice geriatrics, and specialists will have to adapt their specialties to the needs of the elderly and the chronically ill.

A major problem in providing care to the elderly in the industrialized world is the availability of labor. As people live longer, we will find ourselves in a four-generation society with only one generation active in the workforce. The present models of caring for the elderly are labor intensive, and society may conceivably run out of caregivers regardless of price. The response will be to reduce the dependence of this population cohort on hands-on caregivers as much as possible. Thus we will see important advances in more appropriate housing, creative uses of telemedical techniques, and research in geriatric-focused fields, all with the goal of meeting the needs of the elderly and maintaining their independence. The implications of this will be a boom in careers that have not been considered health careers, such as specialized product development, engineering, architecture, and recreation and leisure activities.

In the less developed world, caregiving will be more focused on acute problems, which will be reflected in health careers in those societies. It is unlikely, however, that these societies will go through the explosion of acute health care investment that was typical of the post–World War II Western world, especially as the public health infrastructure improves.

CONCLUSION

The twenty-first century will be a time of almost incalculable opportunity to improve health and functionality, but it will also be a time of constrained global resources and avid competition from other economic sectors. How these resources can best be deployed to seize opportunity and benefit the greatest number of people will require leadership and vision.

The maintenance of health and functionality through all stages of human life is a universal priority for all cultures and societies. It will be no less so in the twenty-first century. Careers that focus on health will therefore be important, rewarding, and of high social value. They will require technical mastery, personal energy and commitment, and great leadership skill.

PART THREE

Organizations, Management, Leadership, and Partnerships

CHAPTER FORTY-THREE

Shaping the Future of Health Through Global Partnerships

William C. Richardson, John P. Allegrante

William C. Richardson, PhD, *is President and Chief Executive Officer of the W. K. Kellogg Foundation of Battle Creek, Michigan. He is former President of the Johns Hopkins University and has served in key leadership posts at Pennsylvania State University and the University of Washington in Seattle.*

John P. Allegrante, PhD, *is a professor of health education at Teachers College, Columbia University, New York City, where he has been a member of the faculty since 1979. He is a past President of the Society for Public Health Education and has served as an adviser to the WHO Regional Office for Europe and the Verona Initiative.*

It is abundantly clear that the world of the near future will be a vastly different place than that of the world we know today. The rapid pace of economic and political change, together with continuing development of communications technologies and biomedical science, are transforming global relations and the possibilities for improving the human condition. Moreover, the devolution of central governments throughout the nations of the world is creating a context of both challenge and opportunity for developing exciting new ways of meeting the needs of people.

Advancing the cause of health in this complex, interdependent, and global society will require a new commitment to cooperation among the private, governmental, and nonprofit sectors. If it can be argued that the world of the twentieth century has been a world of competition and conflict, surely there is opportunity for the world of the twenty-first century to be a world of cooperation and collaboration. Central to this new view of the world will be global partnerships.

This chapter will define the concept of partnership, briefly describe several examples of how partnerships are shaping creative responses to pressing health needs, and conclude by discussing the promise of global partnerships to shape health in the new century.

THE CONCEPT OF PARTNERSHIP

Although we believe that partnerships have the potential to address much of what has been wrong with past efforts to achieve improvements in global health, we must first understand the concept of partnerships. This can be best accomplished by answering three questions: Why do we need partnerships? Where can partnerships be most effective? How and by what principles should a good partnership operate?

Why Do We Need Partnerships?

Simply put, we need partnership because most of the problems we will face in the twenty-first century will require multisectoral, multidisciplinary, and multicomponent efforts. No single sector has either the resources or the capacities alone to work effectively to address the complex problems we confront. Even if health professionals, hospitals, health departments, and ministries of health all did their jobs, we now know that the promotion of health and prevention of disease requires broader efforts to influence the social conditions that determine health. To advance health, we need not only the health care sector but also the synergy that is created when the private sector, government, and nonprofit organizations work together to forge policies that can shape the global economic and environmental conditions that will promote and sustain health. Such synergy is what the World Health Organization (1997) speaks of when it talks about partnerships for health in the twenty-first century making 2 plus 2 equal 5. Put another way, a partnership has the potential to create added value and be greater than the sum of its parts.

Where Should a Partnership Focus Its Energy?

Understanding the *why* of partnerships is not enough; determining where a partnership should focus its energy is equally important. Should a partnership seek to improve the status of a health professions group? Should a partnership seek to improve relations among the community and providers of health services? Should a partnership seek to achieve local change or geographically broader goals when it comes to health?

The answers to such questions are likely to be complicated and will depend on how each participating organizational partner views the value of participation. One of the challenges in forming meaningful partnerships is the extent to which joining a partnership makes sense for any individual organizational entity. Notwithstanding, the focus of a partnership for health should be on filling the gaps that are too often left when government or the nonprofit sector works alone. Most successful partnerships aimed at improving health will, of necessity, need to focus on building social trust, social capital, and the community capacities for change that can be mobilized to meet community needs.

How and by What Principles Should a Good Partnership Operate?

In general terms, how a partnership works should represent a distinct departure from the status quo. By design, a good partnership should provide the freedom and wherewithal to break new ground, challenge accepted wisdom, and advance innovative solutions to solving problems that would not be otherwise solved through the efforts of any single group or sector.

Good partnerships seek out and solicit diverse new voices. Good partnerships are inclusive and strive to achieve consensus and equity. Ultimately, a good partnership should seek to build community capacity and civic trust. This means helping people help themselves and improve their communities by means of solutions that make the most sense to those living in the community. It means empowering people who have been excluded from the democratic process to get a seat at the table and engaging them in vigorous civic discourse that allows them to define the problem and seek practical solutions that they will embrace as their own.

But by what principles should a partnership operate? The Peter F. Drucker Foundation for Nonprofit Management recently convened a diverse group of twenty-eight leaders from public, private, and non-profit organizations at a symposium to discuss the future of public-private partnerships. Despite the wide spectrum of political perspectives represented by the participants, the group reached con-sensus on five key principles that underlie effective partnerships:

- Partners must understand not only the values, goals, and constraints of the partnership itself but also the values, goals, and constraints of the other partners.

- Partnerships must translate broad goals into measurable interim targets and time frames.

- Different issues require different types of partnerships.

- Partnerships rely not just on the clarity of mission but also on a mutual understanding of partners' roles.

- The three sectors of society (business, government, and the nonprofit sector) have different needs and objectives but must work together.

GOVERNMENT AND THE NONPROFIT SECTOR WORKING TOGETHER

Cooperation and partnership between government and the nonprofit sector have a long history. The earliest partnerships between govern-ment and the nonprofit sector enabled institutions of higher learning in the United States to take advantage of special tax provisions; dur-ing the nineteenth century, large cities, such as New York, would not have been able to cope with the poverty of their urban immigrant population were it not for the settlement houses and other nonprofit agencies whose budgets depended heavily on government subsidies; and throughout the history of the United States, Great Britain, and other democracies throughout the world, support from central gov-ernments for social programs administered by nonprofit organiza-tions and quasi-governmental agencies have enabled societies to provide care for the sick and needy. Indeed, great social legislation— the British National Health Service in the United Kingdom and the various other arrangements for the provision of health care throughout much of western Europe, as well as Medicare and Medicaid in the United States—has been possible in part because of the close relationships that have been established between government and the private and nonprofit sectors.

Against this backdrop, partnerships such as the three that follow illustrate the potential and power of alliances between government and both the private and nonprofit sectors to improve health.

Turning Point

In the early 1930s, the United States suffered through the Great Depression. In 1931, the W. K. Kellogg Foundation, a year after it was established, created one of the first partnerships—the Michigan Community Health Project (MCHP), which served seven counties and a quarter million people in south central Michigan. The MCHP served farm counties in an age before much of the population of those counties had electricity or indoor plumbing. Health programs of any sort were practically nonexistent. Schools and libraries were underdeveloped and inadequate. Yet the communities of these counties were rich in human resources. There was no shortage of teachers, librarians, doctors, dentists, nurses, or other community leaders with ideas. Moreover, the local economies of these counties were solid. What the Kellogg Foundation recognized, however, was that what was needed was an organizing focus, a logical way to arrange community resources and the talents of people into a useful system of public health care.

To create such a system, the MCHP brought doctors, nurses, and dentists together with mayors, ministers, well drillers, and dairy farmers. The MCHP opened up county health departments where none had existed. It formed citizens' councils that identified public health problems and engaged in debate to shape practical solutions for schools, hospitals, and libraries. For fourteen years, during which time it was able to create an infrastructure for the delivery of health and human services at the local level, the MCHP also served as a national model for systems change in public health.

The Kellogg Foundation's early success with the MCHP and enduring commitment to partnerships is today being reinvented with a contemporary partnership effort called Turning Point. Turning Point is a new partnership between the Kellogg Foundation and the Robert Wood Johnson Foundation—two of America's leading philanthropies—and forty-one communities in fourteen states. The goals of Turning Point are to help communities assess and determine what health services are best for their populations and to develop a means for communities to work with state officials to ensure better health care and better, more efficient use of community resources. This partnership is creating a framework for communities not only to find their collective voices in expressing needs but also to identify how services can be improved while saving money.

For example, in one location, state officials had assessed a community's health needs and determined that the community needed three new primary care clinics. However, after consulting the community, state officials decided that they did not need new clinics but rather new bus routes so that local people could reach existing facilities.

The Verona Initiative

Another example of emerging partnerships, created to influence health throughout Europe but with global implications, is the Verona Initiative (Bertinato, 1999). The Verona Initiative is an ambitious effort organized by the WHO Regional Office for Europe. The effort has been designed to operationalize WHO's agenda for health by supporting its European member states in taking the practical actions that will be necessary to improve the health of their populations. This partnership was formed to change the debate about health status in Europe in the wake of the political and economic upheavals of the 1990s experienced by many Europeans, particularly those living in eastern European nations.

This new debate has found expression in a strong pan-European dialogue that has brought together political, business, academic, and nongovernmental leaders to explore, develop, and extend what is known about the economic, social, and environmental influences on human health in an effort to implement a new "health investment" approach in Europe. The participating organizations of the Verona Initiative are diverse and include government authorities of the city and province of Verona and the Veneto region; four prestigious universities from the region; and the local health services, the Verona Teaching Hospital, the Italian Ministry of Health, and the Italian Ministry of Equal Opportunity. In addition, the participants of this unique partnership also include locally based private foundations and GlaxoWellcome, a major pharmaceutical concern. WHO and its collaborating centers, together with the Office for Public Management in London, provide organizing assistance.

Together these participants are working to use a set of guiding principles to bring about and benchmark changes in European member states' local, regional, and national policies that influence health. These principles include a focus on health, full public engagement, genuine intersectoral working, equity, sustainability, and a broad knowledge base. The Verona Initiative endeavors to create a political priority for health that focuses on health and not merely health care. Consequently, the initiative focuses attention on agriculture, education, housing, transportation, and other public policies and on how such policies can have an impact on population health. By benchmarking change, the Verona Initiative also seeks to achieve real accountability for population health gains and losses. Thus the agenda for change that this dialogue seeks to achieve includes highlighting the investment potential for health, increasing capacity for intersectoral action, creating new incentives for business and political leaders to make economic decisions that take health into account, and creating a new vision and new infrastructure for the new Europe's health promotion efforts.

In its first two years, the Verona Initiative powerfully influenced the debate about health in Europe and promises to shape how European leaders make health-friendly policy for years to come.

European Partnership Project on Tobacco Dependence

Another partnership that has begun to have a major impact on global health is the WHO's European Partnership Project on Tobacco Dependence. Begun in 1997, the project has been organized to reduce tobacco-related death and disease among dependent smokers. A coalition of numerous private, noncommercial, and public sector partners are currently supporting WHO in achieving implementation of several key strategic activities in four target countries, France, Germany, Poland, and the United Kingdom.

These strategic activities include tracking adult smoking status, regulation of tobacco products and tobacco dependence treatment products, working with private enterprises to promote smoke-free workplaces, supporting the implementation of evidence-based treatment of tobacco dependence, and public education designed to encourage and support smoking cessation.

Although partnerships such as the three just described hold great promise and may indeed be the key to shaping the future of global health, partnerships are not without problems. No private sector organization, nonprofit organization, or government should rush headlong into a partnership without considerable forethought. A good partnership, as we know from friendship or marriage, requires nurturing and compromise. Successful partnerships require full-time care and long-term commitment. Partnerships also require realistic expectations and a clear sense of purpose.

But such partnerships are enabling people to achieve in unison what could never be achieved in isolation or through government alone. Such partnerships are enabling organized collectives of people and their political representatives to speak loudly and effectively because they speak with one voice.

CONCLUSION

WHO's Jakarta Declaration (1997) stated that "we must break through traditional boundaries, within government sectors, between government and non-governmental organizations and between the public and private sector" (p. 55). Partnerships can be a powerful means by which we can achieve the ideals of the Jakarta Declaration. Strategic alliances and partnerships provide a wonderful and exciting way by which social change can be catalyzed.

But partnerships are not for the faint of heart. They require a leap of faith and the willingness to seek new truths, craft new paradigms. If we want to shape the global health agenda of tomorrow, we need to work today to transcend the narrow agendas of individual sectors and regions and create the kinds of partnerships that will strengthen civil society throughout the world. We need multilateral partnerships that bridge nations and peoples.

This means embracing the political devolution of government that has already been set in motion throughout much of the world. It means transferring authority, decision making, and responsibility for health from central governments to governments at the state, region, province, and local municipal levels and to the myriad partnerships that are now emerging to fill the gaps government alone cannot fill. In the end, the essential function of the public-private partnership in the new century is to facilitate that transfer by putting the tools for change and decision making in the hands of the parties closest to the problems and most directly affected by the solutions.

As the philosopher Arthur Schopenhauer once said, "Every truth passes through three stages before it is recognized. In the first, it is ridiculed, in the second it is opposed, and in the third it is regarded as self-evident" (Fitzhenry, 1993, p. 451). If it has not already been recognized, we believe the value of partnerships for global health will soon become self-evident.

References

Bertinato, L. "The Verona Initiative: A New 'Arena' for Debate on Health in Europe." *International Journal of Health Promotion and Education,* 1999, *6,* 19–20.

Fitzhenry, R. I., (ed.). *The Harper Book of Quotations.* (3rd ed.) New York: Harper Perennial, 1993.

Jakarta Declaration on Leading Health Promotion into the 21st Century. Promotion and Education, Vol IV, number 3, 1997, 55.

World Health Organization. *Partnerships for Health in the 21st Century: 2 + 2 = 5. New Players for a New Era.* WHO Jakarta Conference Working Paper. Geneva: World Health Organization, 1997.

Additional Reading

Davies, R. "Mobilising Business Through 'Partnerships for Health Promotion'—New Challenges and New Opportunities". *International Journal of Health Promotion and Education,* 1999, VI, 21–24.

Emerging Partnerships; New Ways in a New World. A symposium organized by the Peter F. Drucker Foundation for Nonprofit Management.

Lorange, P. Interactive Strategies—Alliances and Partnerships. *Long Range Planning,* 1996, *29,* 581–584.

O'Byrne, D. "The Power of Partnership in Health Promotion." *International Journal of Health Promotion and Education,* 1998, V, 7–8.

Richardson, W. C. *The Why, Where, and How of Partnerships.* Presented at Grantmakers in Health National Conference, Los Angeles, California, February 27, 1998.

Trowell, P. "New Partnerships for Health." *International Journal of Health Promotion and Education,* 1998, V, 38.

The Verona Initiative. *Investing for Health: The Economic, Social and Human Environment.* Arena Meeting II, 29 September–2 October 1999, Verona, Italy.

CHAPTER FORTY FOUR

The Role of Governments

Richard G. A. Feachem

Richard G. A. Feachem, CBE, PhD, DSc(Med), *is Director of the newly formed Institute for Global Health at the University of California, San Francisco, and UC Berkeley. He was formerly Dean of the London School of Hygiene and Tropical Medicine and Director for Health, Nutrition and Population at the World Bank. His interests are in international health and in corporate leadership and management. He has served on many boards and committees and has published extensively in health policy, epidemiology, and environmental health.*

> *A wise and frugal government, which shall restrain men from injuring one another, which shall leave them otherwise free to regulate their own pursuits of industry and improvement, and shall not take from the mouth of labor the bread it has earned—this is the sum of good government.*
>
> —Thomas Jefferson, First Inaugural Address, 1801

Jefferson hadn't a clue that two hundred years later, this same government would be the world's largest purchaser of health care for its citizens or would be practicing medicine by legislating lengths of hospital stay for specific conditions.

Two important perspectives should color our thinking about the role of government: the historical and the geographical. Historically, it is mainly in the last century that some governments have come to have a massive direct role in the financing, delivery, and regulation of health care. Geographically, this dominating role of government in the health sector is a feature particularly of high-income and some middle-income countries.

In this chapter, I start by discussing the role of government in health outside the health sector and then turn to various components of government's more direct role in health. Next, I summarize the importance of governments working together to ensure the supply of global public goods. Finally, I speculate on likely and desirable trends for the role of government over the next decades.

IMPROVING HEALTH BY DOING SOMETHING ENTIRELY DIFFERENT

The counterintuitive reality is that the greatest contributions that governments can make to health lie outside the health sector and have nothing to do with doctors, hospitals, or vaccines. Here I outline the four most important of these indirect roles: creating a stable and fair society, providing the conditions for increasing personal incomes, educating girls, and improving the environment.

Creating a Stable and Fair Society

Jefferson was right that "restraining men from injuring one another" is a central role for government and has a major impact on health. More generally, "good government," characterized by democracy, an independent judiciary, and a lack of endemic corruption, is a huge advantage for health. This is not mainly owing to the absence of civil unrest, with its accompanying high levels of injuries and homicides, but because a peaceful and uncorrupted society is a necessary condition for the effective delivery of preventive and curative health services. Regrettably, many countries in the world today do not enjoy good government, and this is a major constraint on advances in global health. This effect is most starkly seen in some disease control or eradication programs; such as those directed against polio, malaria, and tuberculosis.

Creating the Conditions for Increased Wealth

Arguably the greatest promoter of health is wealth. As countries become wealthier, they typically become healthier, although to varying degrees, depending on numerous other characteristics of the particular country. Similarly, at any point in time, richer countries are on average healthier than poorer ones. Although debates and disagreements about macroeconomic policy will always exist, there is clearly a range of policies that is associated with economic growth and poverty reduction and another set of policies (or absence of policies) that is not. Other things being equal, countries applying sound macroeconomic policies and enjoying growth in national wealth and the incomes of the poorest will experience better health outcomes than other countries.

Educating Girls

There is a substantial literature on the strong association between improvement in education and improvement in health. Especially compelling is the evidence that improving education among girls will lead to better health for both them and their families. More educated girls and women enjoy better health, live longer, marry later, and have fewer and more widely-spaced children (which are themselves more healthy) than less educated girls and women in the same society and of the same socioeconomic status. It is widely accepted that governments have a role to play in increasing the enrollment of girls in primary and secondary education and in improving the quality of the education that they receive.

Improving the Environment

Environmental influences on health can be categorized as global (climate change, biodiversity, ozone layer), ambient (generalized air and water pollution), and domestic (water supply, sanitation, drainage around the home, indoor air pollution). In poor countries, it is the domestic environment that has by far the largest impact on health. Governments clearly have some role in this area, although exactly what role remains controversial. Public funds can be used to inform people about the benefits of improving the domestic environment and about the options available. They can also be used to subsidize services for the poorest sections of society—although it is more common in practice for governments to subsidize inappropriately services for the urban middle class. Ambient air and water pollution have public good characteristics, and governments need to be involved through incentives and regulation. (Global environment issues fall into the realm of global public goods, discussed later in the chapter.)

ESTABLISHING A SUPPORTIVE ENVIRONMENT

Government's first obligation to the health sector is to establish an environment in which the public and private actors in health can work in an orderly and effective manner to achieve national, local, and individual objectives.

Setting Policy

An essential ingredient in this environment is a set of policies on the major components of the health sector and the direction of any reforms or changes that may be required. These policies will need to be modified frequently and will benefit from widespread public debate.

Most countries today lack a coherent set of health policies. There are numerous reasons for this, including the following:

- The ministry of health is overwhelmed with operational issues and lacks the capacity to develop policy or to negotiate it with the many stakeholders.

- The ministry of health is concerned only with the (perhaps small) public part of the health care system, and no agency is looking at the health care system as a whole.

- Health policy has become an ideological or political football, beyond rational analysis and debate.

- Health policy is excessively determined by external donors and agencies, and the national government has not managed to exert adequate control.

Various combinations of these circumstances are found in many countries. In the United Kingdom, political polarization has historically impeded an informed debate on health policy. In many smaller, poorer countries, the combined effects of inadequate capacity in the ministry of health and a strong donor role have slowed the development of policy with genuine national acceptance and commitment. In India, a preoccupation with the relatively small public part of the health care system has led to a policy vacuum with respect to the huge private system.

Regulating

In modern societies, government heavily regulates most "free" markets—think of cars, food, air travel, or almost anything else. The degree of such regulation is always controversial. It is arguable that the health care market, with its many failings and flaws, needs more regulation than most.

In an unregulated health system, it is probable that a variety of abuses will occur that are harmful (even fatal) to patients and detrimental to the public interest. Such abuses can include the denial of care to certain categories of people—those who are very poor, those from a particular ethnic or social group, or those having a particular illness (such as infection with HIV). Abuses can also involve providing insufficient, excessive, or inappropriate treatment because it is in the financial interest of the doctor or hospital. Both types of abuse can affect not only the individual patient but also the health of the population. This is particularly the case with certain infectious diseases, where a failure to treat effectively can lead to avoidable transmission to others and to the increased spread of resistant strains of the microbe or parasite.

Most wealthy countries have an elaborate array of regulations and incentives influencing the behavior of insurers and health care providers. They also have established traditions of self-regulation, especially among the health care professions. Arguments in these countries center on the danger of overregulation, as with the current debate around managed care regulation in the United States. For most countries, the situation is typified by a lack of regulation, no tradition of effective self-regulation, and few safeguards for patients. This regulatory vacuum needs to be filled gradually and can move only as fast as institutional and political constraints allow.

Gathering and Disseminating Information

Improvement in health and the fortunes of the health sector are highly influenced by the availability of information and by informational asymmetry between customer (patient) and supplier (doctor). You cannot control malaria if you do not continuously monitor its incidence in humans, its resistance to drugs, the behavior of its vector, or the patterns of treatment and prevention in communities. Patients cannot make informed decisions on choice of doctor or hospital or enter into a discussion on treatment options unless they are reasonably informed about health care and medical issues. Individuals and institutions are unlikely to make optimal choices about health (such as immunizations, diet, smoking, or healthy workplaces) unless they are receiving continuously updated and reliable information about such matters.

Such information is a public good, but without strong government involvement, it will not be efficiently gathered and disseminated. Undoubtedly the surveillance of disease and the identification of epidemics is a government responsibility, even if government chooses to contract some of the work involved to the private sector. Most governments greatly underinvest in this area.

DIRECT ROLES IN HEALTH CARE FINANCING AND PROVISION

At the heart of the debates about the role of government that are under way in many countries lie the issues of financing and providing curative care or individual health care services. This is because the vast majority of health dollars are spent in this area and because it is the aspect of the health sector that individuals (who may be voters) experience most and are most concerned about.

Health Finance

Governments should be involved in health finance in several important ways:

ENSURING ADEQUATE EXPENDITURE. In many poor countries, too little is spent on health; sometimes only a few dollars per capita per year in total—one one-thousandth the amount spent in the highest-spending countries. The majority of this expenditure is private rather than public. Expenditures on this order are insufficient to provide even the most basic package of essential health services for the poor. At this level of expenditure, many people will go untreated, and much preventable disease will not be prevented.

In such circumstances, government has a role to increase both public and private expenditures to a more reasonable level. It is impossible to define precisely what that level is, but 5 to 7 percent of gross domestic product (GDP) may provide a target range for many countries. Governments can increase overall spending by spending more themselves, by mandating others to spend more, and by creating an environment that stimulates the private market.

Governments of poor countries will sometimes ask how they can spend more when the International Monetary Fund is encouraging them to reduce overall public expenditure and to balance their budgets. This problem is magnified in countries that are also heavily indebted. Two partial solutions are advocated. First is the reallocation of public expenditure away from subsidizing money-losing state-owned enterprises. In some countries, such as India, these inappropriate subsidies are massive and dwarf government expenditures on health and education combined. Second is to offer debt relief in exchange for commitments to increase public expenditures on health. Such agreements are in place in countries such as Bolivia, Mozambique, and Uganda.

AVOIDING EXCESSIVE EXPENDITURES. By contrast, some countries expend more than 9 percent of their substantial GDP on health. In one country, the United States, this amounts to nearly $4,000 per citizen per year—far higher than any other country. Countries do and should fear escalating health care expenditures. Even if the increases are in the private health care market ("not our concern," governments might say), they will drive up health care costs in the public sector also because of the interwoven nature of the two parts of the system.

The total health care bill is the result of millions of decisions made by millions of health care personnel (mainly doctors) when interacting with millions of patients. In the long run, the most successful cost-constraining measures will be those that provide incentives to doctors and patients not to overtest, overtreat, overadmit, or overstay and to provide quality care at the lowest level of the system where it can be safely provided.

RISK POOLING AND CATASTROPHIC RISK. If an individual is part of no risk pool, she may face a major illness for which she is unable to afford treatment. She will then either forgo treatment, borrow, or sell assets to pay for treatment. Either of these options may permanently impoverish the woman and her family, and the first option may also kill her. Throughout the world a hundred years ago, and in many parts of the world today (such as rural China), people face exactly this dilemma. The biggest risk pool to which they belong is their extended family; which is far too small and will share certain health risks because of genetics, environment, and income level.

Governments have a responsibility to protect citizens from catastrophic health expenditure by either paying the bill or encouraging or forcing citizens to join large risk pools. A national health service (as in the United Kingdom) is a risk pool of all citizens, financed from general taxation. A social security system (as in much of Latin America) is a publicly mandated risk pool for all employed persons and their families.

Historically, as countries move up the scale of development, the proportion of health expenditure that is risk-pooled rises and the proportion that is paid out-of-pocket shrinks. All the world's wealthy countries are heavily risk-pooled. Most poor countries pay primarily out-of-pocket. The challenge for governments of these poorer countries is not whether to move toward risk pooling—the answer is yes—but how? Should India move from its predominantly out-of-pocket, unpooled current situation by liberalizing the private insurance market or by mandating more social insurance or by providing a national health service with public funds? If it pursues the first option, how will it prevent exclusion of the poor and rapidly escalating costs in a fee-for-service plus indemnity insurance market? Questions of this kind are poorly resolved in most countries and provide the frontier for health policy debate over the coming decade.

REGULATING THE HEALTH INSURANCE MARKET. The private health insurance market requires regulation to avoid some well-documented market failures. In the absence of regulation, the market will exhibit three well-known but counterproductive phenomena:

- *Cream skimming,* in which only the healthy will be able to buy affordable insurance
- *Adverse selection,* in which only the unhealthy will seek to be insured

- *Moral hazard,* in which patients or providers may behave irresponsibly because they know that someone else (the insurance company) is footing the bill

Other aspects of health insurance also require regulation—for example, portability. If insurance is lost when an individual changes jobs, the labor market will be adversely affected.

For these reasons, countries with a history of private health insurance (such as the United States) have elaborate federal and state regulations, and countries that are experiencing a growth in their market (such as Mexico) are developing a regulatory framework.

PAYING FOR THE POOR. Equity is a concern of governments and of citizens. Governments throughout the world recognize a responsibility to buy health care for those who cannot afford it themselves. Some governments manage to put their commitment into practice in a way that benefits the poor. For others, it is mere rhetoric, and the poor are left to pay for their health care as best they are able.

A major debate surrounds whether the primary duty of government is to provide basic health care for common conditions for the poor or to provide expensive hospital care for rare events. The Declaration of Alma Ata and the decades of work on primary health care that followed emphasize the first responsibility. Some governments have decided that their major commitment should be instead to fund catastrophic care. There is no single correct answer, and we may expect considerable divergence among countries in this area over the next decade.

Finally, when a government seeks to subsidize services for the poor, it must figure out how to do so. Typically, the nonpoor capture most of the benefit from a public subsidy, the poor benefit less, and the very poor may not benefit at all. Governments therefore struggle to target their subsidies at the intended beneficiaries. Several approaches are used:

- *Have no target:* subsidize the service for everyone, and the poor will automatically be included (as in a national health service)
- *Target individuals:* subsidize the service to those who have been officially designated as poor or who can prove their poverty
- *Target places:* subsidize services in areas where a high proportion of people are poor

- *Target maladies:* subsidize services for those complaints from which the poor suffer disproportionately

In practice, the first and last of these options may prove more administratively feasible and effective than the second and third.

Health Care Provision

The most vexing questions concerning the role of government relate to provision. Should governments build and own hospitals, employ doctors and nurses, establish laboratories, and supply health care? If so, how much and for whom? We see in the world today governments that own and operate most health care provision (such as the United Kingdom) and governments that do little in this area (such as the United States). Every permutation between these models will be found somewhere.

The arguments in favor of government provision are typically these:

- *Social solidarity:* government service can be made available to everyone irrespective of income, caste, ethnicity, or other factors
- *Efficiency:* by combining government finance with government provision, administrative costs may be minimized
- *Control of costs and quality:* the government has direct control over expenditure and quality of services

The arguments against government provisions are similar but reversed:

- *Inefficiency:* government-run hospitals will have poor management, rampant trade unionism, lack of incentives, and a general disregard for how public funds are being spent
- *Poor control of costs and quality:* the civil service mentality will create a climate that is not cost conscious, is insensitive to patients' needs, and is slow to improve quality
- *Lack of flexibility and innovation:* a hierarchical structure with strong central control will stifle local innovation and improvement

Most governments are heavily committed to providing health services. In some countries they provide a majority (as in Tanzania), and in some a minority (as in India). In both cases, this service provision role is the main preoccupation of the national ministry of health and consumes much of its intellectual and financial resources.

Four trends are evident:

1. To keep hospitals in the public sector but to increase their autonomy by the creation of independent management structures free from some or all central government controls. Such arrangements may include independent boards of directors, freedom to hire and fire, freedom to borrow, accountability for losses, and ability to reinvest profit and carry over surplus to the next financial year. A key reform to enable this process is to ensure that hospital employees are not civil servants.

2. To create some competition among public hospitals, and between public and private hospitals, by separating the government's role as a purchaser from its role as a provider.

3. To auction off some public facilities to the private sector, either to own or merely to operate.

4. To increase the public purchase of private health care services.

These trends are accelerating in many countries. It is likely that the next decade will see a gradual divestiture by the state of the ownership and operation of health care facilities.

IMPROVING THE HEALTH OF THE POPULATION

A distinction, with a fuzzy border, can be drawn between individual health and population health. Population health depends on those activities known in some countries as public health or the public health function. These include the surveillance of disease, the education of the public about disease and its prevention, and disease control and prevention per se. These are in whole or in part public goods because one person's use or benefit does not exclude use or benefit by others. Government plays the lead role in organizing and financing these activities and in many countries will actually carry them out as well. The cost effectiveness of many of these public health investments is high compared to many investments in individual curative health care. Examples include public education on healthy lifestyles, protection of water quality, immunization, vector control, monitoring antibiotic resistance, and food safety. It is arguable that all countries underinvest in these activities, and many poorer countries underinvest greatly. There are few votes in population health until there is an epidemic or other disaster, and then everyone is quick to blame the government. In some countries, the skilled workers necessary to staff a public health system, epidemiologists, for example, are in short supply. Much greater emphasis could be given to this aspect of government's role without risk of inappropriate government activity or unwise use of public funds.

SUPPORTING HEALTH RESEARCH

The health of humankind has improved far more rapidly and more profoundly in the past century than would be predicted by increased wealth alone. For a given GDP per capita, countries are much healthier today than they were twenty or forty years ago, and they will be healthier still in 2010. The reason is knowledge, coming from research.

There are few better public investments than well-targeted and well-conducted health-related research. Although much downstream and product-related research can and will be done by the private sector, there are two important gaps that must be filled by public investment. First is basic research, which does not necessarily lead to a specific product. In all wealthy countries, governments invest in such research, and in some, the research may also be carried out in government laboratories or at public universities. Second is research on products for which the market is ill defined or genuinely small, and so the private sector lacks the commercial incentive to make large research and development investments. Major examples are products related to tropical diseases (which occur in relatively poor countries) and diseases of the poor in wealthier countries. Investment today in research on a vaccine against malaria, tuberculosis, or HIV is woefully small; as is research on a wide range of other products that would make a big difference to the lives of disadvantaged people worldwide. Research into such products is a public good and also a global public good.

COOPERATING ON
GLOBAL PUBLIC GOODS

The foregoing discussion focused on the role of governments at the national level in financing or producing public goods and goods with positive externalities and in addressing issues of inequity and poverty. A similar set of concerns exists internationally. The term *global public good* has been used to describe a public good with beneficiaries worldwide, in all social groups, and among present and future generations. Such global public goods cannot be supplied by a single government. They would be the responsibility of a world government, if one existed. Since it does not, governments have come together, sometimes with nongovernmental organizations and the private sector, to establish transnational structures (agencies, conventions, treaties, and the like) to address the supply of global public goods and the reduction of global public bads.

The world has a century-old tradition of international collaboration to combat the spread of infectious disease. This remains an important global public good, and in this age of drug resistance and emerging and reemerging infections, ever more strenuous multinational efforts are required. However, concerted efforts are also needed to deal with an array of other global public goods with major potential health benefits.

A striking example of the last type of global public good is in the field of immunization. Biotechnology is making available an array of ever more powerful vaccines. Due to international market failures, these new vaccines are not reaching the people who need them most or are doing so only after a gap of ten to fifteen years. Widespread and rapid use of new vaccines is a global public good. All countries benefit from high immunization rates in any country; all sections of a society benefit from high immunization rates in any one section; and future generations benefit from high immunization rates today. This last effect occurs not only when a disease is eradicated by immunization (as with smallpox) but also when immunization causes general improvement in population health and slows the development of antibiotic-resistant microbes and parasites.

Since we lack a world government, global public goods are addressed only when individual governments come together, through the World Health Organization, for example, to create transnational policy and action. The prime movers initiating and financing such international health actions have been a small group of wealthy countries. This is changing and needs to change more. Global public goods in health will be addressed adequately only when *most* countries and governments are proactive and committed to international debate and action.

THE FUTURE ROLE OF GOVERNMENT

Clearly, governments should ensure the provision of public goods (like clean air), but they should also be involved in private goods with major externalities (like ensuring timely and effective treatment of a TB patient), in subsidizing health care and prevention for the poorest, and in encouraging citizens to protect their own health (by wearing seat belts, for example). In practice, many goods in the health sector are mixed goods, with both public and private components. Policymakers have to make judgments, based on economic, scientific, political, and contextual evidence, regarding when and to what extent government should become involved. In doing so, the most influential piece of evidence is the starting point: What is the government doing today? Government roles can in practice move only slowly and incrementally from this de facto position.

Plausible and desirable trends in the role of government over the first decades of the new century include the following:

- Clearer thinking about and better articulation of the essential role of government in the health sector and the public-private interface
- A retreat by some governments from being major providers of individual health services
- A strengthening role for government as a financer of health services, as a regulator of private health financing arrangements, and as a guardian of equity in health financing
- Much greater emphasis on governments as purchasers and providers of population health services
- Continuing development of the role of government in encouraging the appropriate use, and discouraging the inappropriate use, of new medical technologies
- A major expansion in the number and range of governments that are working together proactively on the supply of global public goods

Regrettably, although human health has improved greatly in the past five decades, the gap in health status and access to services between the richest and the poorest has also increased. Governments, alone and together, will have to pay great attention to equity issues in health and health services if irreparable schisms in society are to be avoided. Our ability to achieve greater equity by 2020 will be an important measure of our maturity and the quality of our civilization, nationally and globally.

CHAPTER FORTY-FIVE

The Role of Business

William C. Steere Jr.

William C. Steere Jr. *is Chairman and Chief Executive Officer of Pfizer, Inc. He has been a member of the Pfizer Board of Directors since 1987. He is a member of the Board of Directors of the Mount Sinai–New York University Medical Center, the Business Roundtable, Texaco Inc., Minerals Technologies Inc., the New York Botanical Garden, Metropolitan Life Insurance Company, and Dow Jones Inc. He is also a member of the Executive Committee of the Memorial Sloan-Kettering Cancer Center.*

The twenty-first century will see unprecedented advances in health care, ushered in by an elegant dynamic already at work—a cycle of biomedical innovation that enhances human health and raises human productivity. The greater productivity in turn spurs economic growth, attracting greater investment that finances broadened research and leads to even greater innovation and ever-improving human health.

It is a cycle of high risk and high reward. The risk is financial and borne by the research-based pharmaceutical industry, which in 1999 alone committed well over $24 billion to research and development (R&D). By the year's end, only about thirty new medicines will have received FDA approval, at an average cost of over $500 million apiece.

But the reward is extraordinary. Over the past two decades, we have made tremendous gains in the treatment of cancers, Alzheimer's disease, heart ailments, and diseases of the central nervous system. Pharmaceutical innovation is reducing morbidity and prolonging life. It's also saving money by substituting pharmaceutical therapy for costly therapies such as hospitalization and surgery.

The many slight but innovative differences in the medicines of one therapeutic category are the small steps forward in biomedical discovery that eventually accumulate into giant strides in our understanding of disease and its treatment. The combination AIDS therapies that now make HIV infection a manageable condition for many patients is the result of modest and incremental discoveries.

And it is the pharmaceutical research industry that is producing most of these innovations, not only in the fight against AIDS but in virtually every other disease category. With ever-improving research tools, such as combinatorial chemistry, high-throughput screening, and genomics, novel treatments will continue to be developed. For example, at Pfizer, these tools are allowing us to more than double the number of compounds in early development worldwide.

These new medicines will enhance human productivity. Already we have witnessed the outstanding contribution that innovative medicines have made in the treatment of depression and diabetes, permitting individuals with these conditions to lead normal lives.

Many people once relegated to the economic sidelines because of disease are now able to work, earn a living, and acquire the necessities of life that permit an ever-improving standard of living. Jobs also empower men and women to pursue health improvements and to afford the technologies that improve health. This increase in productivity raises the level of economic activity, enabling more and more businesses to invest in their employees' health.

Healthy workers are a key part of the cycle that increases productivity and leads to greater investment that results in medical innovations and improved human health.

In the United States, businesses that invest in good health are recognized with the C. Everett Koop National Health Award by the Health Project consortium, a public-private volunteer group. Some of the National Health Award interventions have been found to achieve cost reductions within the initial year and to have even greater benefits several years later when improved health habits produce better health and lower costs.

CHALLENGES OF THE
NEW AGE IN HEALTH CARE

But a Golden Age of Medicine is not assured. Before it becomes a real-ity, some daunting challenges must be met.

Infectious diseases must be controlled, an aging population will have to be cared for, and our communities must be strengthened. In meet-ing each of these challenges, sound public policies—policies that encourage innovation, especially biomedical innovation—are essential.

Infectious Disease

None of us is safe from microbes. From developing nations to G-7 cities, the human race fights an ongoing battle with infectious disease. The speed with which infections can spread is a constant concern to health care officials. Considering how many people one person can infect over the course of a few hours in a busy airport, the scope of the problem becomes clear, making the search for novel antimicrobial agents critical. Our challenge is global.

Community

Our challenge is also local. Healthy workers—workers with a stake in the community and a real hope for the future—are the backbone of any business and of every economy. By increasing investments in com-munity health to limit pollution, provide sanitation, ensure safe food, and promote access to quality health care, business helps create a pro-ductive populace. As the new century unfolds, more and more exec-utives will join the already substantial number of business leaders who recognize that the health of their bottom line is linked to the health of employees in their communities and that biomedical innovation is a crucial contributor to employee wellness.

An Aging Population

The population of the world is aging. In twenty-five years, one-fifth of the world's population will be age sixty-five or older. The number of those age eighty-five and older is projected to grow sixfold, and the number of centenarians is projected to grow sixteenfold. In an aging world, chronic diseases will predominate. The global burden of disease will continue to shift in the new century to diseases like ischemic heart disease, depression, diabetes, and cancer—reflecting the aging of the world's population. The new global burden presents a formidable challenge to society that biomedical innovation will play a key role in solving. With that solution will come not only decreased morbidity and mortality but also the expanded opportunity for seniors to contribute to their communities.

ENLIGHTENED PUBLIC POLICIES

In meeting the challenges of an aging population, infectious disease, and productive communities, the pharmaceutical research industry is indispensable. But for the research-based pharmaceutical industry to discover and develop these medicines, a fair regulatory environment is required. Such an environment should include all of the following:

- Strong intellectual property protection and patent laws
- An efficient regulatory and reimbursement process, with an emphasis on free-market pricing, safety, and the dissemination of reliable biomedical information
- A substantial national investment in basic biomedical research

Intellectual property rights must be protected so that those who invest in the painstaking and expensive work of innovation can recoup their considerable investment costs. Where it exists, intellectual property protection has encouraged sustained investment in the research that has improved the human condition. Not only are new medicines developed, but the discoverers of these medicines have been able to reap rewards that are poured back into research, creating even more new medicines that improve worker productivity and stimulate economic activity.

Strong patents also thwart the counterfeiting of drugs, which often results in substandard pharmaceuticals that can harm the world's poorest people. The failure to protect intellectual property (leading to patent theft) in some developing countries also diminishes pharmaceutical companies' incentive to develop new pharmaceuticals for diseases plaguing those countries. If, after an investment of fourteen years and over half a billion dollars, a company is denied a fair return, no investment is likely.

Also essential to the encouragement of innovation is a regulatory and reimbursement environment that strives to improve patient access to innovative medicines. The more efficient the drug approval process, the more encouraging its effect on the development of new products. Unfortunately, moratoriums on the use of a new technology—designed to lower costs in the short term—often impede technological advances that would improve the quality of patients' lives or lower long-term costs.

Regulatory approval for Viagra, for instance, was delayed in a number of countries because of fears that it would mean higher costs for governments that pay for pharmaceuticals. Money drove the issue instead of patient access to a breakthrough pharmaceutical to treat a serious medical condition. As we are learning, however, erectile dysfunction—the disease Viagra treats—is in many cases a marker of some underlying disease such as diabetes or depression. Bringing men with erectile dysfunction into the health care system has resulted in diagnosis and treatment of these and other conditions, easing suffering and lowering health care costs.

In other situations, poor science policy contributes to keeping beneficial medicines off the market. For instance, the European Union's unjustified ban on certain antibiotic feed supplements based on questionable data and unjustified fears of increasing human susceptibility to infection will raise meat prices for Europeans by increasing the cost of hog farming. This leaves fewer resources to be applied to European health care.

The regulatory environment must stress safety and provide adequate resources to regulators that help ensure that safety issues are handled in a timely fashion.

Other policies—related to pricing—may discourage innovation or provide disincentives to long-term investments in pharmaceutical R&D. In Europe and other parts of the globe, regulations that control price and reimbursement put a floor under generic product prices, giving imitators and innovators similar incentives. This has dramatically eroded the strength of Europe's R&D pharmaceutical industry and has contributed to higher overall drug prices for Europeans.

Equally destructive to innovation are the "free riders," countries such as New Zealand and Australia, which discover no new medical therapies yet impose severe price controls on those innovative pharmaceuticals developed elsewhere, especially in the United States. Twenty percent of what Americans pay for innovative medicines is plowed back into research that results in better medicines. America is paying for biomedical innovation, and American companies are providing it, while these countries are not paying their fair share. The effect is to dampen R&D and to make impossible the development of any kind of pharmaceutical research industry within their borders, depriving their national economies of tens of thousands of good jobs. Reasonable market-based prices are necessary to provide an adequate return on investment for the innovation process. The best example of the benefits of free trade on health can be found in the United States, where a market-oriented approach for pharmaceuticals has fueled remarkable innovations and the finest health care in the world.

Quality information to medical consumers is also crucial as patients seek to make informed decisions. Web sites such as Pfizer's, with its links to the Mayo Health Clinic, are examples of the new technology of the twenty-first century, enhancing patients' knowledge and empowering them as health care consumers.

Finally, tax codes should promote research by encouraging investment. I believe that dependable, long-term investments in research are absolutely crucial for the cycle of innovation, health, economic growth, investment, and innovation.

Basic and essential commercial research must be supported. Nations that invest in basic research in government and academic laboratories encourage progress. Nations that support essential industry, academic, and government partnerships to commercialize discoveries reap multiple benefits. One of the most precious national resources is the knowledge encountered in the discovery process. The steady stream of discoveries in university, industry, and national laboratories combines to form a cascade of insights that can find practical and humane expression in a host of applications to improve the human condition.

SHARING THE BENEFITS

The benefits of advanced scientific research must be available to all. This is especially true of pharmaceuticals and vaccines. They are important, cost-effective components of the health care strategies for all countries, since they allow the delivery of safe and effective interventions to large groups of people.

Businesses are eager to participate in a strong global network. As a worldwide community, our ability to share the wealth of technological innovations will enhance human life in the new century. Businesses are ready to stimulate economic growth, improve the overall quality of life, and share technological advances.

For those who want to improve health care throughout the world, I recommend a simple prescription: support policies that encourage innovation, especially pharmaceutical innovation.

New medicines drive down the overall cost of health care, reduce morbidity, and prolong life. They are principal means by which the Golden Age of Medicine in the twenty-first century will be implemented.

CHAPTER FORTY-SIX

The Role of the Nonprofit Sector

Kumi Naidoo

Kumi Naidoo *is Secretary General and Chief Executive Officer of CIVICUS: World Alliance for Citizen Participation. He is the editor of* Civil Society at the Millennium. *A former anti-apartheid activist, he has worked on a broad range of social justice initiatives in the nongovernmental organization (NGO) sector in South Africa.*

T he twenty-first century will bring new challenges for democratic governance and for meeting basic human needs and ensuring the sustainability of our planet. In meeting these challenges, we will need greater innovation and a more serious commitment to creating a more just and humane world. The observations that follow reflect my current work at CIVICUS: World Alliance for Citizen Participation and at the South African National NGO Coalition. Drawing on the approaches of many nonprofit organizations both in the health field and outside of it, we must throw our weight behind the notion of comprehensive physical and civic health for people in a diversity of situations and at different levels of development.

From this perspective, a few themes regarding the nonprofit sector (also variously referred to as the voluntary, NGO, or social sector) deserve special attention, and I would like to develop them here. There is a need for the various parts of the nonprofit sector to understand their roles more clearly and to work together more effectively so as to synergize their efforts. There is a corresponding need for government and the private sector to support the role of the nonprofit sector more concertedly. There is a need to adopt a comprehensive and holistic approach to health, with greater emphasis on primary and preventive care, on self-care within family and community, on access to high-quality health care for all, and on the crucial role of citizens and citizen organizations in making health policy across the voluntary, public, and private sectors.

NEW REALITIES, NEW THINKING, NEW OPPORTUNITIES

New global realities require new thinking and create new opportunities for advancing human health and new challenges for preserving human health. The nonprofit sector has played a unique role by serving as one of the fundamental sources of caring human responsiveness to new challenges and as the impetus for evolution of new and appropriate health policy, processes, and institutions. The nonprofit sector continues to help us see health as a contribution to broader human development—balanced, comprehensive, and sustainable.

The nonprofit sector will have its special contribution to the twenty-first century's paradoxical mix of opportunities to advance human health and threats to human health. The opportunities will arise in the intersection between high-tech health care (technology, pharmacology, management) and low-tech or "appropriate-tech" health care (primary care, prevention, self-care, integration of levels of health support for individuals, families, communities, and societies). The threats will include new diseases, spread in part by new patterns of globalization and cultural interpenetration; as well as possible declines in the effectiveness of current "wonder drugs," with unknown replacement potential. An era of civil conflict could also generate significant new health threats for the world's populations. Advances, as current trends would suggest, might be achievable through the privatization of health care. However, this trend also presents the challenges and dilemmas of sharing health resources equitably and justly and of determining which populations to include, if not all of them, in health care systems.

The nonprofit sector recognizes that human understandings of health have evolved, and will continue to evolve, in more comprehensive directions. Ultimately, health is based on our concept of human life. The conditions for quality of life, in all its dimensions, are the conditions for health. Health is a foundation of all wealth. How will we understand and value human life and health in the future? That, we can hope, will provide the impetus for our renewed health efforts.

The nonprofit sector will be influenced by new research. For example, recent epidemiological studies are illustrative of new thinking about health and suggest that only about 10 percent of potential health improvements in developed societies will come from advances in health technology and management. About 40 percent will come from improved preventive personal health care practices. And the remaining half will come from improvements in the environment we provide for human life. Other analysts correctly observe a correlation between social capital (civic health) and more conventional measures of public health.

The nonprofit sector will undoubtedly be concerned about the broader social impacts of health conditions. When leading social thinkers meet, health threats emerge as a major challenge to the quality of human life and the civility of society. So we can see clearly that the nonprofit sector, with its inherent social capital, must continue to function as the source of adaptive energies and institutional solutions. This will manifest itself in such areas as the creation of awareness, the support of belief systems, and the nurturing of values. It will also serve as the impetus for initiatives on behalf of health inspiration; motivation; incentives; prevention; self-care and mutual care; integrative linkages of individual, family, community, and society; and civil conflict mediation and resolution as a basis for cooperative problem solving.

Important steps are being taken by the international community in the direction of these approaches to health, ranging from the broad civic health concerns of "our global neighborhood" to the "healthy communities" initiatives of the World Health Organization. The United States, with its particular social problems, presents models of collaboration in this area through the work of the nonprofit sector—the National Civic League, the Coalition for Healthier Cities and Communities, the Community Care Network, and the Hospital Research and Education Trust, among others. Strategic planning models will be needed, such as the APEXCPH (Assessment and Planning Excellence Through Community Partners for Health) tool, which is being developed by a coalition of agencies that include the American Society for Public Administration and the Association of Public Health Administrators to assist local communities in undertaking a community health improvement process. Even more broadly, it will be important to develop and link our measures of health, including indices of civic and social health, like those developed by the National Commission on Civic Renewal in the United States. These are the social and analytical foundations of prevention through self-care and mutual care.

More and more, then, the nonprofit sector must contribute to our understanding of the interdependence of biological, physical, mental, and social health. All aspects influence all others, so where one is weak, the others will be weaker, and where one is strengthened, that opens the door to strengthening the others. Physical and mental health are requirements for a functioning society, and vice versa.

INTERSECTORAL AND PARTICIPATORY PARTNERSHIPS

If the nonprofit sector is to continue to perform its traditional functions effectively, its role must be recognized by the public and private sectors—not just in theory but also in practice. Health progress requires healthy intersectoral partnerships, in which the nonprofit sector continues to generate ideas, values, commitments, and support while government provides the necessary enabling environment through policy and regulation, along with funding for services, and the private sector provides a strong system of employer-based health insurance and other types of health assistance. As privatization of the health sector continues, we need ongoing conversation and debate regarding its impact on the quality and accessibility of health care. If we are to have the universal access to health care required for healthy societies, the sectors must work toward that goal as partners.

Such partnerships will come about if the role of the nonprofit sector as the motivating source of intersectoral and intercultural health collaboration is recognized. Historically, new initiatives have emerged from citizens with strong belief systems and humane values, who cared about the common good and its corollary of good health enough to develop ideas and organize efforts. Typically, this was done through religious institutions, which evolved into the voluntary sector, then into public health programs and institutions, then into insured health or medical aid systems, and then into an increasingly privatized health sector.

We cannot know with certainty what mixes of health institutions our various societies will try out and which will survive. But we can be sure that the nonprofit sector, with its "bottom-up" initiatives, will by its nature continue to be the creative source for reinventing the sectors and institutions so that they best meet human needs. In all likelihood, the new century will be characterized by a blend of traditionally competitive health institutions and new kinds of health partnerships across sectors and cultures.

Partnerships among institutions, however, are not enough to create the necessary advances in human health. The required additional dimensions of partnership are participatory—first, through horizontal linkages of individuals, families, and communities, all motivated to care for their own health; and second, through vertical linkages between people in society and larger, more specialized health institutions. These horizontal and vertical linkages will have to be supported by a combination of voluntary self-motivation and institutionalized incentives and rewards.

HOLISTIC APPROACHES: PREVENTION AND CARE

In this context, interdependence and participatory partnerships are crucial supports for any move toward more effective, holistic, synergistic health care approaches. The key to effective prevention is not just more emphasis on primary care, with the reallocation of resources from specialization that implies, but the development of a society that educates its citizens for self-care and mutual care—society itself, through individual, family, and community action, must be the front line of the health care system, its upstream source of effectiveness.

No "top-down" system of incentives and rewards, however necessary, can by itself succeed in achieving the improved health conditions we all envisage. Societies that already enjoy the benefits of strong values and belief systems for prevention and self-care or mutual care—orientations of participation, community, and solidarity—can lead the way in providing models that others can emulate. These crucial orientations are found in societies of various cultural and developmental backgrounds.

The nonprofit sector will be crucial in helping every society, whatever its present status, develop these values and put them into practice. Speaking realistically, it seems very likely that the implementation of such "healthy values" will become an increasingly important factor in guiding investment for development, as investment considerations continue to move beyond the narrowly financial.

CITIZEN DEMAND AND SUPPORT:
TOWARD ACCESS FOR ALL

A core value of the nonprofit sector is inclusiveness of all people in the benefits of the larger society and world. Therefore, the nonprofit sector will always work for universal access to health care for all of humanity, in every society and among societies. The imperative then becomes to create the political will to achieve this, through intersectoral institutional partnerships, and to design these partnerships accordingly. Among rich and poor societies, there are great differences in these designs and in the political will to bring them about. The international nonprofit sector could play a crucial role here, in a variety of ways.

It is the nonprofit sector that works most directly on the cultural, social, and psychological sources or foundations for health and health practices. Furthermore, it provides crucial indirect or secondary support by promoting citizen awareness of health factors, citizen demand for institutional response, and citizen support of collective health practices.

The relationship between citizen participation in self- or mutual preventive care and citizen participation in the formulation of institutional health policies and practices is crucial—its importance cannot be overstated. People who own their institutions make those institutions work.

The implications for institutionalizing participation in health institutions are immense. It will be necessary to break down and transform long-held images of health personnel as authorities beyond question, as having special knowledge that preempts the general experience of people. Health systems, concepts, and personnel will have to be democratized. Ways of doing this include public education, formal advisory groups, informal focus groups, representative governing boards, and cultural diversity of health personnel. These are only illustrations—there is much to be done in this area.

HUMAN HEALTH AND
THE NONPROFIT SECTOR

Thinking about health must include thinking about the health of society. In the new century, the social sector must not only contribute to health in conventional ways but also link our understandings and actions to the interdependent health of individual, family, community, and society.

CIVICUS has taken a first step in this direction by supplementing its reports on the condition of civil societies worldwide with an initiative on the nature and indicators of a healthy civil society, with measures that allow us to compare societies and trace their progress over time. CIVICUS will continue to support new understandings of the role of the social sector in all dimensions of human health; as well as of ways to enhance the health of the social nonprofit sector itself in carrying out these functions.

CHOICES FOR THE FUTURE

My purpose in making the foregoing observations is to prompt analysis of human health conditions, contingencies, choices, priorities, dilemmas, and paradoxes for the future. New concepts such as social capital and their application to health offer prospects for better insights. Health is not just an end in itself; as social capital, it provides the resources for development. Health is an investment with returns for human wealth and well-being that go far beyond financial considerations.

We know that although there are universal health challenges that all societies and cultures share, there are also important differences that need to be acknowledged and more effectively addressed. These differences include the balance of prevention and care; the role of primary care; disease and environment; cultural perceptions of life, health, and health practices; and opportunities for financial and human resource mobilization for better health, both biophysical and social.

Across the diversity of societies and cultures, the nonprofit sector can contribute much to our understanding of the interdependence among levels of health, civility, and development and to participatory partnerships for health and overall human development.

In tackling the health challenges of the future, we need to recognize that probably the greatest challenge we face is ever-greater inequality. While some individuals and societies are securing increasing levels of wealth, others are struggling with distressing levels of poverty. Such inequities exist within nations and between nations. Health practitioners need to ensure that this reality is incorporated into their deliberations and their work so that ultimately a good and decent health care system will be available to all of humanity. If we do not do this, certain communities will become the testing ground for drug research while others will be the beneficiaries. Some communities and individuals will aspire to and achieve Rolls-Royce health care while others—the majority in many cases—will struggle to secure even a broken wheelbarrow standard of care. In meeting these challenges, the nonprofit sector must play a key role, not only in implementing policies and strategies developed by others but also in the development of enlightened policies to create a more just, more humane, and more sustainable world.

CHAPTER FORTY-SEVEN

Business in Partnership with the Nonprofit Sector

Ralph S. Larsen

Ralph S. Larsen *is Chairman of the Board and Chief Executive Officer of Johnson & Johnson, the world's most broadly based health care company. He also serves as Chairman of the Business Council and Chairman of the Corporate Fund for the Kennedy Center; a member of the Policy Committee of the Business Roundtable; and a member of the Board of Directors of Xerox Corporation, the New York Stock Exchange, and AT&T Corp. Prior to his current responsibilities, which he assumed in 1989, Mr. Larsen was Vice Chairman of the Executive Committee and Chairman of the Consumer Section of Johnson & Johnson.*

Nature has found some highly creative solutions to the problems of survival. Mutualism, for example, links two independent organisms struggling to survive in a harsh environment in a win-win collaboration that allows each not just to survive but to flourish under the difficult conditions.

Our global community today faces difficult conditions and enormous challenges, particularly in the health care arena. Our solutions must be as creative and effective as nature's. Win-win partnerships among independent entities—mutualism, if you will—may well be the best way to harness the coming century's explosion of options and technology to improve the lives and health of people worldwide. As in nature's mutualism, partnerships that creatively leverage the unique resources and strengths of each participant add value to society in ways that are transformational.

And make no mistake—transformational change is essential if we are to address the world's health care challenges. Scientific and technological advances have made possible today an extension of healthy life that could not even be imagined a few decades ago. Yet providing those benefits is straining health care systems around the world. Mutualism requires that all sectors reach beyond familiar frameworks to envision and then work toward novel forms of partnership.

BUSINESS IN SOCIETY

Although the business world's involvement in social issues can be traced back only a few decades, the situation has since turned 180 degrees, and now the issues themselves are having a substantial and increasing impact on companies. Environmental concerns, access to health care, quality of life questions, and many other challenges may play out differently—sometimes contradictorily—around the globe, but everywhere they are having an effect on how companies do business and how successful we can be in a given environment.

Enlightened self-interest alone would be reason enough to pay attention, but increasingly businesses also see social responsibility as a way to express their spirit and connect with consumers and constituents on an emotional plane. Leading companies today recognize that efforts to better our world are not just an obligation. They are also an opportunity to knit a business to its community within a framework of human aspirations and to align the company's health with the health of the larger society.

At the same time, the public today expects something more of business than just goods and services. With the fizzling of the cold war and the advent of economic globalization and technological interconnection, business has emerged as one of the most powerful and pervasive forces in the world. As we enter the twenty-first century, business is being asked to fill a leadership void in society and to take on a new and expanded role in communities around the world.

Increasingly, the call is being heard. According to the World Bank, private sector investment in economic development, for example, has expanded from half the size of official assistance to more than four times as much. At the same time, many more companies today are at the table with nonprofit organizations and governments in an effort to address a host of social issues, including illiteracy, sanitation, and environmental protection.

At Johnson & Johnson, we have long believed that business must play an active role in shaping a better society. During the depths of the Great Depression, General Robert Wood Johnson, Chairman from 1932 to 1963, said, "Industry only has the right to succeed where it performs a real economic service and is a true social asset." His view, appreciated more today than when he first articulated it, was that companies must enhance the value of the society in which they operate while they seek to enhance their own value. It is society, ultimately, that legitimizes a company's economic activity.

Our credo, which General Johnson wrote in 1943, clearly sets forth a hierarchy of company obligations, which *begins* with our obligations to customers, employees, and the communities in which we operate and ends with our obligations to shareholders. The credo closes with the line, "When we operate according to these principles, the stockholders should realize a fair return."

As the world's largest and most diversified health care company, we continue to believe that to build and sustain an enduring global franchise in health care, it is *essential* to act in socially responsible ways and to play a role in improving health wherever we do business.

THE PARTNERSHIP MANDATE

Even though shareholder returns will always be a key consideration for any company, we have found that there are plenty of opportunities where financial and credo obligations converge, and most of the time those opportunities involve partnerships. The reasoning is simple: business cannot thrive in an environment of unmet human needs or in the absence of a fair and civil society. It is also clear that in today's interdependent world, to make a lasting difference in just about any domain, partnerships are essential. The fact is that in isolation, no one organization—or economic sector—can have a major impact on a complex issue such as health. The task is too great for any of us.

The National SAFE KIDS Campaign, to reduce childhood injuries caused by accidents, illustrates this point. Founded by the Children's National Medical Center and Johnson & Johnson in 1987, this effort today involves more than five thousand partners just in the United States. They include multinational, national, and local businesses both within and outside of the health industry; schools and local health departments in communities across the nation; scores of nonprofit organizations and community groups; federal and state government agencies; and medical schools. It also boasts the participation of literally hundreds of thousands of volunteers.

The power of this broad collaboration is clear. The first decade of the SAFE KIDS campaign in the United States witnessed a 30 percent reduction in childhood deaths from unintentional injuries. In fact, the effort has been so successful that it has now been expanded, with the help of many hundreds of new partners, to Australia, Austria, Brazil, Canada, China, Germany, the United Arab Republic, and the United Kingdom, and plans are under way to bring SAFE KIDS to Greece and Israel. The campaign is in the formative stages in Japan.

Operation Smile is another example. This effort, which began in 1982 when one of our Ethicon salesmen gave extra samples of sutures to Dr. William Magee, now annually corrects the cleft lips, cleft palates, and other facial deformities of more than five thousand children in eighteen countries. As impressive as the results are the enormous numbers of organizations and individuals contributing to Operation Smile's success. About a thousand volunteer surgeons and other health professionals, two thousand medical personnel on site around the world, and hundreds of nongovernmental, governmental, and private organizations combine their efforts with our $2 million in product donations and the donations and support of many other companies and individuals.

SAFE KIDS and Operation Smile are massive undertakings, but even highly focused interventions require partnerships. Our donation of Vermox, our product to eradicate intestinal parasites, the number one health problem among schoolchildren in developing countries, would not be nearly as effective without the partnership of NGOs, local community groups, health departments, and schools. They administer the medication, test the children, improve sanitation, and offer comprehensive education to teach children and their families how to prevent reinfection.

It is precisely *because* all sectors are interdependent within our common mission in health care that we must cooperate. We need to reach across the boundaries that separate sectors to create new frameworks for action. If we start from our common concerns, we can weave together our individual strengths; if we appreciate each other's unique perspectives, we can form mutually beneficial partnerships that are sustainable and replicable and, above all, deliver for people.

Many other leading companies and organizations concur. The World Health Organization has identified collaboration—meaning the full participation of diverse economic sectors—as a key principle of its health policy for the twenty-first century. The same is true of the European Union, and in the United States, the Healthy People 2010 program relies on a consortium of over three hundred organizations from all sectors. American businesses have traditionally embraced public-private partnerships, and increasingly, so do companies based in many other markets.

MUTUALISTIC PARTNERSHIPS TODAY

Fifty years ago, the role of business in social partnerships was essentially limited to providing funding. We are in a more participatory era today. The most important contributions business can bring to the table are leadership and vision complementary to those of its not-for-profit partners, along with creative leveraging of its considerable connections, resources, and expenditures. Both of these assets can elevate good partnerships that have relatively limited horizons to a new plane, where they can have greater and more lasting effects on many more people and on larger segments of the health care system. It's not unlike the difference between giving a person a fish and teaching that person to fish.

For example, in 1990, we joined forces with the U.S. Health and Human Services Department to create the Johnson & Johnson/Head Start Management Fellows Program. Today more than five hundred Head Start center directors—most without any prior management training—have graduated from an intensive institute at the University of California at Los Angeles where they learned the latest approaches to managing more effectively. The positive impact on the lives of children is almost certainly greater today than had we simply written a check for day-to-day operations.

These kinds of infrastructure investments in local institutions and local people are becoming critically important around the world. In Ecuador, a partnership between Occidental Exploration and Production and the government to train local village "health promoters" resulted in marked improvements in prenatal exams and a reported drop in child mortality from forty-two to zero per thousand.

Leveraging is also the operating principle behind cause-related marketing, an approach that has almost become a way of life for many companies and nonprofits. Cause marketing allows a company to express its concern while giving the cause a level of public exposure through product advertising, packaging, and promotion that is orders of magnitude greater than it could achieve otherwise. A true business partnership, both sides have an entrepreneurial interest in success. American Express and other financial services firms have partnered with hundreds of nonprofits, providing them with incredible reach as well as revenues as a percentage of credit card sales.

The power of these partnerships is illustrated by a collaboration between Kellogg's Rice Krispies and the Zero to Three organization. A single panel on cereal boxes brought Zero to Three's message about the importance of early child development to more people than the combined readership of the nation's thirty major daily newspapers. Some twenty million cereal boxes carried the message and an offer for a Zero to Three growth chart.

Some of the most successful partnerships have involved joint ventures between companies and NGOs that share a common interest. Merck's alliance with the World Bank and other partners to combat river blindness (onchocerciasis) is one example. Merck promised to donate its drug Mectizan "as long as needed" to eradicate the disease, and the World Bank committed to raise $12 million a year for ten years to aid the effort. Today, river blindness has been virtually eliminated from eleven countries in West Africa. Several other companies, including Pfizer, GlaxoWellcome, and Dupont, have initiated similar efforts to combat specific diseases.

Coalitions of companies leveraging their individual resources have delivered some of the most far-reaching results to date. One example is Prescription for Life, to ensure the safety of the U.S. blood supply. Ten pharmaceutical companies joined forces to raise over $20 million in 1995 to help the American Red Cross increase private donations and build new systems and facilities to test blood products. The companies also stepped up their already stellar level of employee blood donations.

Employee volunteerism is another way that businesses are leveraging financial support. The KABOOM! organization solicits funds and, more important, volunteer labor from local corporations to build playgrounds in "child-rich and playground-poor" communities throughout the country. Companies such as CNA Financial, Nike, Kimberly-Clark, and Home Depot have found that building a playground is a wonderful complement to cash contributions and a great team-building experience for employees.

Over time, partnerships that start at one level naturally expand as trust, results, and symbiotic creativity build. Our involvement in the National SAFE KIDS Campaign, for example, now includes philanthropy, membership on the board, communications and management support, a leadership role among participating companies, the volunteer efforts of hundreds of Johnson & Johnson employees, and a very successful annual cause-related promotion of our consumer products. The promotion includes national television advertising and in-store displays featuring practical advice for families on preventing accidents at home, in school, and in motor vehicles.

SUCCEEDING AT PARTNERSHIPS

In spite of the many opportunities for creative partnerships, much of the dialogue between the business and nonprofit communities centers on how difficult partnerships can be. A few approaches can help build effective working relationships.

- Maintain focus on the people who will be served by the partnership. All partners share the common purpose of contributing to people living healthier, more comfortable lives. Individual differences will seem minor in this larger context.

- Articulate shared objectives. Identify early how the objectives of the two organizations overlap, and keep these as a mission statement for the partnership.

- Recognize and use differences. Know your own organization's unique capabilities and those of your partner; let each group focus on what it does best.

- Work with each other as equals and as equally committed to the goal.

- Manage change. Partnerships stretch organizational structures, cultures, and processes and tend to highlight differences in goals and learned experiences. Leading through a positive example, direct communication, support for the partnership's champions, and celebration of its successes can help in managing the process.

- Respect each other's perspectives. NGOs seek funding to help more people. In restrictive markets, corporations may be concerned about property rights, the cost of regulation, or policies that inhibit innovation.

- Develop trust. Trust comes when both sides are honest and deliver as agreed. Although partnerships are rarely anybody's full-time job, a partner is an important focus for your time and attention. Trust also develops with success, so it's important to define success in the particular context and determine how it will be measured.

- Empower the partnership "champions." The handful of individuals who work in the partnership on a regular basis should have the authority to make decisions and lead without having to solicit the input of many others at their organizations.

- Increase participation across the organizations. Over time, successful partnerships become part of the fabric of each organization. Moving into new areas of partnership—employee volunteer opportunities or new business tie-ins—allows more people to contribute and solidifies and enriches the relationship.

- Prioritize strategic partnerships. No organization can be all things to all people. A partnership will be fueled by ongoing support on both sides if it addresses a key strategic need for both parties.

LOOKING FORWARD

Two trends for the future are inevitable. First, many more medical advances will emerge from the laboratories of companies investing in R&D. Second, the resulting extension of life into old age will strain health care payment systems, public and private. It will be virtually impossible for any government to guarantee the best in health care to its entire population. A very high degree of private sector involvement will be necessary.

This suggests many possibilities for partnerships between business, government, and the nonprofit sector. There is no doubt that creative and inclusive partnerships that stretch the boundaries of current thinking will yield the most far-reaching and enduring solutions to the world's health problems. It is also clear that only win-win—or mutualistic—strategies will receive the funding, leadership, and attention necessary for success. Increased investments in both business and society will be made by the private sector in countries that encourage innovation, respect patent and property rights, and create markets that are conducive to investment.

Members of the global health community, which includes fiercely competitive organizations even within sectors, are already setting aside differences as they work together toward common goals. These working relationships will necessarily be a patchwork of large and small, local and global partnerships involving all kinds of companies, all levels of government, and many different nonprofit organizations. Partnership can be as small as a crew of employees spending a few Saturday mornings at a local clinic or as large as a multinational, multiorganization effort to eradicate a disease. Together, they break down isolation and distill the power of individuals to solve our greatest global challenges.

CHAPTER FORTY-EIGHT

The Nonprofit Sector
in Partnership with
Government

Nils Daulaire

Nils Daulaire, MD, MPH, *is President and Chief Executive Officer of the Global Health Council, an international membership organization devoted to improving health around the world; among the council's members are leading nongovernmental organizations, private corporations, foundations, and agencies. Previously, he served as the U.S. government's senior expert on global health issues at the Agency for International Development following two decades of fieldwork as a public health physician in the developing world.*

The closing decade of the twentieth century brought into sharp focus the vast changes under way in the organization and dynamics of global society. Many of these changes derive from the process of globalization, which is itself driven by an unprecedented pace of technological change and innovation. The ways in which health is viewed and health care is accessed and delivered will be profoundly shaped by these dynamics.

The role of governments in directly providing services will be substantially diminished as a result of the systemic changes that will be described in this chapter. It will be crucial for the nonprofit sector to fill this gap, particularly in providing health care to the poor, and to do so with governments' blessing and support.

The overarching paradigm of the postcolonial twentieth century was the global establishment of nation-states as the unifying force for social cohesion, with principal responsibility for addressing the well-being of their citizens. The governments of these nation-states have in most countries assumed the lead role for assuring the provision of health services. They have done this with varying degrees of efficiency and equity, often reflecting the political currents and forces competing for control of the resources and legitimacy, which governments largely monopolized. Clearly, government health services in Norway have meant something quite different from those in Sierra Leone.

CHANGING PATTERN

The twentieth-century paradigm is now rapidly shifting, and nation-states and their governments are destined to play a much smaller relative role in the twenty-first century. The emerging global reality, already coming into view, will instead be characterized by a tripartite dynamic relationship among government, civil society (principally manifested through nonprofit institutions), and the private sector.

The unraveling of Soviet-style communism was emblematic of the reality that governments are no longer sole masters of their financial situations, and in many cases not even the principal actors. Yet the prospect of a world driven exclusively by neoliberal economic forces in a borderless competitive marketplace has led many observers to question whether this is a return to a Darwinian economic jungle rather than an evolution toward a better world. For this reason, the role of the nonprofit sector is more important than ever before: to serve as a balancing force in which the efficiencies of profitability are held up to the light of human need and dignity and in which the resulting gaps are addressed.

However, economic globalization is in some respects directly supportive of the growing role of the nonprofit sector for global health. The dynamics of open markets and open communication lead almost inevitably to a pluralistic network of active partners in which it will be increasingly difficult to monopolize power. Furthermore, the speed with which information can now be widely accessed means that the combined social resources previously mobilized only by governments or very large corporations will no longer be necessary to access information essential for providing adequate health care.

ECONOMICS SHIFTING

At the same time, government's role is diminishing in most countries of the world as the predominant source of financing for health care. In part this is due to the nearly global acceptance of the economic precepts (deficit reduction, open foreign exchange, and so on) that have driven structural reforms, resulting in downward pressure on government budgets around the world. In part it is due to the demonstrated deficiencies in command-style health services provided by many governments, with limited accountability and little competitive pressure to improve services and to innovate.

The increasing role of the private sector has also led to a growing role for nonprofit institutions. With the growth of enormous personal and corporate wealth generated by the rapidly globalizing private sector, individuals and companies have begun to make unprecedented social investments in health through the mechanism of nonprofit institutions. As evidenced by major late-twentieth-century contributions made by Bill Gates and Ted Turner, among others, these investments are made from a growing sense of the importance of good global economic citizenship. They are also driven by a growing recognition in the business community that good health is essential for economic growth and social stability and that health, like commerce, now transcends national boundaries.

Meanwhile, among those billions of people who are themselves achieving some degree of financial sufficiency as a consequence of global economic growth, the perceived importance of the quality of the health services they receive, and their willingness to pay out-of-pocket toward that end, is increasing. This is leading to increased demand and use of services outside those provided by governments and contributes to the growth of both private sector and nonprofit sector health care. In some instances, nonprofit institutions have already demonstrated a nimble response to the marketplace by providing high-quality fee-for-service care to patients able to pay and using revenues to underwrite services for the poor.

In the triangular relationship of government, the private sector, and nonprofit organizations, nonprofits have a number of distinct advantages that need to be mobilized and enhanced to achieve broad improvements in health and to prevent widening disparities. And while the three actors need to maintain the distinct approaches that derive from the difference in their missions and operations, there is enormous scope for cooperation.

The reality of the new century is that governments need the nonprofit sector as a partner in providing health care, particularly to the most underserved, and in maintaining a focus on social need. Most especially in the poorest countries, the generation of additional resources to be applied directly to the health of the poor, both from within the populations being served and from outside, is one of the comparative strengths of nonprofit organizations. This makes them the logical predominant source of health care service delivery for all but the affluent.

CHANGING THE MIND-SET

However, this cannot be achieved in the face of opposition from government officials. In many instances, health ministries look on nonprofit organizations as irrelevant or even a nuisance. This is grounded in the continued perception on the part of many officials that health care is rightfully and exclusively a state service and on the part of some political leaders in poorer countries that the large number of jobs that go along with the health system are a ripe source of patronage. Clearly, this mind-set must change.

The twenty-first century will see an explosive growth of health care provided by the nonprofit sector. For a long time, not-for-profit organizations have shown that they are best able to reach the poor and marginalized, in large part because addressing inequity and social justice is at the core of their values. And the poor and marginalized are the major health challenges the world faces as we enter the new century.

The vast majority of the children born in the closing years of the twentieth century (and therefore the vast majority of the world's citizens by midcentury) were born in developing countries, and a high proportion of them will grow up in slums and impoverished villages. Their adult health and productivity will be enormously dependent on their health as children and on the health of their mothers. This will influence not just the conditions of the societies in which they are born but—thanks to the explosive growth of human migration coupled with globalization—the social conditions of countries all over the world. And who has demonstrated the greatest capacity and commitment to address the health needs of these mothers and children at the community level? The nonprofit sector.

For decades, nonprofits have developed tools for community mobilization, for effective outreach, and for serving the disenfranchised. Not tied to governments, they can avoid the pitfalls of directing resources to where the political pull is greatest; not tied to the private sector, they are not forced to focus on where profit potential is greatest. Operating independently, they are often able to address the needs of those who are deeply suspicious of formal structures of authority. Often satisfied with small-scale operations, they avoid the bureaucracy and inertia of larger systems.

Governments of poorer countries in the twenty-first century would be well advised to take advantage of these strengths and help reinforce them. The greatest source of social and political unrest in these countries is among the poor and the young. Nonprofit organizations that address their health needs will serve a direct social need through the improved health and well-being that they directly engender. In addition, because many nonprofit organizations work across the spectrum of development, their health services become an entry point for a broader range of socially important activities, including nutrition, schooling, skills generation, microenterprise development, and ultimately poverty reduction. Each of these in turn contributes to improved health conditions, creating a virtuous cycle that the vertical structures of government are generally unable to provide.

DEVELOPING ALLIES

Whereas nonprofit organizations are key to health and human development in these poorer countries, health ministries of middle- and higher-income countries would also do well to recognize their potential value. Because government investments are almost universally controlled by ministries of finance, rather than ministries of health, an important potential role of the nonprofit sector—particularly in light of their strong networks of international alliances—is in helping influence and direct both national and multilateral policies and priorities and in advocacy to assure that more resources are directed toward essential health needs. In this context, the nonprofit sector could become a valuable ally of government health agencies, which must generally compete with other government agencies for funds in a political environment.

Governments and multilateral agencies are already beginning to experience the benefits of engaging with nonprofit institutions knowledgeable about health issues and the mechanisms for reaching the underserved in their countries, particularly in national-level needs identification and planning strategies. The result is better, more efficient, and more responsive programs, and this model should be widely followed around the world.

Nonprofit organizations, for their part, need to understand, and be able to make the case, that their work and the investments made in health have enormous potential impacts on national economies. It is increasingly clear that the level of health, particularly among children, youth, and working adults, has a direct effect on economic growth and productivity. Though the motivation underlying most of their activities has to do with equity and justice, they cannot realize their full potential for serving their advocacy mission if they do not use all the tools at their command.

Finally, nonprofit organizations engaged in health pose enormous advantages for those governments willing to engage with them. Because nonprofits are not bound by the same inflexible set of rules and regulations of government agencies, they are far more open to experimentation and innovation. It is natural that a considerable proportion of these efforts will fail, but those that succeed will provide important lessons for the wider health community. And because these organizations do not need to function under the same political and social constraints of government agencies, nonprofits have traditionally been at the leading edge of new and sensitive approaches, such as sexual and reproductive health, in which the people and their desire for effective services and interventions are often ahead of their political leaders. By quietly encouraging these efforts on the part of nonprofits, health ministries can build a base for support for widening those programs to serve important social and health needs.

THE CHALLENGE AHEAD

The world of the twenty-first century could become a world even more deeply split into widely disparate health groups, with the medical "haves" achieving life expectancies approaching a century while the medical "have-nots" struggle to reach and maintain half that. Avoiding this outcome, and its disastrous social consequences in a world in which disparities can no longer be hidden by distance, requires a meaningful partnership between the nonprofit sector and government that respects their differences but recognizes the primacy that both place on social cohesion.

This partnership is essential for the effective tripartite relationship, which also includes the private sector. With a strong voice for equity in health always at the table, the initiative and inventiveness of the private sector can be far more effectively deployed to improve the health of all the world's people and not just its privileged minority. In this way, global health can become a reality in the twenty-first century.

CHAPTER FORTY-NINE

Philanthropy and Global Health Equity

Lincoln C. Chen, Timothy G. Evans, and Margaret E. Wirth

Lincoln C. Chen, MD, *is Executive Vice President for Strategy of the Rockefeller Foundation. He was formerly Director of the Harvard Center for Population and Development Studies and Chair of Harvard University's Department of Population and International Health. His latest publication is "Health as a Global Public Good," written with Timothy Evans and Richard Cash in* Global Public Goods: International Cooperation in the 21st Century.

Timothy G. Evans, MD, *is Team Director in the Health Equity Team of the Rockefeller Foundation. He was formerly Assistant Professor of Population and International Health at the Harvard School of Public Health and currently serves on the Board of Directors of the Global Forum for Health Research and the Global Alliance for Vaccines and Immunization.*

Margaret E. Wirth *manages the Rockefeller Foundation/ Swedish International Development Agency Global Health Equity Initiative, a group of one hundred researchers pursuing in-depth country analyses and fundamental thinking on the gender, measurement, and ethical dimensions of health equity. She previously worked on John Snow, Inc.'s safe motherhood project in Indonesia.*

Τ he early twentieth century in global health was marked by the exciting entree of philanthropists such as Andrew Carnegie and John D. Rockefeller. These pioneers used their substantial personal wealth to support the efforts of the best minds and science to further their vision of improving the well-being of the poor. In health, the dividends have been long-lasting, with landmarks such as the 1910 Flexner Report, a blueprint that revolutionized medical education, the development of a yellow fever vaccine, the eradication of hookworm, the pioneering of new fields such as molecular biology, and the building of schools of public health. Despite this impressive start and further significant expansion of health philanthropies, their relative importance in global health has waned over the past half century. This reflects both a reduction in the purchasing power of philanthropic resources against a trillion-dollar health care industry and a trend toward a more inward focus on domestic health concerns.

As we enter the twenty-first century, new billionaire philanthropists engineering pathbreaking partnerships with civil society and the private sector are heeding the call for greater attention to global health issues (Institute of Medicine, 1997). An exciting new era in philanthropy for global health is upon us.

PHILANTHROPY AT THE DAWN OF THE NEW CENTURY

Philanthropic activity in global health evolved considerably in the twentieth century. It began the century as a surrogate public sector, found a midcentury role as a partner with governments and universities, and evolved into one of the many players in the increasingly heterogeneous institutional landscape of global health.

At the turn of the twenty-first century, sweeping changes in political arrangements, both within and between countries, have spawned an era of governmental retrenchment from the health arena and realigned the partnering potential of philanthropy. A proliferation of nongovernmental organizations (NGOs), coupled with an increased interest in "local community solutions" and "bottom-up development," meant that foundations developed affiliations and direct links at the community level (Renz, and others, 1997). The concepts of "social capital" and of the "social entrepreneur" playing the role of change agent have built on the notions of communities solving their own problems. In an effort to strengthen organizational capabilities, bring programs to scale, and sustain effective social programs, "venture philanthropy" is revolutionizing the way some foundations craft their agendas. Based on a venture capital model, these endeavors "stretch philanthropy beyond traditional grantmaking and into more opportunistic market-based models" (Reis and Clohesy, 1999). Philanthropy is likely to move toward a greater partnership with the private commercial sector and civil society organizations, perhaps allowing greater effectiveness of its funds and faster progress toward common goals.

The dramatic entrance of new players in the global health arena has taken both funding and momentum to a new order of magnitude. In a single year, the Gates Foundation will allocate roughly half a billion dollars for international health, an amount equivalent to the entire outlay of the Rockefeller Foundation for public health and medicine over the past eighty-five years or the annual budget of the World Health Organization. New players, partnerships, and instruments of change are a promising antidote to an increasingly complex set of global health challenges.

An Emerging Global Health Agenda

Health in the twentieth century can be summarized in four words: "spectacular achievements, spectacular inequities" (Foege, 1998, p. 1931). It is remarkable that in some countries, the average person can expect to live to see eighty years of age and deplorable that in others, life expectancy reaches only forty. In the Western world, people can expect to survive with AIDS for twenty years or more, while in eastern and southern Africa, AIDS has precipitated a twenty-year reduction in life expectancy. Maldistribution of health is a challenge both between and within countries. In the United States, the average life expectancy of black men (fifty-eight years) in the least healthy county falls more than three decades short of that of Asian-American men (eighty-nine years) in the healthiest county (Murray and others, 1998). The common challenge for all health systems in the twenty-first century, therefore, is not simply the production of health but its equitable distribution.

These disparities reflect, in part, the failure of global public health to bring the power of science and political will to bear on an unfinished agenda of infectious diseases. Breakthroughs in science today are strongly driven by market incentives, leaving diseases endemic to poor countries or minority populations shamefully neglected. As noted in the example of AIDS, even when lifesaving technologies do exist, they may accentuate rather than diminish health inequities due to issues of affordability and access to health services. To ensure truly global access to scientific advances, development and distribution of health technology for the poor and marginalized therefore requires equity-oriented leadership and public-private partnership.

The ability of health systems to provide equitable health care is being challenged by a global wave of health care reform. Driven by cost pressures, technological advances, and a general weakening of the state, private commercial services are gaining ascendancy in rich and poor countries alike. With the emergence of a second generation of noncommunicable diseases among the middle class, consumer demand is likely to divert health care services away from the first generation of poverty-linked health problems. Thus a weakened public sector and market failures in the private sector are likely to exacerbate inequities in health.

The trend of global health reform is indicative of a new global era, one in which long-present forces are accelerating and broadening their reach. The transnationalization of human interaction is accompanied by potential risks and opportunities that affect health and well-being. Populations that were once quarantined to control disease now move freely across borders. Health risks may spread globally through infectious pathogens, but pervasive economic and social forces are also increasingly seen to affect health and health behaviors. Health advances or setbacks in one place influence health across the globe. The expansion of the tropics, the evolution of species, and even the influence of the media are creating a new set of universal health challenges, making the indivisibility of health and health risks evident.

This set of health challenges is global, not specific to any particular setting or context. Leadership to redress disparities in health, health products for the poor, promotion of equitable health systems, and efforts to confront common emerging threats comprise a common *global* agenda for health. Solutions or breakthroughs in the form of global public goods—goods that are desired and used by everyone without exclusion or competitiveness—are ends for which philanthropy's unique strengths can be marshaled.

PHILANTHROPY'S NICHE

The comparative advantage of philanthropy in global health lies largely in its unfettered resources, which allow it to pursue public health priorities, independent of shifting political tides. Long-term commitments to knowledge-based solutions are cultivated with the intent of distributing benefits to all. This section considers three broad areas in the global health agenda where philanthropic assets might be catalytic: strengthening global leadership, harnessing new sciences, and promoting equitable health systems.

Strengthening Global Leadership

An emerging literature on future challenges of global health has drawn attention to the need to reconsider the world health institutional arrangements (Al-Mazrou and others, 1997; Walt, 1998). In examining institutions such as the World Bank and the World Health Organization, there is consensus that more transparent, flexible, and participatory processes are needed. Shrinking public sectors, increasing private market health care delivery systems, and a proliferation of NGOs are also important trends that diversify leadership for global health. A striking feature of the quickly shifting institutional landscape is that no single institution can be relied on exclusively for solving complex problems. The risk amid this plurality of players is a leadership vacuum—the challenge is to foster leadership opportunities through innovative partnerships and collaborations.

Philanthropy is in an excellent position to catalyze new types of leadership. It is seen by many as a neutral player and can use its convening power to assemble alliances or coalitions of interested parties around a common issue. In addition, it has an unparalleled flexibility of funds, which can be used to facilitate the creation of new leadership forms requiring convening, facilitation, and early seed funding.

The recent efforts toward United Nations reforms reflect a growing desire to remove the institutions from the playground of geopolitics to the forefront of social, humanitarian, and security issues. For example, the philanthropic sponsorship of a fundamental rethinking of global health governance called the "Pocantico process," was not only an important contribution toward the blueprint for a renewed World Health Organization, but also brought a degree of accountability to the process of selecting the new Director-General

(Al-Mazrou and others, 1997). The arrival of the new Director-General at WHO was accompanied by a catalytic injection of philanthropic resources for a Global Health Leadership Fellows Program aimed at infusing the institution with fresh talents to accelerate reforms and priority programs.

Another important future issue in global leadership is vigilance regarding the health consequences of other global phenomena—environmental, economic and social—including, for example, scrutiny of the health effects of trade and intellectual property rights agreements. Central to health leadership will be the imperative of fostering the role of civil society as both partner and leader in mobilizing for health equity.

Harnessing New Sciences

We are on the cusp of an explosion in new knowledge in health technologies based on unprecedented power to understand the basic mechanisms of human function embedded in the genetic code—genomics. The health products industry's primary incentive of market returns, however, constrains the application of this tremendous scientific potential to solve the diseases of the poor. Economically orphaned diseases, such as tuberculosis, are unable to draw the requisite research and development investments from private industry to ensure a prospective flow of new drugs and vaccines. The global health challenge, therefore, is to harness the new sciences for orphan diseases afflicting populations that cannot command the attention of private markets.

Philanthropy is well positioned to take up this challenge. Its long-standing commitment to knowledge-based solutions provides a global set of contacts and healthy respect in both the private and public sectors. This scientific credibility, along with convening power, allows philanthropy to assemble a diverse set of actors with complementary assets around the problem of orphan diseases. With strategically placed investments aimed at unleashing latent corporate goodwill, innovative partnerships may emerge. A philanthropy-brokered partnership between a start-up biotechnology company and a large pharmaceutical company for applied research on malaria drug discovery is one such example of a business opportunity that neither company might have embarked on on its own.

Innovative partnerships for new products and their distribution have often been stimulated by philanthropy. The International AIDS

Vaccine Initiative (1999), for example, has linked novel vaccine technologies for AIDS vaccines with clinical trial partners in developing countries. This view of the need for more applied or translational research signals a dramatic departure from a previous era when scientific investments earmarked for new technologies were directed largely toward more basic academic research. Such a shift requires new philanthropic tools and skills. A promising example is provided by the Wellcome Trust, the world's largest scientific philanthropy; in 1998, it launched "Catalyst Biomedica," a unit dedicated to facilitating the translation of its basic research toward product applications.

Promoting Equitable Health Systems

Success in strengthening global leadership and developing technology for the poor must ultimately find its expression through a viable health system. Integrating these health opportunities into fragile and underresourced health systems may run the risk of exacerbating inequalities in health. Even when an impressive arsenal of health technologies exists, health inequities may be created where health services are inaccessible because of constraining factors such as gender, geography, infrastructure, or economic development. Time and again, the lifesaving benefits of new breakthroughs like oral rehydration therapy for diarrhea or childhood vaccines, remain largely unrealized because political will, resource allocation, and health care delivery systems are unable to ensure universal access to scientific progress.

The inequitable processes and outcomes of health systems are encapsulated by the following set of maxims: (1) the healthiest often consume most health care, (2) public subsidies for health are highest among the highest-income groups, and (3) prevention services for diseases that disproportionately affect the poor are greatest among the wealthy (Hart, 1971). Research has demonstrated the almost universal existence of these "inverse care laws." Not only are the poor less likely to receive care, but they are more vulnerable to impoverishment due to the medical care and other expenditures associated with catastrophic illness. As first steps, health systems must develop more equitable financing policies and priority interventions. In the longer term, health systems research and development must generate new pathways for a cadre of public health professionals and dynamic institutions that safeguard the needs of the poor in the complexity of the global health environment.

The comparative advantage of philanthropy in the realm of health systems lies in its ability to transfer knowledge and lessons across national boundaries, engage in networking, and promote a paradigm that provides alternatives to standard prescriptions. The Henry J. Kaiser Family Foundation's funding of the Equity Gauge in South Africa (a project directed by Health Systems Trust) is an exceptional example of philanthropic interest in the equity of health systems (Franklin, Harrison, and Sinclair, 1998). The project works directly with provincial legislators to develop indicators of health equity and to monitor trends and successes within and between South African provinces. This program may serve as a model for other countries, given its promise in introducing accountability and an equity focus to evolving health systems. Though the problems are similar, solutions for health systems will vary by country, culture, and region. Through partnership with civil society, "laboratories" of creative experimentation and strategic thinking can contribute to the reclaiming of public health systems by the populations they ought to serve best.

Envisioning the Way Forward

The conditions that favored a prominent role for philanthropy in health at the beginning of the twentieth century—unusually concentrated industrial wealth being made available for social good at a time of major social transformation—have in essence reemerged at the beginning of the twenty-first. Likewise, the awareness of a new set of universal health challenges and the recognition of the indivisibility of health emphasize the imperative global perspective. The global health agenda for the twenty-first century is staggering—environmental insults, mental health issues, ethnic conflicts, displaced populations, infectious threats, economic volatility, and decentralization, to name but a few. Amid these myriad issues and concerns, philanthropy can blaze a path toward global health security by catalyzing leadership, channeling scientific know-how, and reorienting health systems around the health needs of the poor and excluded.

What would success look like?

- Revitalized global health institutions that are open and accountable to the health needs of the poor

- The integration of health concerns into diverse arenas that influence health, including institutions such as the World Trade

Organization and the International Monetary Fund

- New and innovative community-based partnerships that monitor progress toward equity in health
- A global surveillance and early-response capacity for emerging and reemerging health threats
- Promotion of individual agency in health via access to knowledge and resources through the new information technologies
- A flow of new drugs and vaccines for orphaned diseases drawn from the frontiers of science and technology
- Funding that ensures global access to orphan vaccines and drugs
- A children's health trust that ensures that all children enjoy the benefits of a universal package of essential health interventions
- Sustainable health care financing mechanisms that insure against medical care impoverishment
- Clear evidence of ways to redress health disparities in a range of interventions, both within and beyond the health sector
- A Flexner Report equivalent, representing a consensus on global public health training and education for the twenty-first century

With the unique confluence of new partners, dramatically increased resources, more global reach, and a commitment to equity in health, philanthropy is poised to make contributions to world health that will surpass those of a century ago.

References

Al-Mazrou, Y., and others. "A Vital Opportunity for Global Health: Supporting the World Health Organization at a Critical Juncture" (letter to the editor). *Lancet,* 1997, *350,* 750–751.

Foege, W. "Global Public Health: Targeting Inequities." *Journal of the American Medical Association,* 1998, *279,* 1931–1932.

Franklin, L., Harrison, D., and Sinclair, M. *A Travelling Seminar on the Attainability and Affordability of Equity in Health Care Provision: Workshop Proceedings, the Philippines, June 28–July 5, 1997.* Durban, South Africa: Henry J. Kaiser Family Foundation, 1998.

Flexner, A. *Medical Education in the United States and Canada*. New York: Carnegie Foundation for the Advancement of Teaching, 1910.

Hart Tudor, J. "The Inverse Care Law." *Lancet,* 1971, *1,* 405–412.

Institute of Medicine. *America's Vital Interest in Global Health*. Washington, D.C.: National Academy Press, 1997.

International AIDS Vaccine Initiative. *IAVI Report: A Newsletter on International AIDS Vaccine Research*. New York: IAVI 1999, *4,* 1, 12–13,

Murray, C.J.L., and others. *U.S. Patterns of Mortality by County and Race, 1965–1994*. Cambridge, Mass.: Harvard Center for Population and Development Studies, 1998.

Reis, T., and Clohesy, S. *Unleashing New Resources and Entrepreneurship for the Common Good: A Scan, Synthesis, and Scenario for Action*. Battle Creek, Mich.: W. K. Kellogg Foundation, 1999, 3.

Renz, L. J., and others. *International Grantmaking: A Report on U.S. Foundation Trends*. New York: Foundation Center, 1997.

Additional Reading

"Balms for the Poor." *The Economist,* August 14–20, 1999.

Franklin, L., Harrison, D., and Sinclair, M. *A Travelling Seminar on the Attainability and Affordability of Equity in HealthCare Provision: Workshop Proceedings, The Philippines, June 28–July 5, 1997*. Durban: Henry J. Kaiser Family Foundation, 1999.

Letts, C. W., and others. "Virtuous Capital: What Foundations Can Learn from Venture Capitalists. *Harvard Business Review,* 1997, *75,* 2.

Walt, G. "Globalisation of International Health." *The Lancet,* 1998, *351,* 434–437.

World Health Organization. *The World Health Report: 1995: Bridging the Gaps*. Geneva: World Health Organization, 1995.

CHAPTER FIFTY

The Role of Public Health Associations

Mohammad N. Akhter

Mohammad N. Akhter, MD, MPH, *is Executive Director of the American Public Health Association and Adjunct Professor of International Public Health at the George Washington University School of Public Health and Health Services. He is also a member of the Executive Board of the World Federation of Public Health Associations and a member of the U.S. delegation to the WHO World Health Assembly.*

W hat will be the future role of public health associations? In answering this question, it is helpful to consider what public health associations (PHAs) are doing right now. Once we know and understand their present role, it is easier to forecast what their future role will be.

PUBLIC HEALTH ASSOCIATIONS: THEIR PRESENT ROLE

Public health associations vary greatly in the world today. They range from small, primarily social groups to large, diverse organizations that carry out a host of functions such as publications, advocacy, and policy development. The smaller groups are more commonly found in the developing world and are often centered on just a few individuals—family members or friends—and their social networks. The larger, diverse associations exist more in the developed world, in such countries as Canada, the United Kingdom, and the United States. Most of the associations fall somewhere in between. Educational development of their members is a key component. These associations, a number of which are in Africa, Asia, and the Middle East, are often project-based organizations and receive assistance from donor agencies.

The larger, more developed associations currently participate in a wide variety of activities. In the United Kingdom, for instance, the Royal Society for the Promotion of Health is an accreditation body for programs dealing with food safety, and it is empowered to qualify public health workers in certain specialties.

In Canada, the Canadian Public Health Association, in partnership with the federal government, has been involved in disease surveillance and control, health promotion, and environmental health at home and in activities to strengthen public health associations in other countries.

In the United States, the American Public Health Association (APHA) places a high priority on policy development and advocacy. By using current technologies such as e-mail, listservs, and broadcast faxes, APHA is able to rapidly marshal member positions on pending legislation and regulations through its network of membership groups.

THE DEVELOPMENT STAGES OF PUBLIC HEALTH ASSOCIATIONS

Judging from experience in the field, we know that PHAs typically progress through four distinct stages of development: the social stage, the professional stage, the policy formulation stage, and the policy implementation stage.

Social Stage

In this first stage, a group of public health professionals, most often known to each other from the workplace, become better acquainted and seek a social outlet as their mutual professional interests become clear. Thus develops a core group of like-minded health professionals with a growing commitment to professional interests, strengthened by social contacts and blossoming friendships. At this stage, the group is a proto-organization, its functions loosely structured and informally carried out. Leaders emerge, but they are not elected, and functions are understood rather than being written down. This type of PHA will continue to exist in the twenty-first century, mostly in the less developed countries.

Professional Stage

As the professional health interests of the group strengthen and become more focused, interests begin to diversify among the group's members—for example, some may be more interested in continuing health education while others may be more motivated by policy issues and advocacy. At this point, the organizational structure of the group is likely to become more formalized, possibly with elected officers and written rules for the organization's activities. These are the hallmarks of the professional stage—the stage PHAs in most of the developing countries will be at in the coming decades.

Policy Formulation Stage

At this stage, the PHA reaches maturity: it becomes fully conversant with the broad range of public health issues in its country and is recognized by the government as an authority on these issues. It is therefore positioned to help shape the policy debate on these issues in the broader context of national public policy. As a result, PHAs will often initiate the policy debate and help influence policy outcomes that protect the health interests of the public. Developing countries at the upper end of the social and economic development process will be in this stage.

Policy Implementation Stage

This is the most advanced stage of PHA development; it is also in some sense the most challenging, for it calls on PHAs to commit their resources to a lengthy and sometimes difficult process of policy development and implementation. The successful attainment of this stage is well worth the effort, as it invariably imparts the benefits that come from active participation in the nation's health agenda. It also entails advancing human rights and social justice, of which health policies form an integral part. One of the most salient characteristics of this stage is the role of the PHA in generating public support to encourage policymakers to make decisions that are consistent with the best public health practices. This becomes increasingly possible as the world's governments grow ever more democratic.

These stages may be seen as benchmarks along a continuum that gauge progress in the professional development of PHAs. Such a continuum may be used over time to analyze the development of PHAs and to enhance the understanding of their roles, scope, and effectiveness.

THE FUTURE ROLE: MAXIMIZING UNTAPPED POTENTIAL

Increasingly, PHAs are being seen as key players in future organized efforts to improve the health status of the world's population. In such scenarios, PHAs that reach their full potential by developing and advocating policy, translating research findings into practice, and providing public and professional education will make a very substantial contribution to improving health outcomes.

Any discussion of the future role of PHAs must also take into account the role of government in the public health arena. Governments have historically been seen as the principal funding resource for public health, but many have allocated relatively little funding for this purpose. With the trend toward democratization, PHAs will have a significant role in creating public support for the use of expanded governmental resources for public health programs. This is exemplified in many democratic countries today in which without PHA advocacy, only a small portion of the countries' budget would be made available for public health. The American Public Health Association's key role in advocating for passage of the U.S. public health budget is a case in point. In the international arena, too, PHAs or NGOs are being looked to as agencies that can make an important contribution to public health. International organizations such as the World Health Organization and the World Bank have demonstrated that they wish to go beyond focusing on governments to reach out to the private sector and involve institutions such as the PHAs in the development process.

In many countries, PHAs will play a catalytic role in bringing together other nongovernmental associations to address common public health problems and issues.

The approach of PHAs will be to take a leadership role in forging links with the government and to develop productive public-private partnerships that become models for others to emulate.

TRANSCENDING POLITICAL BOUNDARIES AND CULTURAL DIFFERENCES

Furthering productive partnerships between governments and PHAs is an important means of improving the health status of populations. There may also be situations where PHAs can move beyond the bounds of these relationships and make positive contributions to global public health. PHAs can also pursue initiatives in areas and move in directions where governments have found it difficult or even impossible to make headway.

For example, in the South Asian region, recent collaborative efforts have begun bringing together public health officials and professionals to discuss and identify cooperative actions to deal with emerging and reemerging infectious diseases. PHAs everywhere have an important role to play as emissaries creating understanding and goodwill among the peoples of different nations and facilitating regional collaboration to address specific public health concerns.

PHAs are positioned to play an increasingly important role in the years ahead not only in global health but also on the broader stage of national and international policies and programs. This also suggests several important roles for the World Federation of Public Health Associations (WFPHA), a global federation with more than sixty active members drawn from national public health associations around the world. For example, the federation can help strengthen its member associations in a variety of ways. Also, along with its national members, the federation will continue to shape a global agenda on public health problems and issues of key importance and chart a future course that helps resolve those problems.

THE FUTURE ROLE OF PUBLIC HEALTH ASSOCIATIONS

In summary, PHAs may be expected to play the following roles in the twenty-first century:

- *Fulfilling professional obligations*—educating members of the general public about public health issues and transforming them into advocates for effective resolution of these issues
- *Fulfilling national obligations*—translating research findings into public health practice and educating health professionals to use

these findings in the most cost-effective manner; also, creating public-private partnerships by providing an environment in which governments and NGOs can establish productive partnerships

- *Fulfilling international obligations*—creating regional collaborations among PHAs and other NGOs to deal with major public health issues that cross political and ethnic boundaries; taking a leadership role through WFPHA in exploring and addressing global health concerns such as environmental health concerns; and serving as major advisers to international agencies working on global health issues, such as WHO and the World Bank

Public health associations are rapidly evolving as a force in public health and over time will undoubtedly play a significant role in the improvement of global health.

CHAPTER FIFTY ONE

The Mandate: Transformational Leadership

Gary L. Filerman, Clarence E. Pearson

Gary L. Filerman, PhD, *is Senior Health Adviser at the Academy for Educational Development. He has been President of the Association of University Programs in Health Administration and Associate Director of the Pew Commission on the Future of the Health Professions. He has served as a consultant in three dozen countries to foundations; bilateral and multilateral development agencies; and government agencies including ministries of education and health.*

Clarence E. Pearson, MPH, *is the Founding President and Chief Executive Officer of the National Center for Health Education, established in 1975 at the recommendation of a special presidential commission. He is currently Senior Adviser to the World Health Organization and the United Nations' Task Force on the Tobacco Free Initiative. He has served as an executive and public health and management consultant to nonprofit organizations, global corporations, and governmental agencies in the United States and abroad.*

From a wide range of perspectives, the chapters in this book present a thorough assessment of the state of global health at the turn of the century and propose an agenda for the progress of health sciences and prognostications for how the sciences will contribute to improved global health status. There is considerable consensus on health objectives and increasing agreement on the means of accomplishing them. The question is, given the realities of resource constraints, political will, and resistance to change, is the existing health service infrastructure up to the job? Are we organized to apply the knowledge, information, and data in the right way, in the right place, and at the right time to achieve the objectives?

Clearly, existing resources and knowledge are not invested or deployed optimally now. From the standpoint of access, quality, and cost, not a single health system is achieving its objectives. Some health systems are more effective than others, and many have relatively effective research, education, public health, service provision, and financing components. But every system has significant and measurable gaps in health status, and despite the expansion of knowledge and resources, many of the gaps are widening.

Every component of the health enterprise is being empowered by the knowledge surge. Progress in preventive, therapeutic, and rehabilitative technologies, communications, nutrition, genetics, and many other fields is providing an armamentarium that is continually changing the ideal of an effective health care system. At the same time, poverty, with all its implications for health status, remains entrenched. Income disparities within and among nations is intractable. Environmental degradation continues to expand threats to health. Disasters of both natural and human origin continue to impose huge burdens on limited health resources. There is a wide gap between even the existing health system and the needs it is intended to address. The gap will not narrow in the foreseeable future.

Positioned between the progress and the needs is the health infrastructure, the myriad of people, organizations, systems, and public policies that societies have crafted to protect and improve the public health. It is not performing adequately. The largest gap of all is the inability to apply existing knowledge.

That is not a new disclosure; the history of health systems is a history of efforts to increase resources and to employ them more effectively. From the perspective of international development, these efforts have been incremental and have in large part consisted of attempts to transfer relatively successful experiences among very different cultures, with uneven results. These efforts have also been characterized by fidelity to a handful of health organization models, driven by a belief that with more authority, staff, and resources, these models will cost-effectively lead to improved health status. But have these models of organization, derived in conditions that are changing rapidly, now become more confining than empowering?

Take, for example, departments or ministries of health. Is the ministry of health the instrument to achieve the fundamental public policy objective of closing the gap? Given what is known about the determinants of health status, what is the most logical way of organizing a country's efforts to improve the productivity and health of the people? Some students of organization development would argue that the structure prevents, or least does not encourage, learning. The case can be made that coherent public health policies and investments can best be achieved through innovative approaches to organizing many of the education, health, nutrition, and economic functions of modern government. Perhaps the answer is a ministry of home and family or a ministry of community development. Can such an approach raise the status of the health function, institutionalize inter-sectoral collaboration, improve the process of prioritizing resource investments, attract and retain more top talent, and reduce the silo mentality of many health bureaucrats?

Who will challenge the conventional wisdom of health service policy and organization by raising such questions and proposing such options? We are certain that individuals will ultimately rise above the current frame of reference to envision different ways of achieving the goal of health for all. Leadership development in health has stressed mastering the current frame of reference and has focused on management process. Much has been achieved, but progress has been confined by learning the old models rather than challenging them; it has also been constrained by credentialism.

The surge of knowledge mandates the health infrastructure to reach for new leadership (rather than management), empowered to lead change in how we think and how we organize the work of health and ultimately to reengineer health systems to address the gap between what we know and what people need. It must be transformational leadership.

Transformational leadership is driven by vision. A vision is a preferred future, reduced to its component specific objectives, and an agenda for achieving them. A vision is useful only if it is transformable into action. What differentiates the transformational health leader from the typical health manager is a synthesis of vision and skills in translating the agenda into policies, practical applications, benchmarks, accountabilities, assessments, and revisions. Perhaps visioning cannot be taught or learned, but it can be nurtured.

The surge of knowledge suggests that the vision of transformational leaders must first be predicated on results—quantifiable or qualitative outcomes against which the wisdom of policy and the value of investments can be measured. The crescendo of insights into the determinants of health status makes it clear that results depend on coherent health policies, many, if not most, of which lie beyond the traditional scope of health policy. Thus the transformational health leadership role reaches across many policy domains.

The vision recognizes the strengths and limitations of government and those of the private and the voluntary sectors and weaves them into a practical, realistic, and appropriate health system. Such systems will rationalize the existing vertical, competing programs. They will seek strategic partnerships opportunistically with any entity that is best able to contribute to achieving the objectives.

Systems with transformational leadership institutionalize continuous adaptive change to improve quality, both in structure and in people, who constitute the core asset. It has been difficult for many health organizations to put new knowledge to work because of the tendency to make it conform to the organization instead of adapting the organization to the knowledge. If there is any lesson in the inability of extant systems to capitalize on the surge of knowledge, it is that the vision must embody a learning environment invigorated by the synergistic energy of decision makers who bring different disciplines, experiences, philosophies, and talents to the table.

Transformational leadership requires specific skills to operationalize the agenda for change. The first is strategic thinking on a large (political) scale and on a small (individual patient) scale. To think strategically is to identify options for achieving the objectives of the vision and to evaluate their consequences for all of the stakeholders. Second are the political skills to shape priorities and objectives, such as the healthy development of children and mothers and coping with the income maintenance needs of an aging population, and to advocate successfully for the resources to accomplish the objectives. The leader will know how and when to encourage policymakers to build health in to the full range of social policy objectives. The third essential skill is in using new knowledge to reorganize health care processes—how health professionals and their colleagues work—and to constantly promote restructuring to maximize outcomes.

Transformational leaders understand the importance of carefully framing the issues and asking the right questions. To identify and clarify those questions, they must be comfortable managing ambiguity and complexity. The most central questions are directed to large databases to assess performance in terms of indicators that the leadership has established for purposes of assessment and benchmarking. The answers are in terms of cost-benefit ratios and epidemiological profiles. It is the responsibility of leadership to translate complex data into information that can be applied to drive decision making and change at all levels of the system. Skills in questioning and not answering, if the goal is to create a transformational organization that is not dependent on the leader, are particularly crucial to the success of governmental efforts to guide partnering with other sectors to achieve public health policy objectives.

There is a growing recognition that there are limits to the ability of the state to meet the social needs of the citizenry. Resolving this dilemma requires a shift in the way that many governments think about how people's needs are to be met and the public's expectations. The ministry of health knows it cannot do it alone, and the health sector is struggling with the implications of that reality. There are fundamental issues of equity to be resolved. The fact is that achieving public health goals by applying new knowledge will require all of the resources, skills, and energies of the government, private, and voluntary sectors that can be mobilized.

Transformational leadership will guide the recognition of the interdependence of all of the sectors and create new configurations that protect their interests while meeting public health objectives. The process is certain to bring forward values that are strongly held and often conflicting, so the transformational leader must be able to generate and tolerate disequilibrium and conflict. Clarity of the vision will be essential for the leader to steer through the whitewater created by such issues as appropriate forms of regulation, incentives for research and development, the role of the for-profit sector in service provision, the privatization of public assets, the independence of the NGOs, and private versus public financing. In this context, skills to articulate the core vision concepts of improved quality of life, maximum health gain, and value for money are extremely important.

The NGO community is expanding rapidly, moving these organizations into the center of national and local health policy development and implementation. The growth of NGOs in numbers, size, variety, and influence is in part attributable to the limits of the state and to the failure of existing structures to meet the challenges of learning. It is also attributable to responsiveness, innovation, and flexibility. In many countries, NGOs have demonstrated the ability to provide high-quality services and their potency as advocates for public support of research, education, and health services. The most serious constraint on NGOs' realizing their full potential is a shortage of qualified leadership—transformational leaders who will envision new roles, gain recognition, and create new resources. The public and private sectors can make no better-leveraged investment in achieving public health policy objectives than in enabling the development of transformational leadership for the NGO community.

Among the distinctions between many current health system leaders and transformational leaders is breadth of perspective, comfort in bridging into adjacent policy domains, and the ability to influence based on broadly informed judgment rather than technical competence and credentials. The evidence is overwhelming that greater health gains can be made by improving the quality of life than by refashioning health services. To that end, the vision, agenda, and skills of transformational leaders will engage public policy in its broadest sense, be it at the community, city, or national level.

In a practical sense, that means being conversant with the issues, politics, and the health implications of economics (for example, poverty, income security, employment), education (access for girls, health literacy of teachers and in school systems), agriculture (food security, environmental impact, rural nutrition), infrastructure (transportation, water supply), and environment (industrial development and behavior, pollution regulation). These issues converge at the level of cities, which are in some respects the key political level because they can enable or impede community-based health improvements. Transformational leadership in the community will educate, build trust, foster communication, and develop partnerships in support of community development, always reaching for a vision of a better way to get there.

The most potent tool for improving health is changing behavior. The individual is, potentially and logically, the coproducer of health along with all of the factors that contribute to the quality of life. There is an urgent need for health leadership to shake out the preoccupation with traditional health education processes and focus on accountability for outcomes. It is a daunting challenge both technically and politically. The technical problem is that the science and art of social marketing is immature. The highest priority for health services research is designing behavioral change interventions that work and are sustainable over time. Yet some people do not believe this to be a legitimate research investment. The political problem is that there is a tremendous vested interest in present approaches despite the reservations about their cost effectiveness. It is clear that more of the same will not accomplish the health objectives that are central to the vision. Transformational leadership is required to establish the importance of developing new and more effective social marketing strategies to effectively encourage lifestyle modification.

Leadership, like learning, is expressed through communication. Transformational leadership employs communication both to drive the system or organization and to shape its environment. It is an essential tool for sharing the vision, rallying people behind it, and creating the political, public, and professional forces that will sustain it. The specific skills are knowledge of media and how to develop and target messages that are in the public interest. That includes the diffusion of knowledge that supports public health objectives, such as appropriate public expectations, appropriate use of health services, policy option trade-offs, and information on quality of care. It also includes the skill of confronting, through policy and exposure, the exploiters of communication, who employ the media to convey deadly messages. There is risk in transformational leadership, particularly when it entails confronting politically powerful interests through communication with the public.

Read the job descriptions for executive leaders of complex health organizations such as international agencies, integrated service delivery systems, ministries of health, research centers, HMOs, public health departments, NGOs, hospitals, academic health centers, and long-term care or home health or rehabilitation agencies. Or ask the incumbents to describe their mission and their vision. What you will discover is that there is little emphasis on the role or the skills associated with transformational leadership. There is not a hint of stimulating debate regarding whether this is the appropriate way to organize resources for the knowledge-driven future. This is not an indictment of current leadership; it is a call to action.

What is required is a bold, even presumptuous response. The premise is that transformational health leadership can be deliberately and systematically nurtured, that talented and motivated individuals can be attracted to assume the mantle, that they can be placed where they can make a significant difference and be reinforced over time. A critical mass of such individuals, sharing visioning and exchanging implementation experience, will be an agency of change. It will be essential to use the network to cross-fertilize with successful executive leadership in other sectors. In particular, we must learn from the businesses that are thriving on adaptability to new knowledge.

We have a wealth of leadership development experience, much of it from other sectors, to build on. It should be assembled and evaluated by a multidisciplinary and multinational team that does not represent the interests of any agency, university, or vendor. A second team should at the same time assemble the evidence in practice to define the essential skill needs; again, it is important to reach into other sectors, especially the research and knowledge-driven business community, for relevant insights. A third team should search the world for examples of transformational health leadership in action to provide case studies and living laboratories and to identify role models.

Then a small planning committee should design a program plan that would be circulated widely for comment and ratification. A small global policy board, working through contracts aimed at avoiding the creation of a new bureaucracy or reinforcing an old one, would implement it. To refresh the process, the policy board would be designed for continual turnover. Every donor agency has a stake in the success of this venture; all decry the shortage of transformational leaders in whom to invest. This should be an appealing investment, but it must be insulated from the pulls of donor self-interest.

The mandate is transformational leadership that is capable of integrating the wealth of knowledge expansion reflected in this book into a vision of a more effective global health system. The challenge is to envision a system with that leadership, establish concrete objectives to nurture it, and to pursue them aggressively.

Name Index

Subject Index